English Delftware Drug Jars

English Delftware Drug Jars

The collection of the Museum of the Royal Pharmaceutical Society of Great Britain

Edited by Briony Hudson

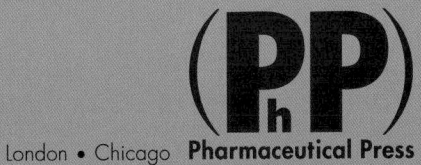

London • Chicago **Pharmaceutical Press**

Published by the Pharmaceutical Press
An imprint of RPS Publishing

1 Lambeth High Street, London SE1 7JN, UK
100 South Atkinson Road, Suite 206, Grayslake, IL 60030-7820, USA

© Pharmaceutical Press 2006

(**PP**) is a trade mark of RPS Publishing

RPS Publishing is the wholly-owned publishing organiastion of the Royal
Pharmaceutical Society of Great Britain

First published 2006

Text design and typesetting by Champion Design, Dartford, Kent
Printed in Great Britain by The Bath Press, Bath

ISBN-10 0 85369 643 8
ISBN-13 978 0 85369 643 8

A catalogue record for this book is available from the British Library.

In memory and admiration of Agnes Lothian Short.
The Royal Pharmaceutical Society's historical collections, and the English delftware collection in particular, are founded on her hard work, enthusiasm and expertise.

Contents

Foreword

Apothecary delftware has fascinated pharmacists and other collectors for at least 150 years. However, it has generally been overshadowed in museums by other, more decorative, wares in general collections of tin-glazed earthenware. This book is based on one of the major exceptions – the extensive and comprehensive collection of the Royal Pharmaceutical Society.

As Briony Hudson explains in her history of the collection, the core of the collection is that of Geoffrey Howard, which consists of some 65 jars acquired by the Society in 1957. This has been expanded to its present size of 172 jars and six pill tiles, largely through the enthusiasm and keen eye of Agnes Lothian, but also through the generosity of other collectors.

Although it is not quite the largest collection of such material (see the table below), the Society's collection does contain a very good representative selection of the different designs, drug names and jar sizes used by apothecaries in the 17th and 18th centuries. There are several unique items, such as the 1647 dated display jar (Cat. 50) and the 1670 Fautrart pill tile (Cat. 219), but there are also many other gems.

Comparison of English apothecary delftware collections		
Collection	**Number of jars**	**Number of pill tiles**
Colonial Williamsburg	140 (3 dated)	3
Private collection, London	173 (11 dated)	4
Private collection, New Zealand	26 (1 dated)	1
Private collection, Scotland	116 (7 dated)	1
Royal College of Surgeons	36 (6 dated)	0
Royal Pharmaceutical Society	172 (40 dated)	6 (3 dated)
Society of Apothecaries, London	11	13
Thackray Museum (Wilkinson collection)	436 (419 in Wilkinson Collection) (32 dated)	11 (10 in Wilkinson Collection)
Wellcome Collection (in the Science Museum)	136 (4 dated)	18
Total in these collections	1,246 jars (104 dated)	57 pill tiles (3 dated)
Total of English delftware jars and pill tiles traced to August 2005	**1,992 jars (175 dated)**	**162 pill tiles (7 dated)**

All of the figures quoted for the numbers of jars in existence or in particular collections are based on a database compiled over the last 7 years.

These massive display jars (the Society's collection holds two of the three known mid-17th century examples) must have been proudly displayed in the shop windows of the apothecaries who first owned them, an indication of their opinion of their status within the profession.

Similarly the pill tiles, although in actual fact a purely practical item rather than the 'qualification certificate' sometimes suggested, must have given their users a glow of pride as they displayed the arms of the professional association to which they belonged.

Alongside these special items, there is a good range of the practical vessels that were the mainstay of the apothecary's day-to-day dispensing needs, both as stores of the ingredients for the recipes and for the finished products. One of the few reliable pointers to the dating of the various types and styles of jars and tiles is the dated pieces. The Society's collection is particularly rich in these, with three of the eight known dated pill tiles, and 40 out of the 175 known dated jars (the larger Wilkinson Collection has only 32 dated examples, the Colonial Williamsburg three and the Wellcome Collection just four). Most of these dated pieces also bear initials, assumed to be those of the apothecary who had the jars made.

There has been much written about apothecary delftware, some of it quite fanciful, but Bill Jackson distils the more sensible writings to give a good general introduction to the wares. The addition of a contemporary recipe for the contents, together with indications of the purpose of the medicines, will add greatly to the usefulness of the catalogue entries. Another advantage of this catalogue is that all the items are illustrated, rather than just representative examples: one can be certain of the exact design of every item.

What is the significance of the collection? It forms an invaluable resource for studying the jars themselves from an art-historical point of view, but also enables us to study the production methods and styles of the delftware potters by giving an overview of the designs and styles used over the production period of these wares. It also provides a wide range of the different forms and presentations used by the apothecary, and provides a basis for studying the use and development of the different organic and (later) inorganic substances used in 17th and 18th century medicine.

Alan Humphries
Librarian, Thackray Museum, Leeds
September 2005

Preface

"These are all obsolete Contrivances, and are no where else now to be heard of, but upon the Titles of some very old Shop-Pots."

John Quincy, 1718.

The English delftware collection at the Royal Pharmaceutical Society provides a fascinating insight into the practice of pharmacy in the 1600s and 1700s in a tangible and beautiful way. Like so many of the Society's Museum collections, the appeal is multi-layered. The tin-glazed jars, pots and tiles provide an insight into the social history and the practice of pharmacy, while also representing a moment in time in the fashion and production of ceramics. They provide a link with an individual painter or potter, perhaps sitting not far from my desk in Lambeth High Street today, working to produce a practical storage vessel or a stunning show jar for a demanding and successful customer. The weird and wonderful contents of the jars evoke a different age and approach to treatment, although sometimes the parallels with current practice are as intriguing as the differences. The acquisition of the jars by the Society also reflects the development and changing collecting policy of its Museum.

The rows of jars on display today at the Society's headquarters stop visitors in their tracks because of their visual appeal and impact, in the same way that they must have impressed customers in an apothecary's shop in the 17th or 18th century.

The opportunity to share some of this impact and interest has been a long time coming. Agnes Lothian, in charge of the Society's historical collections from 1940 onwards, and author of many articles on English delftware, turned down the suggestion of writing a complete catalogue, claiming that she found writing for publication difficult. There is no way that I could ever hope to rival her massive expertise. My role has primarily been as a facilitator and collector of other people's knowledge, past and present. This publication is an attempt to draw together the information we have about the English tin-glazed items in the collection. The hope is that the introductory chapters will set the collection in context, and that alongside the detailed illustrated catalogue, we will have provided readers with a means of enjoying and appreciating all of the many layers. By raising awareness of this collection, just one amongst many here, we also hope to prompt further interest and research into the objects, so that our knowledge of them will continue to grow. Correspondence from any readers who have additional comments or insights, would like to share findings or research, or have spotted errors or omissions will always be extremely gratefully received.

Briony Hudson
Keeper of the Museum Collections, Royal Pharmaceutical Society, London
September 2005

Acknowledgements

This publication is the culmination of many decades of effort and represents the tip of a very large iceberg.

Without Agnes Lothian Short, there would have been no collection, and this book draws massively on her work. All of the Museum staff who have looked after the collections and added to our knowledge about them since have played an important role. I would particularly like to thank Caroline Reed, my predecessor, who (with the assistance of grant aid from the South East Museums Service) had the collection surveyed and photographed, and had conservation work carried out on all the objects. Penelope Fisher carried out the condition survey and the subsequent conservation work. Rod Tidnam has taken all the photographs for the catalogue section and the majority of the additional illustrations. Peter Arney of Sotheby's provided additional information. Diane Hudson carried out supportive proofreading. Charles Harmer provided life outside delftware. Peter Homan helped greatly with research, especially into the contemporary sources. Roy Allcorn and all of the Information Centre and Museum staff unfailingly provide help and support for all of my work, and this book is no exception.

The greatest thanks must go to Alan Humphries, Librarian at the Thackray Museum. His name only appears as the author of the foreword, but he has been a peer reviewer *par excellence* of all aspects of the publication. Part of his job, and a large part of his spare time, is spent researching both the largest collection of pharmaceutical delftware in the UK and English pharmaceutical delft beyond the Thackray's walls. Both Bill Jackson and myself have found his advice and expertise invaluable, and the catalogue section in particular has benefited immensely from his research and input.

About the editor

Briony Hudson studied History at Clare College, University of Cambridge, and Museum Studies at the University of Leicester. Having worked for short periods at museums as diverse as the Hereford Cider Museum and the Victoria and Albert Museum, she became Assistant Keeper of Social History for Wakefield Museums and Arts, during which time she co-wrote *Liquorice* (WMDC, 2003) with Richard Van Riel, Curator of Pontefract. She joined the Royal Pharmaceutical Society in September 2002 as its Keeper of the Museum Collections, and she heads the team responsible for collections of around 45,000 objects.

Contributors

W A (Bill) Jackson, MSc, FRPharmS, is a retired pharmacist who is a member of the International Academy of the History of Pharmacy, a past President of the British Society for the History of Pharmacy, and a past President of the Manchester Pharmaceutical Association.

Alan Humphries is Librarian at the Thackray Museum, Leeds. He has been researching pharmaceutical delftware, particularly their Wilkinson Collection, for several years, and is currently trying to trace all other English apothecary jars and pill tiles.

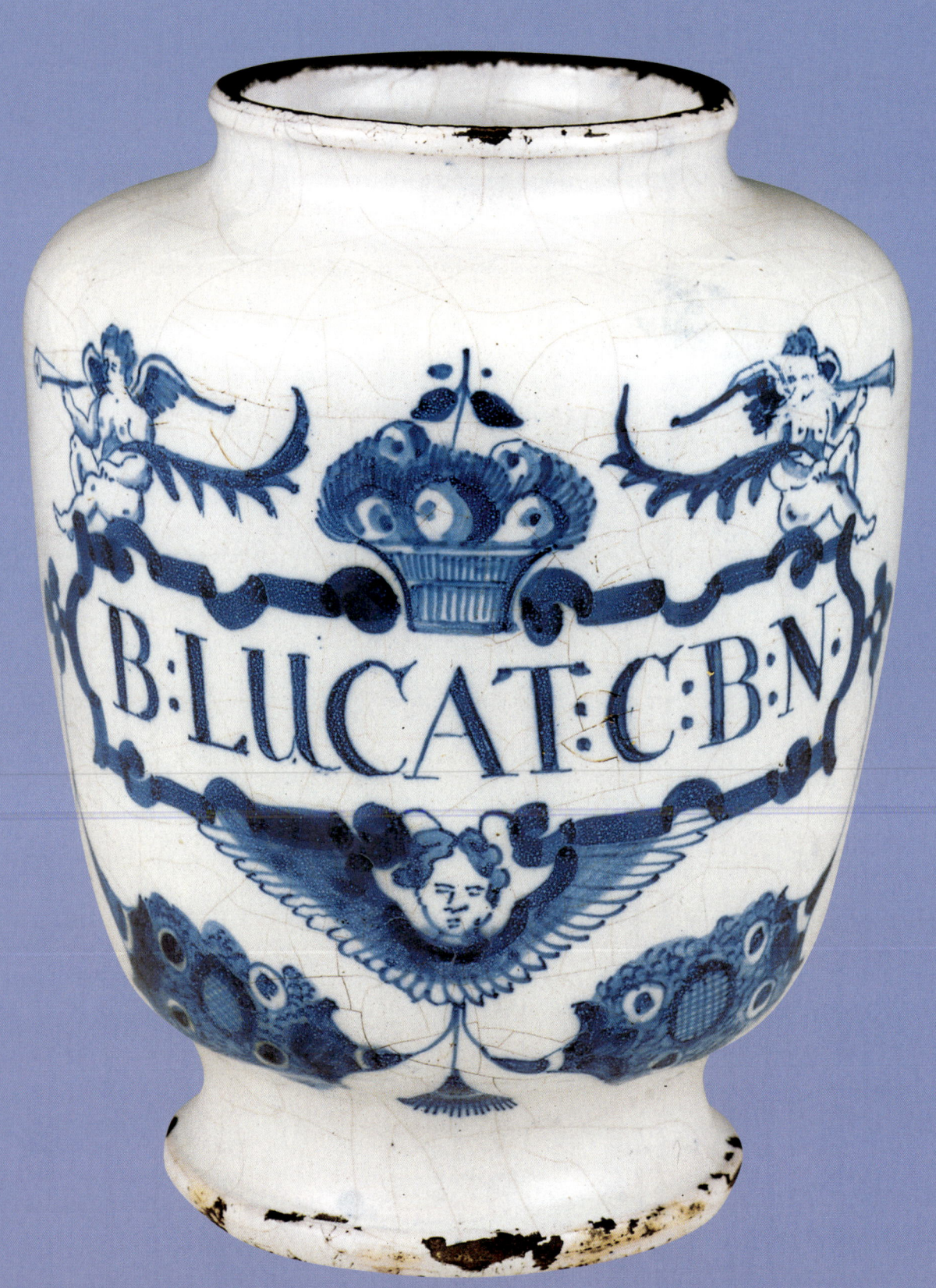

The English delftware collection at the Royal Pharmaceutical Society

Briony Hudson

The Museum

The Museum of the Royal Pharmaceutical Society was founded in 1842, a year after the Society itself. It was intended as a reference collection for the students of the newly formed School of Pharmacy. William Allen, the Society's President, wrote in his first President's Address that the purpose of the Museum, alongside the Library, lectures and pharmaceutical demonstrations, was "to facilitate the acquisition of knowledge by the rising generation".[1]

Jacob Bell, the Society's founder, described the Museum soon after it was set up:

"The museum is a front room on the ground floor, 26 feet by 20, containing not a vestige of furniture. The bare boards are well-scoured, the ceiling and walls are in a perfect state of repair, but there is not even a chair or table to invite the student to sit down and contemplate what alterations are likely to take place in the apartment within the next six months. On the floor at one corner is a small heap of brown paper parcels, containing a few donations from two or three members, and on the mantel-shelf are about a dozen glasses and bottles, in which are sundry crystals, roots and other substances. These objects form the nucleus of the MUSEUM OF MATERIA MEDICA OF THE PHARMACEUTICAL SOCIETY OF GREAT BRITAIN."[2]

Dry drug jar showing cherubs with trumpets, manufactured in London between 1700 and 1725 (Cat.159).

There was no intention for the Museum to attempt to collect historical material, or items that reflected the profession's past. Theophilus Redwood (1808–1892), the first Museum curator, therefore appropriately set the trend for the men in charge of the collection to be experts in pharmacy, or more accurately pharmacognosy,

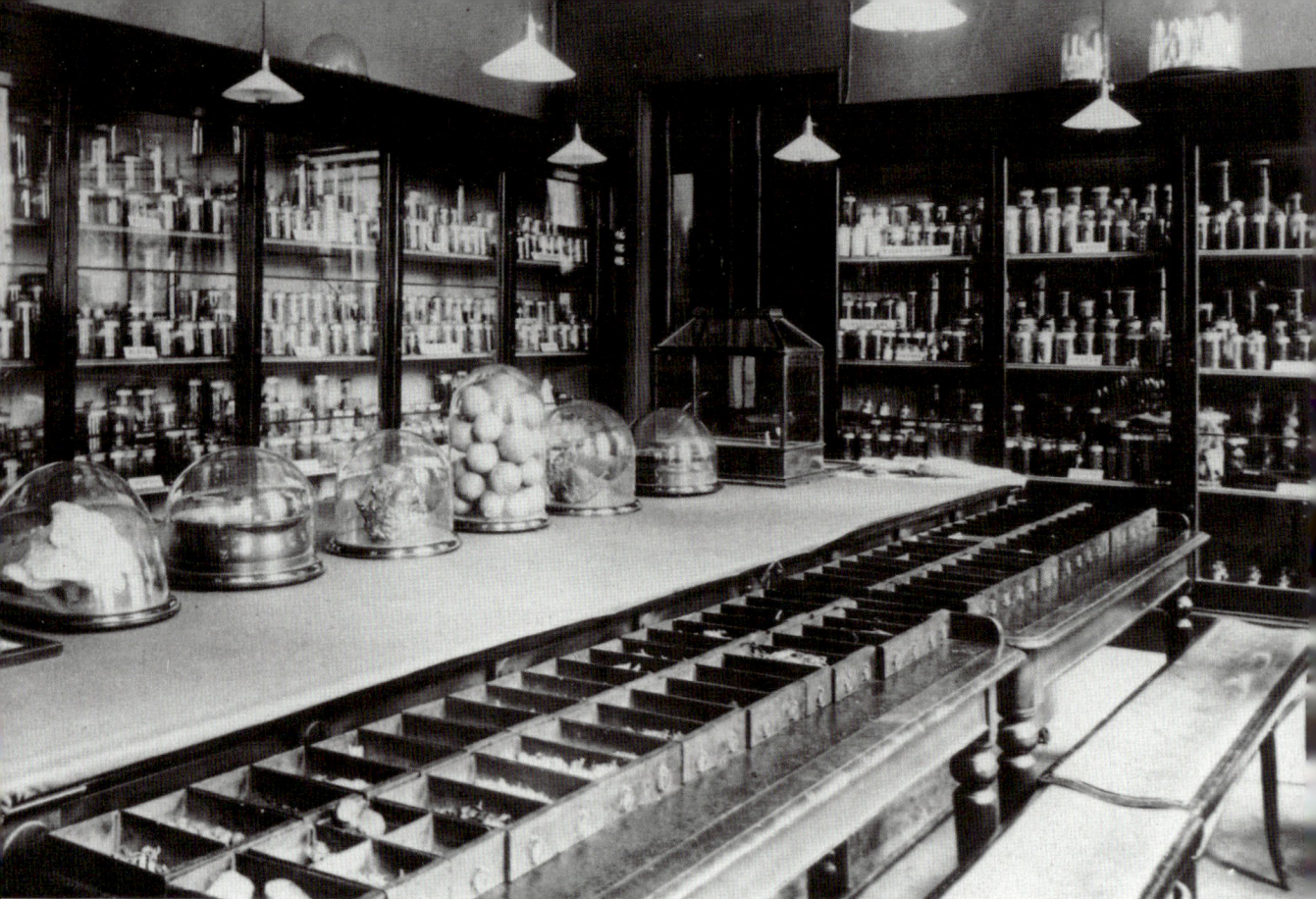

not in history. An academic pharmaceutical training made them best qualified to collect, research and interpret the specimens. The appointment of Edward Morell Holmes in 1872 was a significant turning point in the Museum's history. Holmes (1843–1930) was curator for 50 years until his retirement in 1922, by which time he had built up the Museum collections to over 20,000 specimens.

Museum Room 1, with materia medica specimens on open display in drawers for study, 1903.

The collectors

A new chapter in the Museum's history began in 1937, when the decision was made to establish a historical collection, to coincide with the Society's move to a new headquarters. Although this move was abandoned for financial reasons, the Museum collections expanded as intended. Agnes Lothian, the librarian from 1940 to 1968, was also put in charge of these historical collections, and carried out an ambitious purchasing programme, particularly in the areas of ceramics, caricatures and proprietary (brand name) medicines. Her particular passions were delftware and mortars.

However, she did not arrive at the Society with this enthusiasm about tin-glazed drug jars. Following in her father's footsteps, Agnes Lothian qualified as a pharmaceutical chemist in 1926, having studied at Heriot-Watt College, Edinburgh. After 3 years working for Mr W H Fowler, Redhill, Surrey, a short time as a representative for a baby food manufacturer, and 10 years at Allen and Hanburys

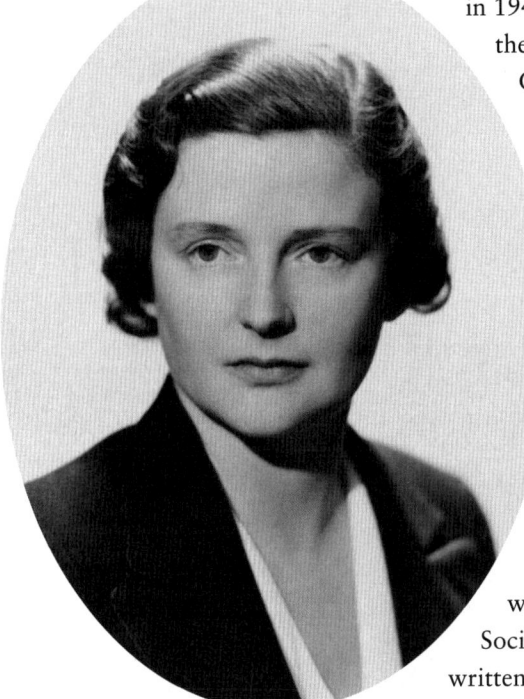

Agnes Lothian, around the time of her appointment by the Society in 1940.

Ltd, she was appointed by the Pharmaceutical Society as its Librarian in 1940.[3] Something or someone must have encouraged her to join the English Ceramic Circle, and about the same time she met Geoffrey Howard. This seems to have marked the beginning of her interest in delft, and also the beginnings of the collection at the Society. However, she had to convince those that held the Society's purse strings:

"It was hard work getting even a small budget approved for purchases...What made it harder was that some members of the Council of the Pharmaceutical Society saw no purpose in such expenditure."[4]

Her first publication was 'Drug jars and their inscriptions' in *The Chemist & Druggist* in June 1950. In spite of the many articles that she wrote on tin-glazed earthenware, she confessed that writing for publication was not an easy task for her. This was her response whenever the idea of a catalogue of jars and mortars in the Society's collection was proposed, and hence one was never written.[5]

She retired on 31 December 1967, but was retained by the Society to catalogue the historical collections, and was made "emeritus Keeper of the Society's historical collections" in March 1969.[6] Her achievements in the field of pharmacy history were impressive: she was the first female member of the International Academy of Pharmacy, and with Hugh Linstead, one of the first two British members; the recipient of the Fritz Ferchl medal from the German History of Pharmacy Society in 1973; the recipient of the Schelenz-Plackette of the International Society of the History of Pharmacy (ISHP) in 1977; and she addressed meetings of the ISHP in Germany, Austria, Yugoslavia and Greece.[7]

On her death in October 1980 she was described by Desmond Lewis, then Secretary and Registrar of the Pharmaceutical Society, as a "world authority on drug jars and mortars".[8] Quite correctly it was remarked that: "Nan will be long remembered...not least by every visitor to the Pharmaceutical Society's Headquarters in Lambeth who appreciates the Historical Collection there. Many will regard this as her permanent memorial."[9]

Agnes Lothian herself wrote in 1960:

"The nucleus of the Society's collection of English delft was formed in 1938 when Mr J T Appleton presented to the Society three 18th century syrup jars. During the next 20 years many items were added by both gift and purchase. Of these the most important is the Howard Collection of English delft drug jars which was acquired in 1957."[10]

We have no record of the first time that Agnes Lothian and Geoffrey Howard met, but by 1946 she was asking to visit the delftware collection at his company's offices. Because Howards of Ilford Ltd were having new offices built at the time, Lothian didn't see the collection until 1949.[11] If there was anyone who was going to enthuse a newcomer to delftware, it was Geoffrey Howard. In his book, *Early English Drug Jars*, written about his own collection, he waxes lyrically:

> "Just as Pepys' Diary brings us adorably into touch with the everyday life of our ancestors, so, as we shall see, do these fat, smug, comfortable little vessels with their dates, initials and inscriptions."[12]

Howard was clearly addicted, and had managed to track down related jars from all over the country.[13] However, he was not knowledgeable about the jars' inscriptions, and continually called on Agnes Lothian's help to decipher the Latin abbreviations.[14] By June 1950, Lothian had collected nearly 300 inscriptions, and had visited a number of collections, such as those at the Royal College of Surgeons, to see their jars.[15] Her growing enthusiasm extended to her building up a personal collection. She wrote to Howard in May 1950: "I have now got twelve nice pieces

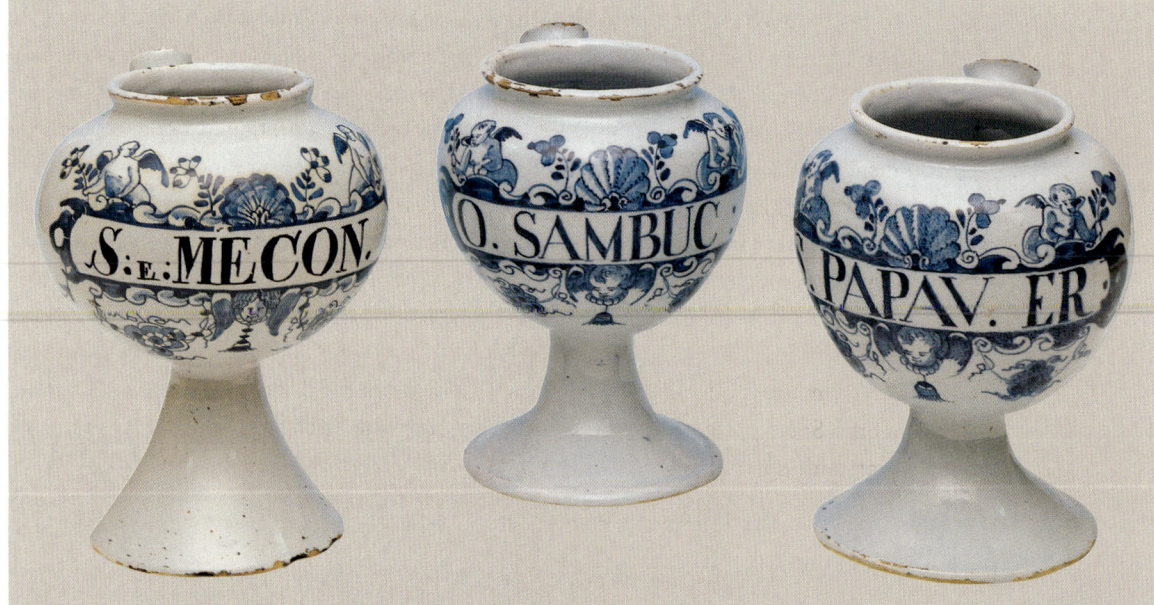

Mr Appleton's delftware donation of 1938
(Cat. 201, 192, 195).

John Thompson Appleton

John Thompson Appleton was responsible for donating the first three delftware drug jars to the Society's Museum. He registered as a chemist and druggist on 3 January 1900 in his native Sheffield, and continued to take a very active part in the profession: he was Secretary of the local Pharmaceutical Committee from 1934 onwards, Chairman of the Sheffield branch of the Society, co-opted onto the Society's Council in 1940, and was Chair of its Public Services Committee. Having opened his own pharmacy in 1902, he retired from retail practice in 1921, and retrained as a dentist. He died on 25 August 1945, aged 68.[16]

of Lambeth and will soon be insufferable!"[17] Howard also encouraged her to build up the Society's collection, and the two often compared notes about the delftware being sold by one particular dealer, Archibald Frith Allbrook:

> "I was pleased to hear from Allbrooke [sic] that you have finally got the dated and named Pill slab for the Society and that the latter were willing to fork out so much money – a great feather in your cap."[18]

They were both collecting in an era when delftware was rapidly gaining in popularity amongst collectors. Howard remarked in 1951: "Drug Jars are fast disappearing from the market, they have become a kind of craze." One possible explanation was that momentum had built after the publication of Howard's book in 1931.[19] This collecting craze was certainly not evident earlier in the century – Henry Walker wrote in *The Connoisseur* in 1908: "The collection of old pharmacy jars does not appear to have received the attention of connoisseurs to any appreciable extent."[20]

In view of their constant correspondence and mutual support, it therefore seems entirely fitting that Agnes Lothian was able to persuade the Society to acquire Howard's collection on his death in January 1957. Howard had left his collection to his three sons, but Dennis Howard wrote to Agnes Lothian in May 1957 to ask her advice about finding "a home for the complete collection where it would be cared for and cherished".[21] The Society's Council agreed to purchase the collection at its June meeting, and by December the Howard Collection was on permanent display in the Society's Reception Room at its headquarters in Bloomsbury Square.[22]

During this period, Lothian was also corresponding with Dr John F Wilkinson, another voracious collector of drug jars in Manchester and Mobberly, Cheshire. Again, the two of them compared notes on pots, discussed what was available in the sale rooms and at Allbrook's. Lothian also bought jars on Dr Wilkinson's behalf.[23]

A smaller collection, but still significant, was the 26 jars and one pill tile left to the Society by its past president, Ernest Saville Peck, in 1955. Peck's first love was undoubtedly bell-metal mortars, but he also collected delftware drug jars:

> "My collection now is about 60 mostly Lambeth Delft. I have had two shelves put up in my offices and they look rather well."[24]

Peck acquired a core of his collection from James Prior of Stamford, whose jars were illustrated in an article in *The Connoisseur* in 1908. He wrote to Agnes Lothian:

> "You will be interested to hear I have acquired the small collection of Drug Pots made by my old friend Mr Prior of Stamford who very much wanted me to have them when he died. I saw them some years ago – they are somewhat of a mixed lot but many are Lambeth Delft. I have not seen them lately but expect them to arrive here this week."[25]

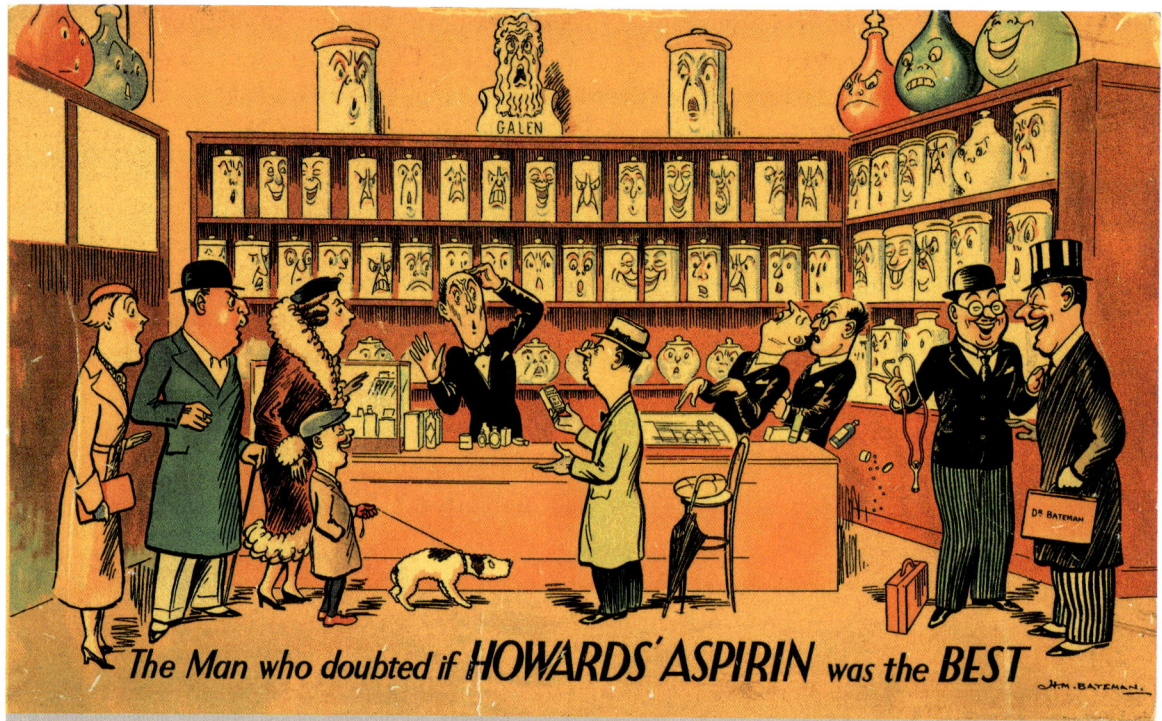

The Man who doubted if HOWARDS' ASPIRIN was the BEST

Geoffrey Howard

An advertisement for Howard's Aspirin, by cartoonist H M Bateman.

Geoffrey Howard was born in Walthamstow, educated at Marlborough, and studied in Germany. He started at the family firm, Howard and Sons, in 1897, and was made a partner in 1901. He became Director of Howard and Sons Ltd in 1903, when the company was formed, and was made Chairman of the Company in 1941.

He also held a number of posts in the wider pharmaceutical world. He was Chair of the Fine Chemicals Group of the Association of British Chemical Manufacturers from 1929 to 1931, a member of its council from 1933 to 1955, and was elected Honorary Member and Honorary Vice-President in 1955. He was also a Council member (including Chair) of the Association of British Pharmaceutical Industries from its time as the Drug Club until 1953. He also travelled extensively, and was a keen mountaineer, and a member of the Alpine Club for more than 40 years. He collected more widely than delftware, particularly fine art: "His taste was catholic and embraced, without any change of critical standard, English delftware of the eighteenth century and Matthew Smith's paintings of the twentieth."[26] He died on 17 January 1956, aged 78.

Agnes Lothian seems to have cultivated Peck's enthusiasm for his drug jars, and certainly sent him reading material on the subject.[27] He admitted to her in February 1952: "I am getting to appreciate more my Drug Pots!"[28] Peck was also instrumental in helping Lothian to acquire one of the most important jars in the Society's collection (see Cat. 50). The large show jar with the coat of arms of the Worshipful Society of Apothecaries on the front, and Chinese designs on the reverse, is the earliest known dated delft drug jar – 1647. It was Peck who put the owner of the jar, a Reverend Willimot, in contact with Agnes Lothian in the first place.[29]

In 2002, the transfer of Peck's drug jar collection to the Society was finally completed when four additional jars, which had belonged to Peck's daughter, were bequeathed by her to the Museum (see Cat. 106, 114, 145, 180).

The Society also received a significant donation of delft jars collected by John Austen of Sheffield. His widow presented his wide-ranging collection, which included 33 drug jars of varying types, in 1960.[30] These were well-travelled jars, having been exhibited at the St Louis Exhibition in 1904.[31] In fact, one of the jars still has an American customs sticker on its base.

Some of the earlier examples of cylindrical, unlabelled delftware pots came from the large collection of pharmaceutical antiques amassed by H E Brocksom.

Ernest Saville Peck

Ernest Saville Peck began his career as an apprentice in his father's chemist shop in Trumpington Street, Cambridge. He studied in the science schools in Cambridge for his Minor examination, which he passed in 1888, and for the Major, which he achieved in 1889. He also found time to study for a BA (1896) and an MA (1897), before taking over the family business in 1904.

After qualifying, Ernest Saville Peck was active in pharmaceutical affairs. He was a founder member of the Cambridge Pharmaceutical Association. He was a speaker at the British Pharmaceutical Conference (1898), its Secretary for 11 years (1901–1912), and President twice. He served on the Pharmaceutical Society's Board of Examiners, as Chairman of the Education Committee for several years, as a member of the Society's Council from 1922 to 1943, and as President from 1935 to 1936.

As a territorial officer Peck was called up on the outbreak of war in 1914. He was promoted to Major in 1915, and a year later formed the Anti-Gas School at Halton Camp. Through experience he developed a speciality in defence from gas warfare and he went on to organise a larger school at Crowborough. In 1918 he went to America to assist in organising and training troops in anti-gas technique in the US Army Gas School.

He was keen to promote pharmacy as a career in its own right and after the war was appointed to the Civilian Advisory Board under the government scheme for the education of men within the Army. In addition, he assisted in establishing new schools of pharmacy and advised the Society as to the approval of teaching institutions for the retraining of demobilised troops.

He also found time to be involved in civic affairs, as a founding member of the Cambridge Rotary Club, a founder of the Cambridge County Folk Museum and mayor of the city in 1937–1938.[32]

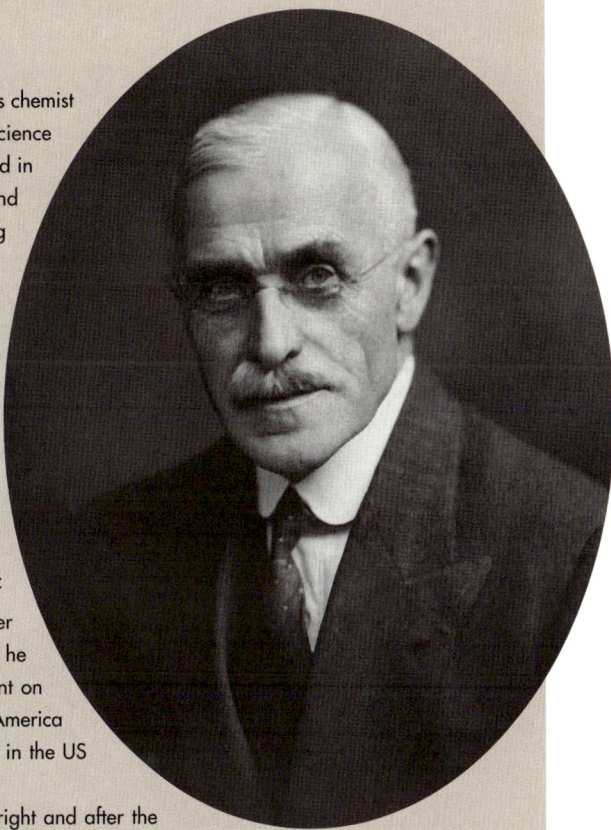

Ernest Saville Peck, 1935.

John Austen

John Austen, originally from Sussex, went to work in Sheffield, aged 19, as an apprentice of G T W Newsholme. Austen qualified as a chemist and druggist in 1892, and as a pharmaceutical chemist in 1899, and eventually became managing director of the firm. As a president of Sheffield Pharmaceutical and Chemical Society, the Literary and Philosophical Society, and the Microscopical Society, and a founder member of the Hunter Archaeological Society, and the Sheffield Rotary Club, he was well known and respected in historical and scientific circles in Sheffield. "One of the kindliest of nature's gentlemen...",[33] his widow presented his collection to the Pharmaceutical Society after his death on 29 November 1952.

John Austen, c.1900.

However, some of the smaller and earlier examples were bought from archaeological digs. Tantalisingly, the Museum's documentation does not reveal the full provenance for many of these acquisitions. For example, the record card for a purchase of a group of ointment pots in September 1961 reads:

"An important collection of 34 Lambeth delft and other early unguent pots recovered from various excavations in London circa 1926."

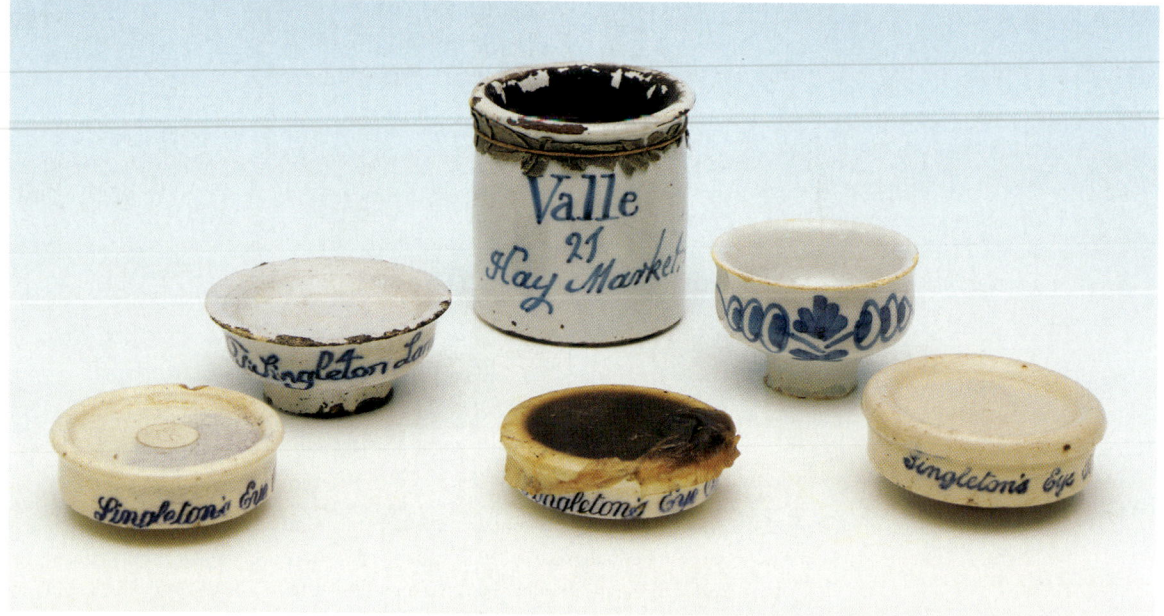

The Museum's collection also includes a number of other smaller tin-glazed items including ointment pots for Singleton's Eye Ointment, made on Lambeth Road from the 16th century until the 1970s. Other small containers show the manufacturers' name, such as this one marked 'Valle 21 Hay Market' (with some contents remaining), and there are simpler decorated pots, some with floral decoration.

The Society's tin-glazed drug jar collection has now grown to encompass both British and European storage jars, smaller ointment pots, pill tiles and barber's bowls.

What seems entirely appropriate is that so many of the tin-glazed jars, originally made on the banks of the Thames, are still here in Lambeth. An archaeological dig in 1968 at Norfolk House, on a site next to the Pharmaceutical Society's current headquarters, was the first delft production site to be excavated in Britain.[34] The jars are still impressing and fascinating people with their striking designs and intriguing contents, just as they did when they were first made.

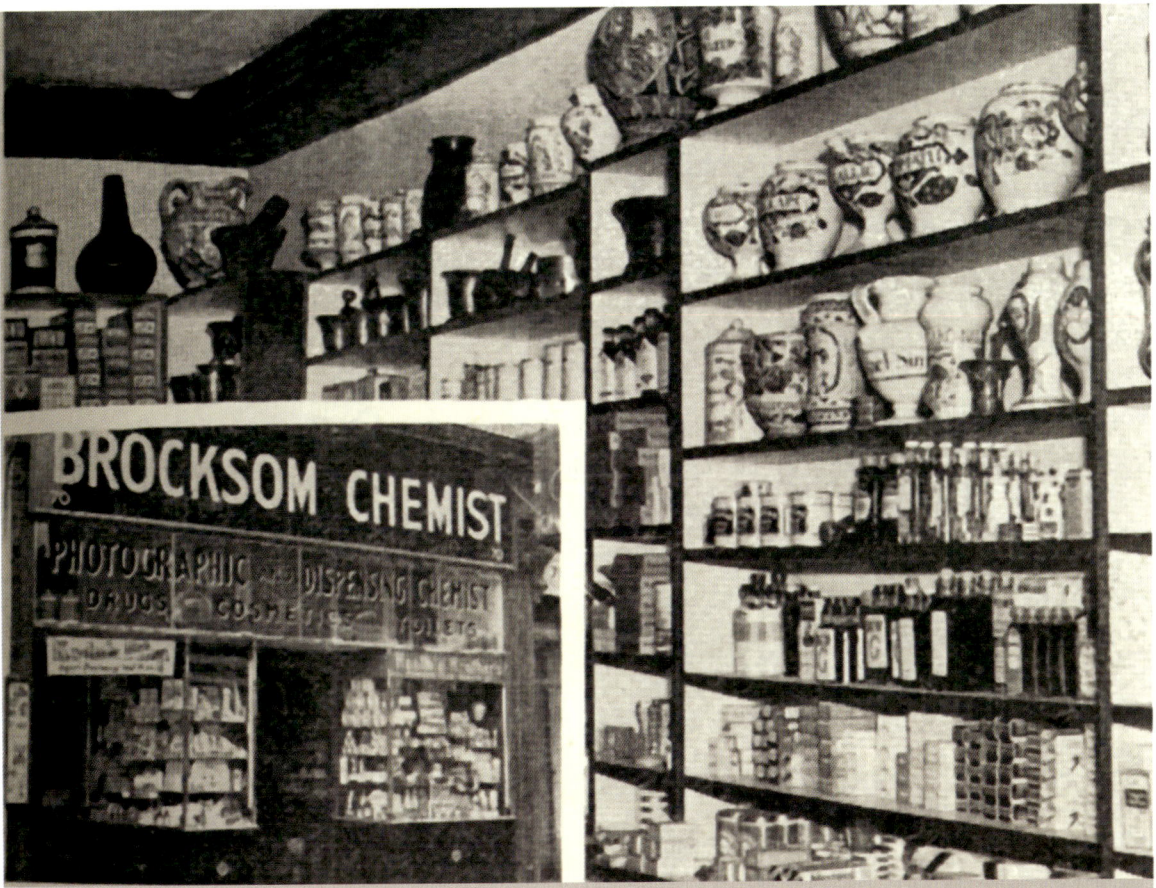

Henry Everatt Brocksom

Mr Brocksom's pharmacy at 70 Chapel Market, Islington, c.1953.
Reproduced with permission from *The Chemist and Druggist* 1953; 160: 399.

Henry Everatt Brocksom was a keen collector of pharmacy antiques and an active member of the British Society for the History of Pharmacy. He qualified in 1928 and initially worked in the pharmaceutical industry. In 1948 he bought the pharmacy at 70 Chapel Market, Islington, and worked there until his retirement in 1968.[35] His large collection of English and continental delftware and mortars was all displayed in his shop, in and amongst the proprietary medicines. On his death in 1985, the Society acquired more than one hundred items from his collection, including tin-glazed jars, but also dispensing equipment, bottles and proprietary medicines.

References and endnotes

[1] The President's Address. *The Pharmaceutical Journal and Transactions* 1(number 8, February 1st 1842): 393.

[2] The Library and Museum. *The Pharmaceutical Journal and Transactions* 1 (number 8, February 1st 1842): 437.

[3] Personalities. *The Chemist and Druggist* Jan 20th 1968; 189: 50, Agnes Lothian Short. *The Pharmaceutical Journal* October 22nd 1983; 231: 475, Obituary. *Pharmaceutical Historian* December 1983; 13 (4): 4.

[4] Obituary. *Pharmaceutical Historian* December 1983; 13 (4): 4.

[5] Obituary. *Pharmaceutical Historian* December 1983; 13 (4): 4.

[6] Personalities. *The Chemist and Druggist* Jan 20th 1968; 189: 50, About People. *The Pharmaceutical Journal* July 9th 1977; 219: 39.

[7] Agnes Lothian Short. *The Pharmaceutical Journal* October 22nd 1983; 231: 475.

[8] Obituary. *Pharmaceutical Historian* December 1983; 13 (4): 4.

[9] Leslie Matthews' appreciation, reported in Obituary. *Pharmaceutical Historian* December 1983; 13 (4): 4.

[10] Lothian A., *English delftware in the Pharmaceutical Society's Collection*, (reprinted from the Transactions of the English Ceramic Circle, volume 5, part 1), 1960.

[11] Lothian, A., *Letter to G.E. Howard*. Dated 4.12.1946; Lothian, A., *Letter to G.E. Howard* Dated 30.6.1949.

[12] Howard, G.E., *Early English Drug Jars*, London: The Medici Society, 1931: 6.

[13] Howard, G.E., *Early English Drug Jars*, London: The Medici Society, 1931: 17.

[14] For example, Howard, G.E. to Lothian, A. 13.7.1949.

[15] Lothian, A. to Howard, G.E. 20.6.1950.

[16] Death notice. *The Pharmaceutical Journal* September 1st 1945; 155: 112.

[17] Lothian, A. to Howard, G.E. 25.5.1950.

[18] Howard, G.E. to Lothian, A. 19.5.1951.

[19] Howard, G.E. to Merck, G.W. 23.5.1951.

[20] Walker, H. Ancient Pharmacy Jars. *The Connoisseur* April 1908: 251.

[21] Howard, D. to Lothian, A. 15.5.1957.

[22] Lothian, A. to Howard, A. 6.12.1957.

[23] Dr Wilkinson's extensive collection is now owned by the Thackray Museum in Leeds. The Thackray Museum also holds Dr Wilkinson's archive relating to his collection, and there are numerous letters between Dr Wilkinson and Agnes Lothian.

[24] Peck, E.S. to Lothian, A. 4.8.1948.

[25] Walker, H. Ancient Pharmacy Jars. *The Connoisseur* April 1908: 251-254. Peck, E.S. *to* Lothian, A. 9.8.1948.

[26] Leslie Matthews' appreciation, reported in Obituary. *Pharmaceutical Historian* December 1983; 13 (4): 4.

[27] Peck, E.S. to Lothian, A. 23.3.1952. She sent him a copy of F.H. Garner *English Delftware*, London: Faber and Faber, 1948.

[28] Peck, E.S. to Lothian, A. 2.2.1952.

[29] Confirmed in Peck, E.S. to Lothian, A. 4.12.1953. First mentioned in Peck, E.S. to Lothian, A. 10.10.1953.

[30] Monthly Meeting of Council. *The Pharmaceutical Journal* 1960; 185: 382.

[31] Brede yeoman who became a druggist. *Sussex Express and Community Herald* August 25th 1961: 1.

[32] The Late E. Saville Peck. *The Pharmaceutical Journal* January 22nd 1955; 174: 55, The Late E. Saville Peck. *The Chemist and Druggist* January 22nd 1955; 163: 85, Candidates for the Council. *The Pharmaceutical Journal and Pharmacist* May 6th 1922; 108: 377-378.

[33] Obituary. *The Pharmaceutical Journal* December 6th 1952; 169: 399.

[34] Gower, Graham with Tyler, Kieron. *Lambeth Unearthed. An archaeological history of Lambeth,* London: Museum of London Archaeology Service, 2003: 43-44.

[35] Death notice. *The Pharmaceutical Journal,* August 31st 1985; 235 : 272.

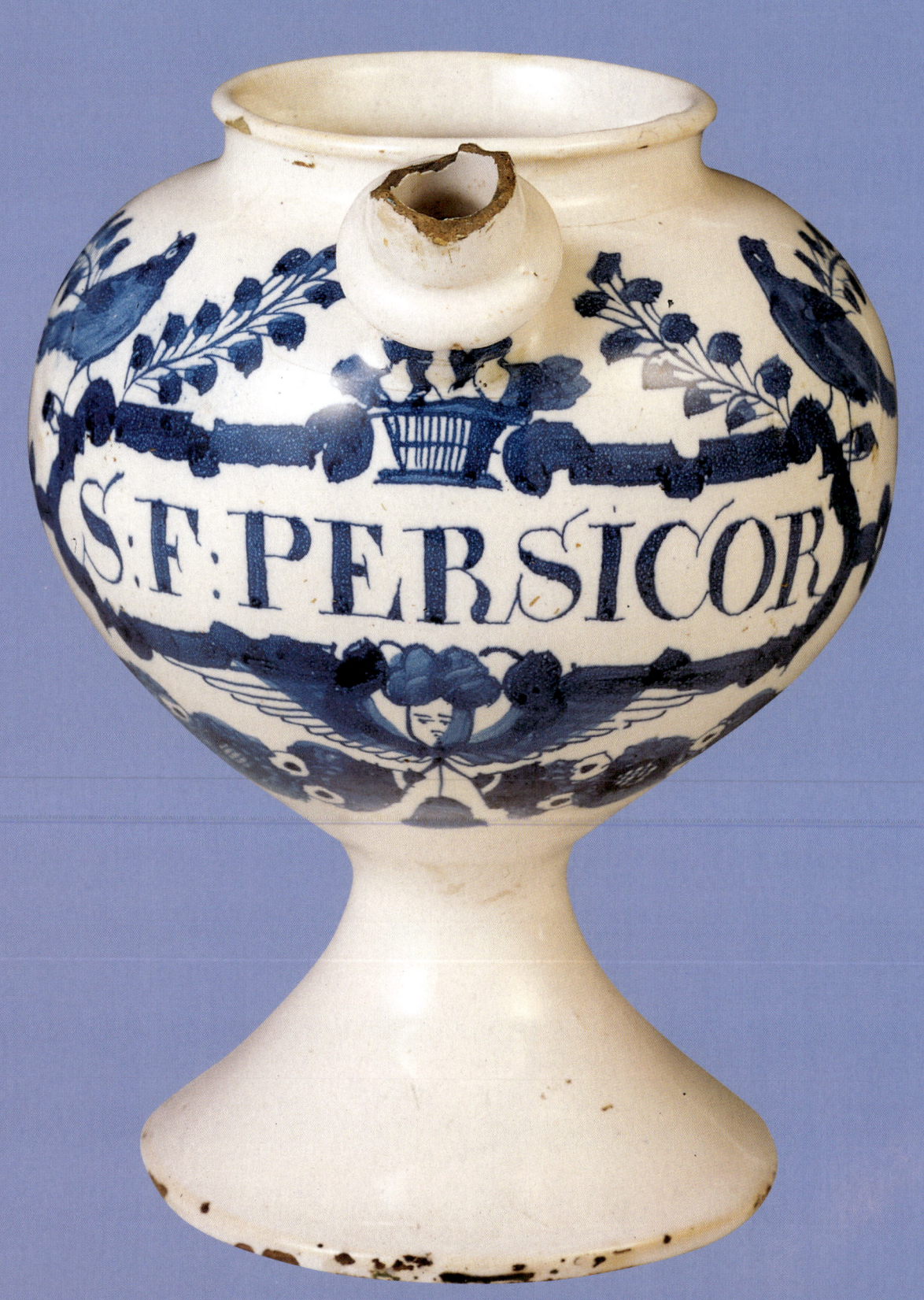

English delftware drug jars

Bill Jackson

Apologia

Some excellent books have been written on the type of pottery known as delftware, majolica, faience or tin-glazed (enamelled) earthenware, but the only one that is devoted exclusively to English delftware drug jars and related items is Geoffrey Howard's *Early English Drug Jars*, published in 1931.[1] Much has been learned about them since then, but the information is scattered throughout a number of books and articles written by scholars such as Rudolf Drey, Agnes Lothian, John Wilkinson and John Crellin, as well as items in books dealing with British delftware in general. In this chapter I hope to assemble much of the information available from these sources in the hope that it will serve as a useful introduction to the fine collection of drug jars owned by the Royal Pharmaceutical Society of Great Britain, and provide references for those who might wish to study the subject in more detail.

Medieval pottery in England[2]

During the period from AD 1100 to 1500 pottery was made at many sites in England but, apart from crucibles and retorts, there seems to be little or no evidence of wares produced specifically for apothecaries. We know of no storage containers from this time labelled with the names of drugs or medicines, although jars with everted lips, over which a cover could be tied, and spouted jars suitable for storing oils and syrups, were made. Some jars with lead glazes that were coloured yellow by the addition of lead sulphide or oxide, or green by adding copper compounds, are known. These are often referred to as 'Tudor Ware', and it is probable that these could have been used by apothecaries to hold drugs. In

Wet drug jar with glazed rim and flanged spout, depicting song birds. Manufactured in London between 1700 and 1730 (Cat. 149).

Shakespeare's *Romeo and Juliet* (Act V, Scene I), Romeo visits a penurious apothecary to buy poison, and speaks of:

> "A beggarly account of empty boxes, Green earthenware pots, bladders and musty seeds...."

Early drug containers

There is a surprising lack of information about the containers that were used to hold stocks of drugs and medicines in England before the middle of the 17th century, but some idea can be obtained from the will of the apothecary, Thomas Baskerville, which was proved in Exeter in October 1596.[3] Among the items in the shop this listed:

> "2 dossen of syrup pottes with pipes, ...; 16 oyl pottes with pipes, 18 dossen & halfe of other gally pottes, ..."

The term "gally pottes" probably referred to tin-glazed earthenware,[4] and presumably the "pottes with pipes" were spouted jars.

An inventory of 1665 of the contents of Thomas Needham's shop in Chesterfield[5] included:

> "25 'syrup potts,' 21 'conserve potts,' a gross and a half of 'gally yellow potts,' two dozen and a half 'stone bottles' (probably Rhenish stoneware), 'two pound potts Holland mettle,' 18 'w(hi)t(e) Galley potts' and an 'oyle pott.'"

I am tempted to think that here the "gally yellow potts" were of lead-glazed 'Tudor Ware', while the white ones and the pots of "Holland mettle" were of tin-glazed earthenware.

Tin-glazed earthenware

Tin-glazed earthenware is so called because tin oxide was added to the lead glaze in order to make it white and opaque. Sometimes a little cobalt oxide was added to counteract a tendency towards yellowness. Usually, the bisque (unglazed) object was fired at a low temperature, then dipped in the glaze and allowed to drain and dry. Designs

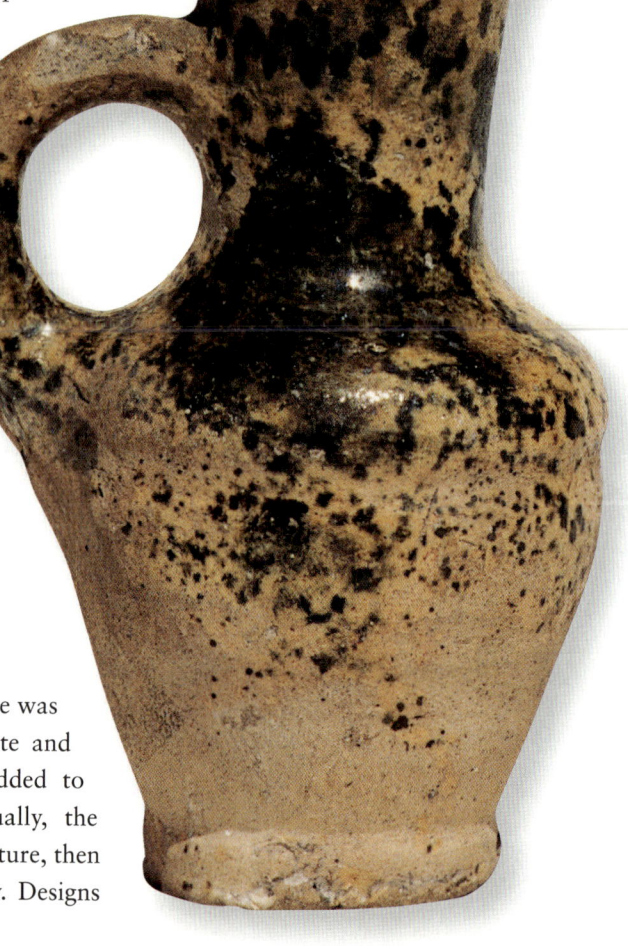

Jug with green glaze, late 14th century, author's collection. Photo by W A Jackson.

could be painted on the resulting powdery surface, often using cobalt oxide to produce a blue colour when the second (high-temperature) firing took place to vitrify the glaze. Other colours that are found on early delftware are green (from copper), purple or purplish-black (from manganese), brick-red (from iron) and yellow (from antimony).[6] Tin glaze tends to craze and flake with the passage of time.

It is known to have been used from about 1000 BC by the Assyrians, and to have been revived in Persia in the 8th century AD. It was introduced into Spain in the 11th century AD by the Moors (Hispano-Moresque pottery), to have been exported from Spain to Italy, and to have been manufactured in Italy from the 14th century. It reached France, Germany and Holland in the early 16th century, and was produced in England about 50 years later.[7] It is also known as enamelled earthenware; maiolica (or majolica), perhaps from the belief that some of the pots were made in Majorca; faience, after Faenza in Italy, a centre of production; or delftware. The latter name became popular because great quantities were produced in Delft, Holland. That made in this country is usually called 'English delftware' (note the lower case 'd'), although British delftware would be a better term as a certain amount was made in Ireland and Scotland.

British tin-glazed earthenware

Tin-glazed earthenware was produced at a number of different locations in Britain.

Norwich

During the second half of the 16th century a considerable number of Protestant craftsmen left Antwerp because of religious persecution. In or around the year 1567, Joris (George) and Jasper Andries fled to England, but apparently Joris did not remain there long as he is recorded as a resident of Middleberg, Zeeland, in 1568. Jasper Andries and Jacob Jansen (or Janson) established a pottery producing tin-glazed "Galley Paving Tiles, and Vessels for Apothecaries and others" in Norwich, one factor for this choice being the proximity of clay that was particularly good for producing pottery.

London

Andries and Jansen were said to have moved to London in 1570 to the parish of Aldgate, but Andries could not have stayed there long as he is recorded as living in Colchester in 1571. The pottery in Aldgate was operated by Jansen until his death in 1593.[8] Among the items produced at this time were untitled drug jars, including albarellos (jars that were more or less cylindrical but with a slight waist), which were decorated with horizontal lines or bands of dashes, chevrons or intertwining curves.[9] It is not surprising that these are difficult to distinguish from similar jars being produced in the Netherlands at this time.[10] Other potteries were

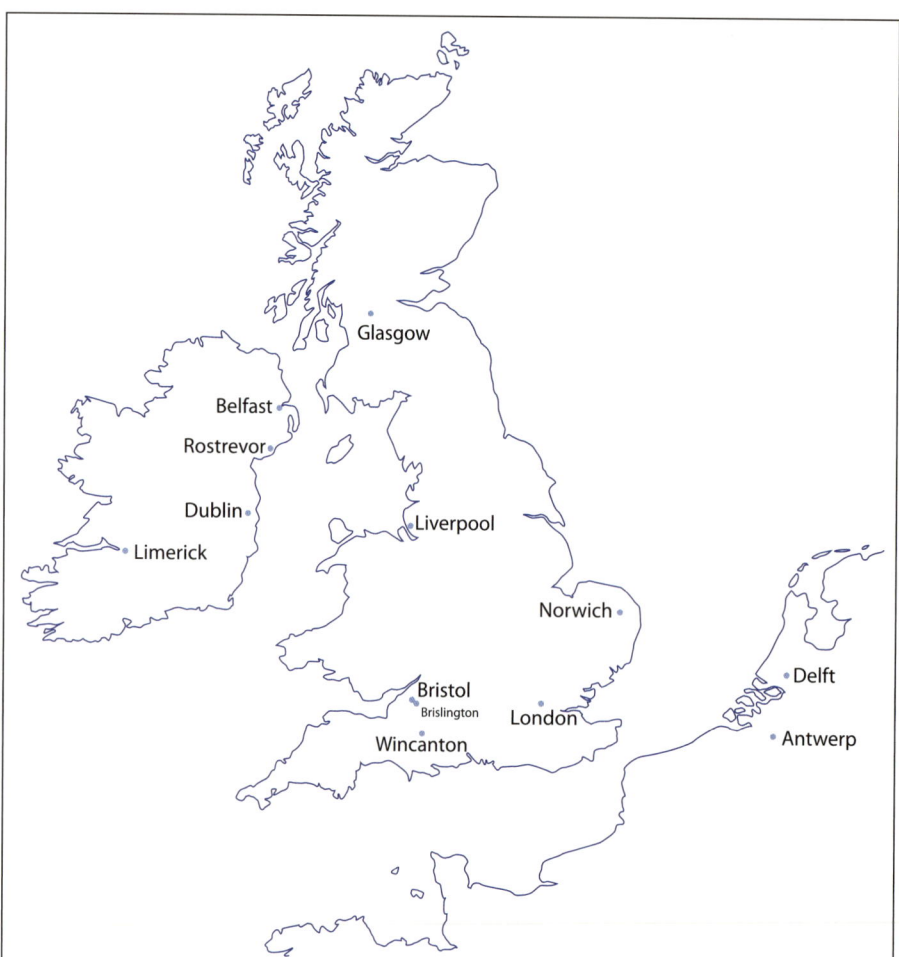

Map of the British Isles and the Low Countries, showing major centres of delftware production.

soon established along the banks of the Thames in Lambeth, Southwark and Vauxhall, and produced tin-glazed earthenware until about 1780.[11] We know of no English drug jars bearing the names of their contents before the middle of the 17th century, and it seems a reasonable assumption that the unlabelled jars decorated with geometric designs date mainly from 1567 to 1650, and that the different designs on the jars would enable the apothecary to locate the drug he required. No doubt jars such as these were used to hold commodities other than drugs. In all, 19 factories in the London area produced delftware, some of them surviving into the first half of the 19th century.[12]

Brislington and Bristol

Later, provincial potteries made tin-glazed wares, and a factory was established at Brislington, near Bristol, in the 1640s. At the time Bristol did not permit strangers to trade within its boundaries, but by 1683 a pottery had been founded in the city itself, and soon more of them were in existence.[13] Bristol, being a thriving port, was an excellent site for these activities because suitable clay could be imported and the finished goods exported.[14] The clay almost certainly came from Boyton (Norfolk) up to about 1680, when supplies from Aylsford in Kent started.

Wincanton

A pottery was founded at Wincanton in Somerset in about 1730 and manufactured delftware for approximately 20 years. It made two plates dated 1738 decorated with Apollo standing over a dragon, a motif taken from the arms of the Apothecaries' Society.[15] They also made a posset pot with the date 1744,[16] but I do not know of any drug jars that can be attributed to this factory with certainty.

Liverpool

A great deal of delftware was made in Liverpool from 1710 to 1780. According to Wilkinson[17] there were approximately 23 potteries, the most important being that

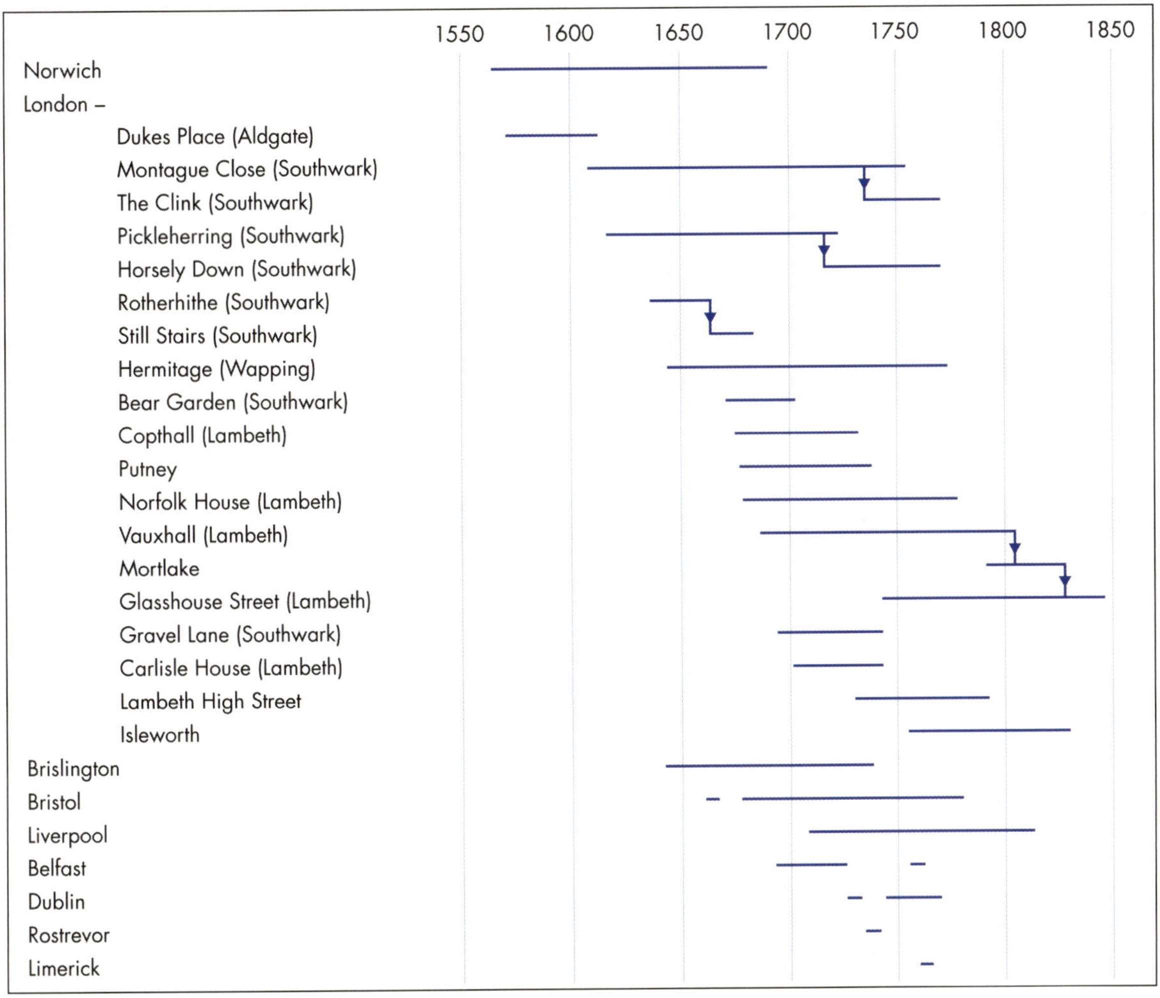

Dates for delftware factories in Great Britain and Ireland, thought to have produced drug jars (adapted from Britton, *London Delftware* and Archer, *Delftware*).

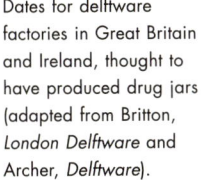

	1550	1600	1650	1700	1750	1800	1850
Norwich							
London –							
Dukes Place (Aldgate)							
Montague Close (Southwark)							
The Clink (Southwark)							
Pickleherring (Southwark)							
Horsely Down (Southwark)							
Rotherhithe (Southwark)							
Still Stairs (Southwark)							
Hermitage (Wapping)							
Bear Garden (Southwark)							
Copthall (Lambeth)							
Putney							
Norfolk House (Lambeth)							
Vauxhall (Lambeth)							
Mortlake							
Glasshouse Street (Lambeth)							
Gravel Lane (Southwark)							
Carlisle House (Lambeth)							
Lambeth High Street							
Isleworth							
Brislington							
Bristol							
Liverpool							
Belfast							
Dublin							
Rostrevor							
Limerick							

of Zachariah Barnes, but both Britton[18] and Garner and Archer[19] only list 13. There can be no doubt that delftware was a very important product of the Liverpool pot-banks. In fact Alan Smith, an expert on Liverpool ceramics, observed:

> "The Liverpool delftware is considered to be its most typical pottery, as it was made on a tremendous scale for almost a hundred years. All the pot-banks made their tin-glazed delftware...."[20]

Again the value of being based in a port is demonstrated as the clay used was imported from Ireland, and it was easy to export the finished pottery.

Ireland

There was a working pottery in Belfast in 1688. It is thought that delftware was being produced there in the early 18th century, although its history is rather nebulous, and it is not known when it closed. It is likely that tin-glazed pottery was also made at Limerick and Rostrevor, but by far the greatest quantity was produced in Dublin between 1735 and 1771. The clay used came from Carrickfergus, and it is probably because of this that it is difficult to distinguish Belfast pottery from that of Liverpool, which used clay from the same source.[21]

Scotland

In 1784 the Delftfield pottery was established in Glasgow to produce tin-glazed earthenware, largely for export to America and the Caribbean Islands,[22] but I am not aware of any drug jars that were made there.

English jars

Compared with the beautifully decorated polychrome drug jars produced on the continent, the majority of English jars are very simply painted. However, they have a naive charm and amply repay time spent in studying them.

Although polychrome delftware was made in England, drug jars with this type of decoration are extremely rare, almost all the designs being executed in cobalt blue of varying shades. Sometimes the name of the drug might be in black or manganese purple, and in a relatively small number, the blue design is outlined in black. When one looks at large collections it is difficult to avoid the impression that the painters with greater skill were employed in decorating large items or high-quality tableware, while those with less ability worked on utilitarian articles such as drug jars.

Unlike many foreign jars, very few carry marks to show where they were made, but Wilkinson illustrates some marked with an underglaze blue 'R' that he believes were made by Woodes Rogers at Limekiln Lane, Bristol, and some with an 'X', made at Bristol or Wincanton.

Other identifying letters were:[23]

'B' Edward Bye, Brislington
     Thomas Baddy, Brislington, Wincanton
'F' Thomas Frank, Brislington (1689–1706)
     Michael Frank, Bristol (Redcliff) (1706–1777)
'I' (Ireson) Wincanton
'P' Pines, Brislington, Bristol (Temple Pottery)
     Seth Pennington, Liverpool (Shaws Brow) (1750)
'R' Richard Riley, Bristol (Redcliff) (1741–1750); puce or manganese purple
'R' Woodes Rogers, Bristol (Limekiln Lane) (1706–1746); cobalt blue 'R'
'W' Wincanton
'X' Bristol or Wincanton.

However, Alan Humphries, Librarian at the Thackray Medical Museum, and an acknowledged expert on delftware drug jars, is very sceptical of most of the suggested links, and has supplied the following list of base marks on those jars that he has traced:

'B' One blue and two manganese, made in London (Lambeth)
'F' One black and one blue made in London (probably Mortlake)
'I' Fifteen marked with an 'I' or a single stroke, one possibly made in Liverpool and the remainder in London.
'P' Three made in London, and one possibly in Liverpool.
'R' Two, both probably made in Liverpool, but possibly Bristol.
'W' One, and one lower case 'w', both probably made in London.
'X' Twenty-eight, two with names in black and the rest blue, probably London.

Other marks that he has noted are 'AM' (or possibly 'AN'), 'C', 'G', 'H', 'J', 'N' (possibly 'Z' or '2'), 'O', 'Q', 'S', 'V' (or possibly '7'), 'VX' (or 'XA'), and a lower case italic 'g' that resembles '6', '11', '29', '38' and '50'. An arrow, an eye, a star, a maypole, a pothouse and a sketch for chinoiserie decoration are also known.

Shapes

Early unlabelled jars

Generally, the earliest (unlabelled) jars either had straight or slightly convex sides or were albarellos. They were probably used mainly for holding such things as ointments, confections and pill masses. They usually had an everted rim so that a piece of parchment or chamois leather could be tied over the top (see, for example, Cat. 1).

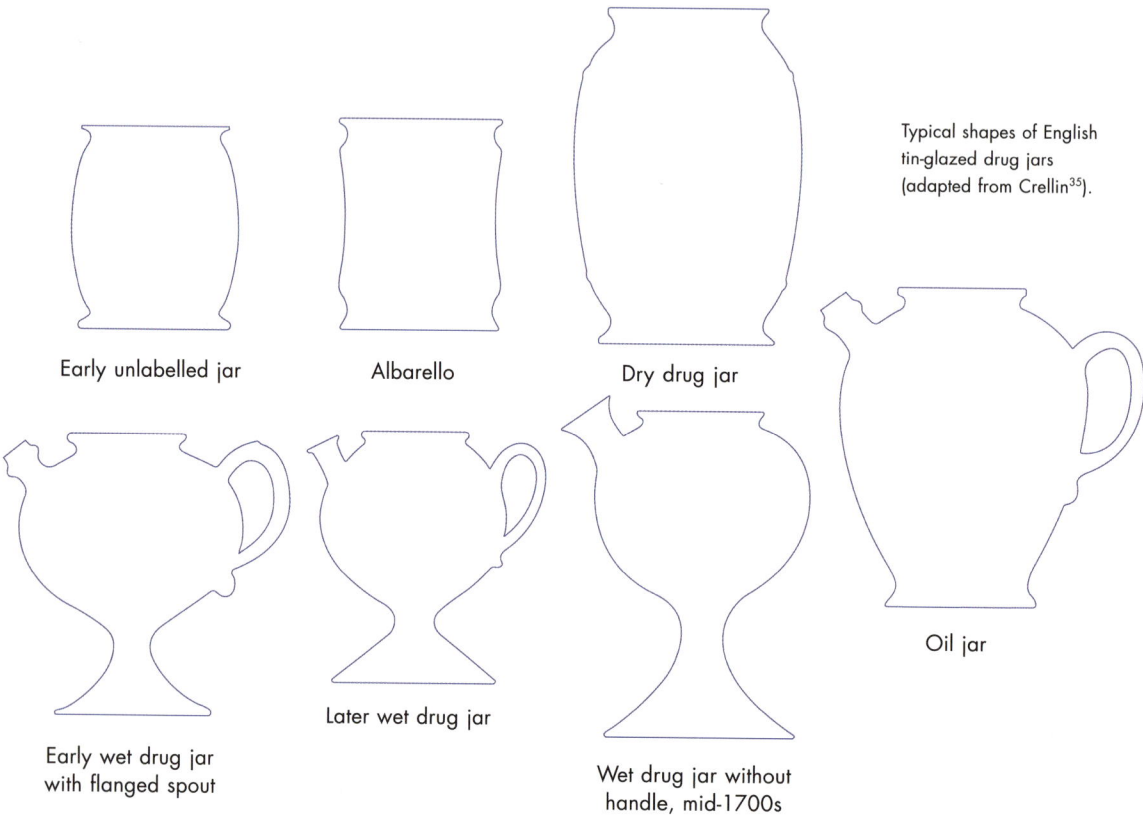

Early unlabelled jar   Albarello   Dry drug jar

Typical shapes of English
tin-glazed drug jars
(adapted from Crellin[35]).

Oil jar

Later wet drug jar

Early wet drug jar
with flanged spout

Wet drug jar without
handle, mid-1700s

Later jars for dry drugs and ointments

Jars for holding herbs, powders, ointments, conserves, confections, electuaries and lohochs had wide mouths, and were roughly barrel-shaped, ovoid or (rarely) baluster-shaped or cylindrical, with openings that had everted rims (see, for example, Cat. 37). Pill masses, lozenges and extracts were held in jars of this shape, but these were only 8–12 cm in height, rather than the more usual 17 cm or more (see, for example, Cat. 39).

Jars for syrups and oils

Syrup jars usually had a spherical body on a hollow pedestal foot. In early jars, a flanged spout (sometimes known as an 'onion spout'), was placed near the top of the body, above the name of the drug, and there was usually a strap-shaped or, less commonly, a rounded handle on the side opposite the spout (see, for example, Cat. 55). Later the flange was replaced by a thickened rim at the end of the spout (see, for example, Cat. 163). From the middle of the 18th century, they were also made without handles, and this type of jar usually had a taller, narrower pedestal, making it easier to pick up the jar and pour from it. They stood on splayed feet, which were almost always hollow. In jars of this shape the name of the contents is found on the opposite side to the spout (see, for example, Cat. 154).

Early oil jars are simply dry jars with the addition of a spout and handle (see, for example, Cat. 66), while later ones were similar to those for syrups, although the bodies were more cylindrical or ovoid, and they had splayed feet, not pedestals (see, for example, Cat. 164). Both oil and syrup jars had wide mouths for convenience in filling them, and were designed to have tie-on parchment covers. It is thought that the mouths of the spouts were covered in the same way.

Towards the end of the 18th century, the everted lips of both the wet and dry drug jars were replaced by straight necks, and they were covered with slip-on metal lids instead of parchment (see, for example, Cat. 197).

Foreign jars used in England

As early English delftware jars were not inscribed with the names of their contents, it is probable that a few labelled jars may have been imported. In 1970 a previously unrecorded jar labelled 'LOHOCH E PVLMONE VULPIS' (Lohoch of fox's lungs)

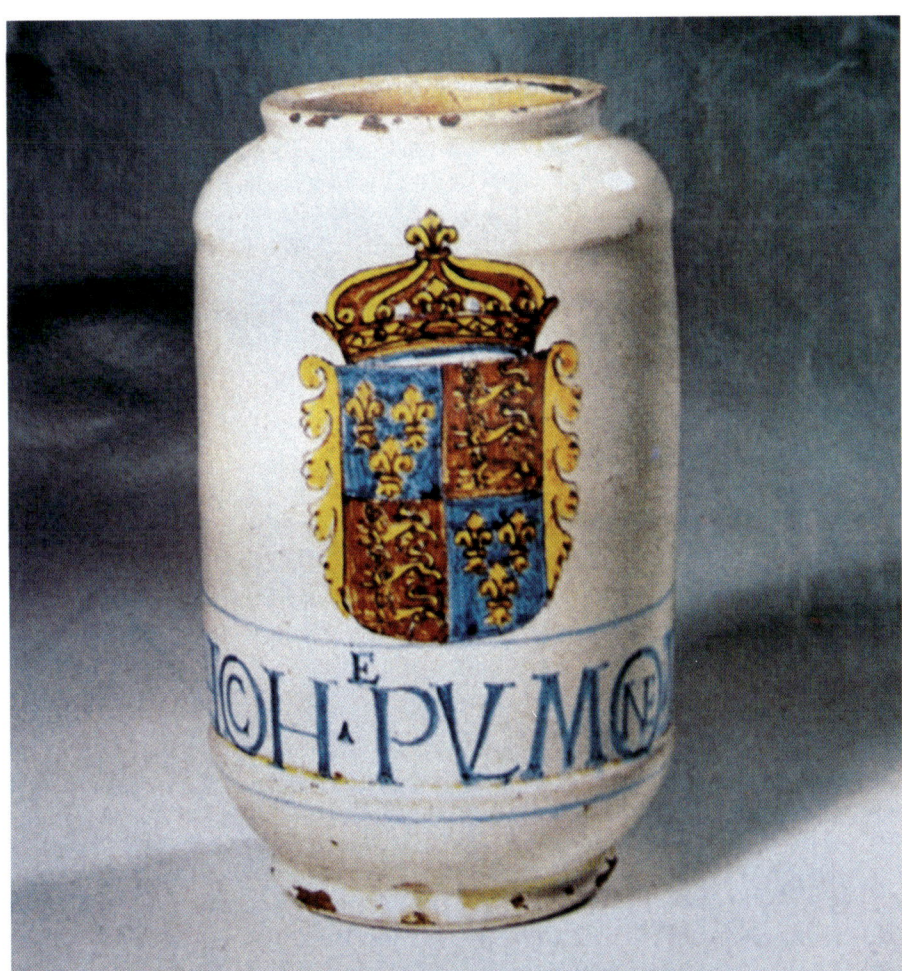

Tin-glazed jar decorated with the Royal coat of arms, probably made in Deruta, Italy, before 1603 (by kind permission of Sotheby's).

was auctioned at Sotheby's. It bore the Royal coat of arms, painted in yellow ochre, blue and manganese, which were in use before the accession of James I in 1603, and was probably made at Deruta in Italy.

Designs on English jars

Unnamed jars with geometric designs (Cat. 37–49)

As mentioned previously, jars decorated with horizontal and/or geometric designs were made in this country for almost a hundred years before it became customary to label them with the names of their contents. These jars are virtually indistinguishable from those made in Holland during the same period.

Jars labelled with the names of their contents

From the first appearance of English named drug jars in the middle of the 17th century, different designs surrounded the cartouche carrying the name of the jar's contents. These help to establish the period in which they were made, and to distinguish them from Dutch jars of the same period. However, it was not a steady progression from one design to the next. Different designs were in use at the same time, and the same designs were produced by different potteries at varying times so, although they are helpful, these designs can rarely establish the date of manufacture or the individual pottery where they were produced without taking other factors into account.

In the following list the approximate dates in which the designs were used are given in parentheses.

Pipe-smoking man: 1650–1670 (Cat. 53–57)

The first English-made jars labelled with the name of their contents appeared about the middle of the 17th century. There are existing examples dated 1652 and 1665. Below the middle of the straight cartouche, typically edged with scrolls, there is a usually a satyr's head, and at each end, a larger grotesque head in profile, with something protruding from the mouth. Originally suggested by Howard,[24] this is usually accepted as being a pipe, giving the name 'pipe-smoking man' to the design, but it could be argued that it is a protruding tongue. The noted collector, the late Dr Wilkinson, supported the pipe theory, pointing out that tobacco had originally been introduced into Europe towards the end of the 16th century as a medicinal herb, and that in 1665/6 the boys at some schools were required to smoke a pipe a day as a prophylactic against disease.[25] However, this theory does not explain the elf-like appearance of the heads or the fact that the 'pipes' bear a greater resemblance to 19th century briar pipes than those made from clay in the 17th century, and I put forward the idea that the design might have been inspired by the 'Green Man' or the Dutch 'Gapers'.[26] The 'Green Man' is also known as 'Jack-in-the-Green', 'Green George', 'The King of the May', 'Robin Goodfellow' and 'Robin Hood', a pagan deity whose image, often in the form of a male head made from or surrounded by leaves, can be found in many churches, both in England and on the Continent.[27] Often he is represented with vegetation emerging from his mouth, and I suggest that it could be foliage rather than a pipe that is depicted in the pipe-smoking man jars. Another possibility is that the design was introduced by an immigrant potter who had memories of the 'Gapers'. These were large carved wooden heads, many with a protruding tongue (often with a pill on it), found outside the shops of Dutch apothecaries from the 16th century onwards.[28]

The Royal Pharmaceutical Society of Great Britain possesses a magnificent collection of English jars, including many originally belonging to Howard, which it purchased after his death. This collection includes a fine pipe-smoking man with touches of yellow and red enlivening the main design of blue. It is rare to find English jars of any design with polychrome decoration, so this is a particularly desirable specimen (Cat. 53).

It has been suggested that many of these jars were destroyed in the Great Fire of London in 1666, but we must remember that labelled jars of this type were an innovation that had not had time to become popular, and few provincial apothecaries would have been likely to own such expensive items at this date.

In addition to drug jars, this design is also found on a posset pot (a spouted cup) dated 1653, and caudle cups of 1644 and 1658.[29] Posset is a spiced, hot drink made from milk mixed with ale or wine. Caudle is warm gruel mixed with spice, sugar and wine.

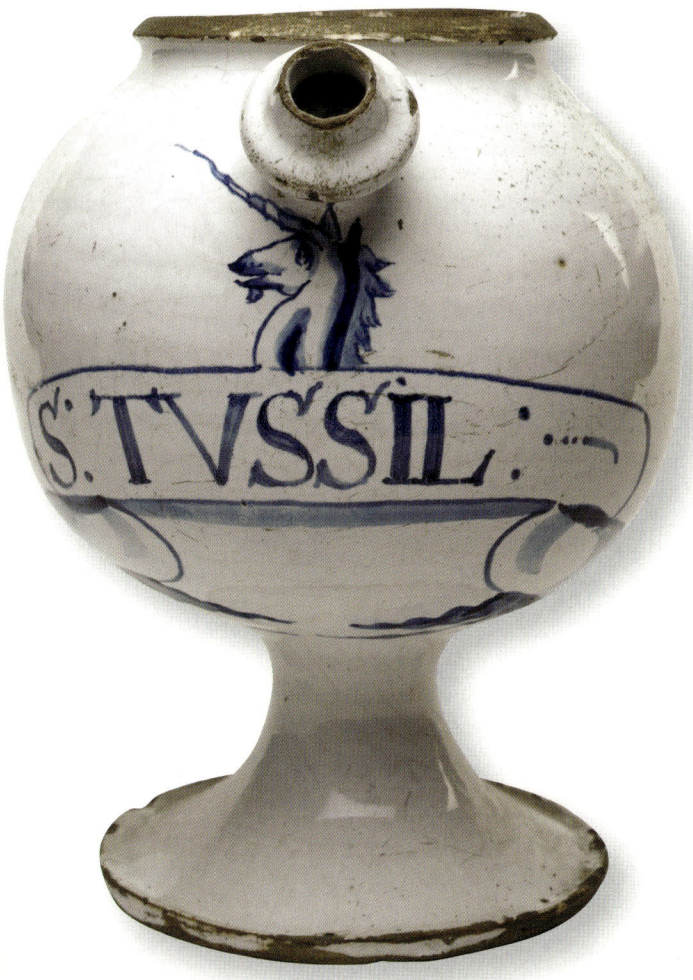

A variation on the ribbon cartouche design, with a unicorn's head (by kind permission Museum of the London).

Ribbon cartouche: 1655–1670 (Cat. 58–62)

Another Commonwealth design had the cartouche in the form of a ribbon with swallow-tail ends. As well as undated examples, there are dated ones from 1655, 1658 (Cat. 58), 1659 (Cat. 59), 1661 (Cat. 60 and 61), 1662 (Cat. 62), 1664, 1665 and 1666. In addition to the dates, all these carry initials, presumably those of the apothecary for whom they were made. The dated jars show that this design was being produced at the same time as the 'pipe-smoking man' jars. There is a rare variation of this design that held Syrupus Tussilago (coltsfoot syrup, a cough mixture) in the Museum of London, in which the cartouche is surmounted by the head of a unicorn.

A transitional design

In December 1977, a rare jar for 'LINIMENT : ARC' (Liniment of Arcaeus), which had a cartouche with a satyr's head below, and terminating in the pipe-smoking man design, but surmounted by an angel with outspread wings, was sold at Sotheby's.[30] A similar jar, but without the satyr's head, labelled 'E : DIACATHOL' (Diacatholicon electuary) is also known.[31] These form a link between the pipe-smoking man and the design found on many English drug jars, the 'Angel with outspread wings', often abbreviated to 'Angel'.

Angel with outspread wings: 1659–1725 (Cat. 68–117)

This design was introduced about the time of the restoration of the monarchy, with the first known dated jars having been made in 1659. It was produced throughout the rest of the century, and into the 18th century, one jar being known with the date 1722. This means that initially it must have been in production at the same time as the other two designs, although, to the best of my knowledge, it has not been established whether one pottery made more than one design concurrently. Basically, this is the ribbon design with the addition of a head, flanked by outspread wings, resting on the top of the cartouche. The folding of the ribbon made two compartments, and the left-hand one might contain the initial letter indicating the type of drug it contained, for example 'S' for Syrup or 'V' for Vnguentum, 'V' normally being used instead of 'U' at this time (see, for example, Cat. 69).

Howard states that the angel's head is a valuable guide to the date of the jar, varying from early examples with "scanty locks after the manner of the puritans" to angels wearing fashionable wigs similar to those worn at court, and that in later jars these change following the fashion of the day.[32] Lothian observes that in some jars the angel's head appears to resemble that of the reigning monarch.[33] Wilkinson said that the angel showed "the gradual change from the puritanical style through the humorous and Florentine appearances to the luxuriant William III style".[34] However, Crellin, pointing out that the wigs were freely drawn and that there is a considerable variation in jars that are all dated 1684, advises caution and says, "dating on the basis of the wig must be used with extreme care".[35] There are two distinct styles of the 1684 jars. Fifteen have the initials MH and six VP, both of which seem to be from the same pottery. The wet jars have a young 'puritan' head (see, for example, Cat. 79), but most of the dry and oil jars, five in number, have a 'James II' style wig (see, for example, Cat. 83), with the other two having the young face. There is one dry jar where the face has been repainted, but the wig is in the young style as well. There are four other 1684 jars, which have an intermediate style of wig. A jar with the same design, dated 1661 and with the initials 'R S', decorated in blue, brown, green and yellow, is in the Colonial Williamsburg Collection in Virginia.[36] In spite of the date this has an older style wig, of the type worn in the 1680s.

One cannot help but agree with Crellin that extreme care should be taken in trying to assign the relative dates of manufacture for these jars on the basis of the style of the wig.

Slipware jar, 1692

Horsham Museum in Sussex possesses a curious jar that has a rather primitive angel with outspread wings above a rectangular cartouche labelled 'V : RUB :

Slipware drug jar, angel with outspread wings design, 1692.
Photo by W A Jackson.
By kind permission of Horsham Museum.

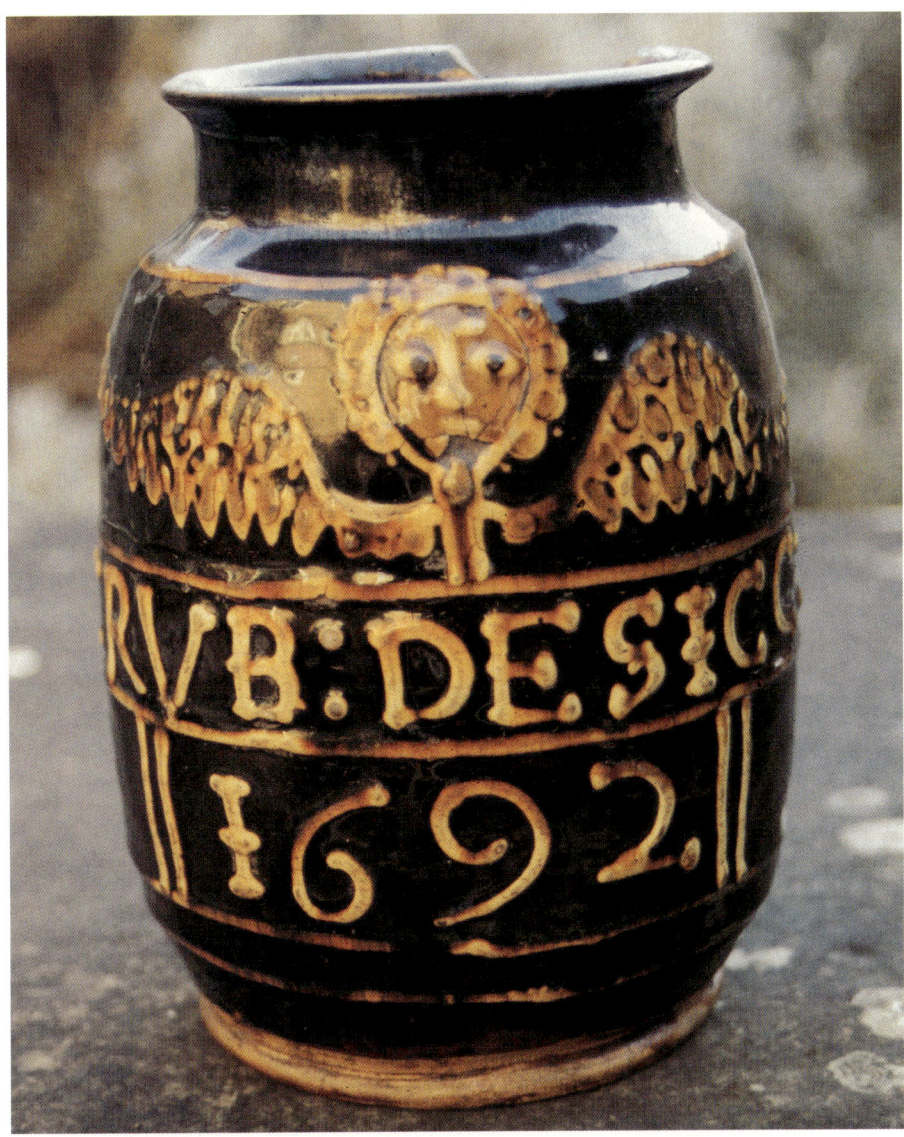

DESICC:' (red drying ointment) and the date '1692' in a panel below.[37] It is 21 cm high, and is exceptional in having been made from slipware, not tin-glazed earthenware. It was probably made in Staffordshire and decorated by trailing lines and dots of semi-liquid slip onto the jar, which was then covered with a transparent lead glaze. It is not known whether it was one of a set or whether it was a trial piece that did not come up to the potential customer's expectations. For many years it was in the possession of the Gudgeon family of Towcester.[38] There is another jar of this type in the Weldon collection.[39]

Angel transitional designs: 1700 (Cat. 118–121)

Two jars of 1700 are unusual in having a heraldic rose between the ends of the ribbon[40] (Cat. 118 and 119). Among the last of the angel jars made were a few in which the scallop shell of Saint James of Compostella is found below the cartouche (see Cat. 120 and 121). There are 15 of these recorded, and they form a distinct group because the cartouche has become more like a banner or heraldic mantle. By the end of the century the swallow-tails were replaced by scrolls. We shall see that this shell motif was used on many jars during the 18th century.

Fleur-de-lys: 1665–1690 (Cat. 63–67)

Unfortunately, as I mentioned previously, the story of English drug jars is not a straightforward one in which there is a steady progression from one design to another. We have already seen that at one time the 'pipe-smoking man', 'ribbon cartouche' and 'angel' jars were all in production at the same time. Now we come to a small group of jars, also from the second half of the 17th century, dated specimens of which were made in the period 1667 to 1690, just after the 'angel' jars first appeared.

Here the name of the drug is surrounded by a thick wavy line, and this incorporates a fleur-de-lys in the centre at the bottom, and a stylised flower, flanked by what I believe to be two leaves at the top, although Wilkinson thought that these were stag's antlers.[41] Three swags, separated by pendant tassels, hang below the label, and a tassel or a stylised flower rises from each end.[42] Two distinct sizes of flower are known.

Early songbirds: 1670s (Cat. 122)

Lothian illustrates another 17th century jar made in 1672 that has a cartouche with a similar thick surrounding line, but a basket of fruit replaces the stylised flower, and a pair of songbirds the fleur-de-lys below it. In addition, there is a songbird perched on top of either end, and these are flanked by upturned tassels.[43] This type is sometimes referred to as the 'early songbird' design. It is extremely rare, the only other known example being in a private collection in London.

Apollo and peacocks (1675–1700) (Cat. 123–137)

Apollo, the central figure in the Apothecaries' Society coat of arms, was the Roman god of medicine, and his head figures prominently in the next design we examine. Placed centrally above a straight-edged label, it is flanked by a pair of peacocks – a common motif on Dutch jars. An angel's head above a pair of wings is placed centrally underneath, and the earlier swags are replaced by two peacock feathers and three tassels. One jar with the initials 'C W' is dated 1679, and another three with the same date are usually considered to belong to this group, although the head of Apollo is replaced by the date 1679 and the initials 'I P' (see, for example, Cat. 123).[44] Two jars from 1694 have a cock immediately above the angel's head.[45]

Apollo and serpents c.1717 (Cat. 138–139)

Two jars have a label bordered by scrolled leaves and two sea-serpents, and surmounted by a bust of Apollo and a shield bearing the date 1717, but have no peacocks.[46] Another ten undated jars of this type are known. One undated ovoid

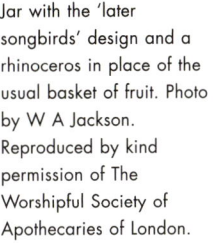

Jar with the 'later songbirds' design and a rhinoceros in place of the usual basket of fruit. Photo by W A Jackson. Reproduced by kind permission of The Worshipful Society of Apothecaries of London.

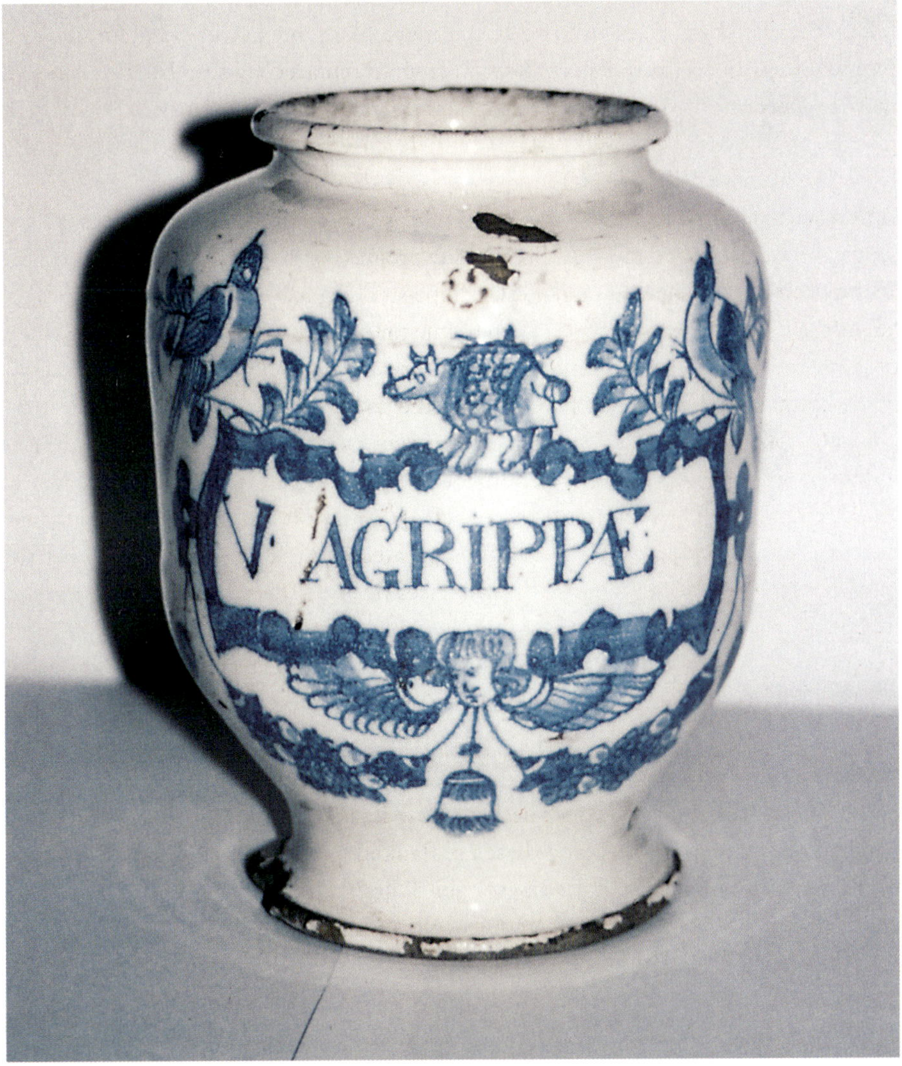

jar is in the Wilkinson Collection,[47] and Lothian noted two undated large cylindrical jars in the dispensary of St George's Hospital, London, which were obviously decorated by the same artist.[48] Unfortunately, these were stolen from the hospital in the mid-1970s and have not surfaced yet.

Later songbirds: 1700–1770 (Cat. 140–158)

The beginning of the 18th century saw the introduction of a large group of jars, known as 'later songbirds' or 'birds and baskets', which had features from both the early songbirds and the Apollo and peacock designs. The wavy, thickly outlined label with the songbirds and basket of fruit above it had the angel and peacock feathers below. In some jars the peacock feather swags become more like stylised flowers, or baskets of fruit. Leslie Matthews had a rare jar in which the basket of fruit was replaced by a rhinoceros, the crest from the coat of arms of the Apothecaries' Society.[49] This jar was bequeathed to the Society of Apothecaries and is now on display there.

Dated examples range from 1702 to 1763. One large jar, dated 1724, has the arms of the Apothecaries' Society on the back. Another made in 1741 is unusual, not only because it is baluster-shaped, but also because it has a peacock amongst foliage and flowers on the side opposite the name.[50] Four jars have the date 1763 with the initials 'W N' on the opposite side to the cartouche.[51]

About the middle of the 18th century, syrup jars without handles and with the name of the drug on the opposite side to the spout were introduced (see, for example, Cat. 154).

Cherubs with trumpets: 1700–1725 (Cat. 159–163)

In the next design we consider, 'cherubs with trumpets', the basket of fruit, angel and peacock feather swags have all been retained, but the songbirds have been replaced by winged cherubs. They are sitting on top of the label and playing trumpets. This group contains 49 jars, and no dated jars are known, but because it appears to be a transitional design, linking the songbirds and the cherub and shell pattern, these jars are thought to have been made in Bristol during the first quarter of the 18th century.[52] Another 11 jars are of the same basic design, but in a far finer style. They include two cylindrical jars, suggesting that they date from 1740–1780. It is possible that these later jars were made in Liverpool.

Cherub and shell: 18th century (Cat. 164–211)

This design is the one most commonly encountered on 18th century tin-glazed drug jars. Here the cherubs have exchanged their trumpets for a sprig of foliage, and the basket of fruit has been replaced by a scallop shell. Below the cartouche the angel's head is now flanked by folded rather than outspread wings, and the tendency for the peacock feathers to be replaced by stylised flowers, which we saw in the later songbird jars, is confirmed. For some reason, which has never been explained, very few jars of this design were dated.

Only two dates are recorded, eight from 1723 (see, for example, Cat. 164 and 165) and four from 1738 (see, for example, Cat. 167 and 168). Jars from the earlier set are extremely unusual in having polychrome decoration, and there is one undated polychrome jar in the Royal Pharmaceutical Society collection, almost certainly made at the same time, and decorated by the same artist (Cat. 166).

Miscellaneous designs

Although most tin-glazed jars we encounter fall into one of the groups described above, a number can be seen in which the basic design has undergone a significant modification, and others that do not seem to fall into any established category. For example, there is a unicorn on a jar in the Museum of London, thought to date

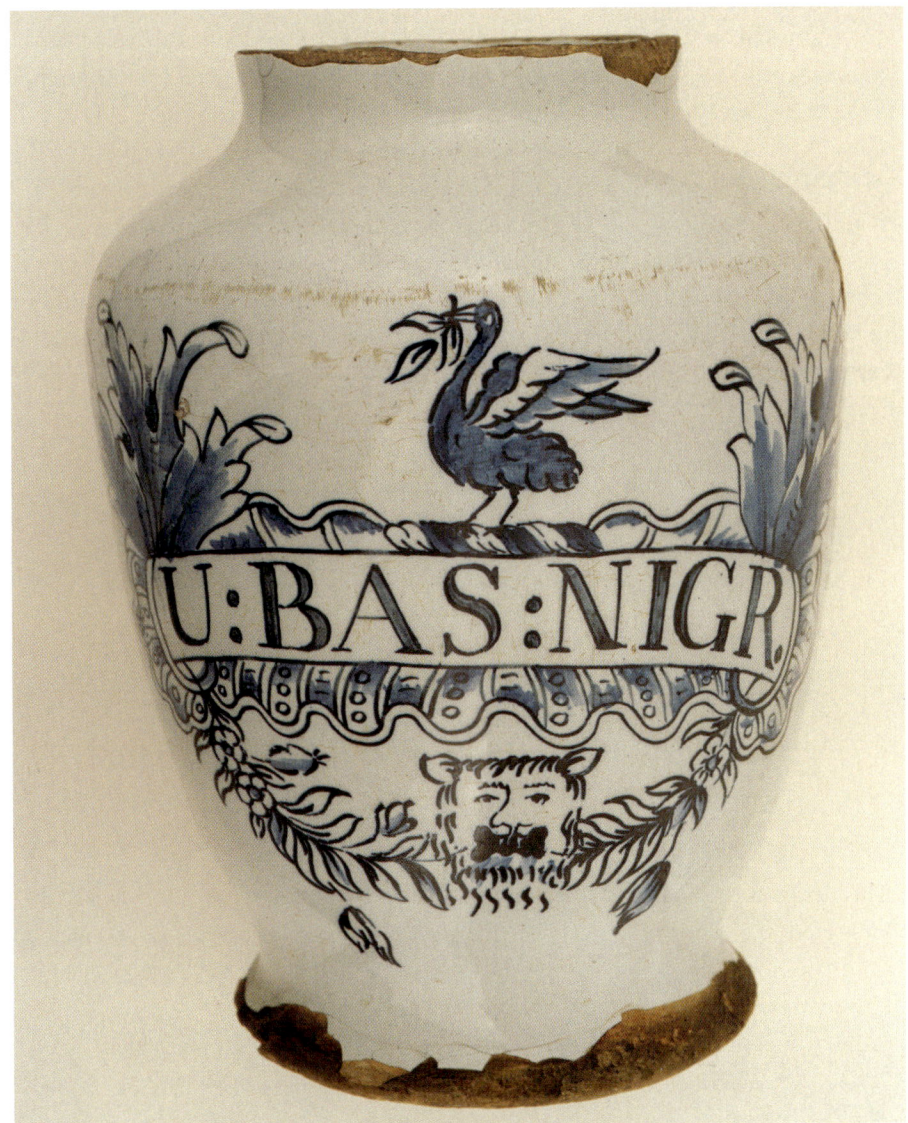

Jar decorated with the symbol of Liverpool, the 'liver bird', holding a sprig of liverwort in its beak and, below the cartouche, a grotesque head, apparently eating a bow tie. The statues of the two liver birds on the towers of the Liver Building are reputed to flap their wings whenever a virgin walks past. Photo by W A Jackson. Hunterian Museum at the Royal College of Surgeons.

from the middle of the 17th century; a group of 24 show a flying wyvern (a winged two-legged dragon with a barbed tail); a jar with a straight neck, almost certainly made in Liverpool, with the symbol of the city, the 'liver bird' holding a sprig of liverwort in its beak and, below the cartouche, a grotesque head, apparently eating a bow tie;[53] the jar with a crescent moon on the spout and the sun and some leaves below the title,[54] another in which a basket of fruit is flanked by two dolphins (Cat. 215), and one in which the cartouche is surrounded by scrolled leaves and has the initials 'W M' and the date 1764 on the reverse side.[55] Another 21 jars of this type, all undated, are known (see, for example, Cat. 217). Lipski and Archer record a jar dated 1675 labelled 'C. CICHORI' (sic), which has the cartouche over a tulip flanked by simple sprays,[56] and another specimen, labelled 'S.DE.POM.PVR. 1675' exists in a private collection in London.

An unusual jar, labelled 'S. DIAMOR' (syrup of mulberries), now in the Royal Pharmaceutical Society's collection, has a diagonal cartouche, and decoration that can only be described as abstract (Cat. 213).[57]

Armorial jars

In addition, there are a number of very fine large polychrome decorative jars bearing the coat of arms of the Society of Apothecaries of London. One example, from 1647, is the earliest known dated English drug jar, and is in the Museum of the Royal Pharmaceutical Society of Great Britain (Cat. 50). Another, which is in

Dated English delftware jars	
Design	**Dated jars known**
Pipe-smoking man	1652, 1665
Ribbon cartouche	1655, 1658, 1659, 1661, 1662, 1664, 1665, 1666
Angel	1659, 1660, 1661, 1664, 1665, 1666, 1667, 1668, 1669, 1671, 1672, 1673, 1674, 1675, 1677, 1678, 1679, 1680, 1681, 1682, 1683, 1684, 1689, 1690, 1695, 1697, 1700, 1722
Fleur-de-lys	1667, 1669, 1670, 1675, 1677, 1690
Early songbird	1672
Apollo and peacocks	1679, 1694
Apollo and serpents	1717
Later songbirds	1702, 1706, 1714, 1724, 1741, 1763
Cherub and shell	1723, 1738
Scrolled leaves	1764
Tulip	1675
Display jars	1647, 1656, 1658

the Longridge Collection, is illustrated with a number of objects, such as birds, flowers, insects and a dragon.[58] It seems likely that such jars were intended for display rather than for storage purposes. The Glaisher Collection contains a jug decorated in blue with the initials 'EV' and the date '1650'. The lip has an 'eye' on either side of it, giving it some resemblance to an owl. Underneath it the arms of the Apothecaries' Society are on the side opposite to the handle, and on the sides and neck are seashore scenes depicting ships and buildings. There are silver mounts with the hallmarks for 1844 on the rim and the foot.[59]

Significance of the designs used

Little has been written about the origins or significance of the designs used to decorate English drug jars: individual pot-banks seem to have used different designs, and similar designs have been used by different potters.

It is tempting to think that there might be a religious theme, although not necessarily a Christian one, linking some designs. Images of the pagan god, the 'Green Man', are to be found in many old churches, both in England and on the Continent, Apollo was the god of healing, the scallop shell was the emblem of Saint James of Compostella (and the badge of those who made pilgrimages to his shrine)[60] and the religious significance of angels is well known. However, unlike some Continental jars, no portraits of saints are depicted,[61] and how do we account for the presence of peacocks, songbirds, baskets of fruit, antlers, fleur-de-lys, unicorns, wyverns and dolphins?

The only obvious evidence for drug jars following the wider trend in delftware for Chinese-inspired designs is a small number of the most decorative armorial jars, having beautiful Chinese-style scenes on their reverse (such as the 1647 dated jar in the Royal Pharmaceutical Society's collection). However, Matthews suggests that the songbird design was also inspired by late Ming Chinese porcelain.[62]

It is with some regret that I must confess to being unable to see any connecting link between the various designs used, and this is probably why nothing seems to have been written on the subject. They may have been partially inspired by the wood carvings used on furniture or architectural features, and angels with outstretched wings are found on gravestones and on memorials in churches. Perhaps they were originally devised by the owner of the pottery or commissioned by an apothecary. Unless some documentary evidence is found to offer an explanation I fear this is likely to remain a mystery.

Later types of drug jar

There can be little doubt that most collectors find these 17th and 18th century tin-glazed jars by far the most interesting group of English drug jars, a point of view that is difficult to dispute when one looks at their great variety in shape and

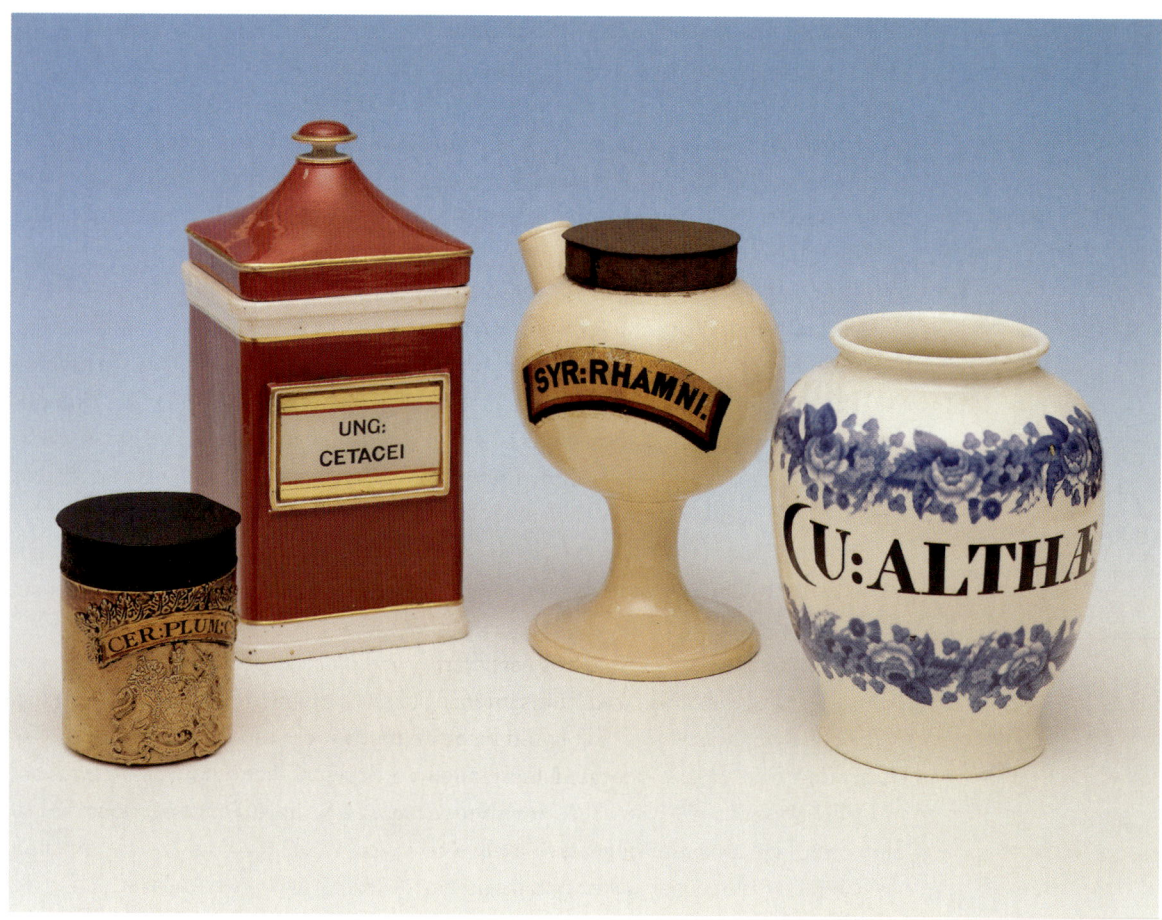

decoration. Advancing technology in methods of manufacture and simplification of decoration resulted in increasing standardisation of jars as time progressed, and later jars lack much of the charm of the examples we have been considering. Nevertheless, each later group has its own appeal, and should not be neglected by those with an interest in pharmaceutical artefacts.

Creamware[63]

As the 18th century progressed, tin-glazed earthenware was largely replaced in England by cream-coloured earthenware, which later became known as creamware. These articles were thinly potted with a brilliant, transparent creamy glaze. Creamware first made its appearance in the years preceding 1740, and before the end of the century had virtually replaced tin-glazed earthenware in this country, although the latter went on being produced on the Continent.

Pearlware

Originally known as pearl-white ware, pearlware was a type of earthenware introduced by Josiah Wedgwood in 1797. The glaze contained a little cobalt oxide,

A group of later English ceramic drug jars from the Royal Pharmaceutical Society's collection: stoneware ointment jar embossed with the Royal coat of arms, early 1800s (Ceratum plumbi compositum, compound cerate of lead); earthenware ointment pot with lid and removable lining, late 1800s/early 1900s (Unguentum cetacei, spermaceti ointment); creamware wet drug jar, late 1700s/early 1800s (Syrupus rhamnus, syrup of buckthorn); apothecary jar with a 'Union Wreath' design, made by Spode c.1825 (Unguentum althaeae, marshmallow ointment).

producing vessels with a bluish-white cast, and in early specimens the bluish glaze had a tendency to accumulate in folds and near the base. It is not always easy to distinguish later creamware from early pearlware, and the Wellcome Collection contains two rare jars that are probably pearlware, but are decorated with cherub designs similar to some found on tin-glazed earthenware.[64]

White earthenware

Eventually it became possible to produce earthenware with a body that was really white. Decoration became less important, and was often limited to the name of the drug on a cartouche, usually ending in ribbon scrolls, but a particularly attractive set of jars was made at the Spode factory. These were decorated with blue and white transfer prints of their second 'Union Wreath' design, which was introduced about 1825, and the names of the drugs were painted over the glaze in black. This probably unique set of jars were used by Corbyn, Stacey and Company until 1895.[65]

Earthenware with coloured glazes

Probably the reason so few drug jars were made from white earthenware was the increasing use of coloured transparent glazes, making it possible to produce attractively coloured jars that could be made much more quickly and cheaply than ones that had to be decorated individually. Although such jars continued to be made and used until the 1950s for some drugs, often having recessed glass labels from the end of the 19th century, only a few were made for liquids – for example a syrup jar listed in a Maw's catalogue dated 1839.

Stoneware[66]

As I said earlier, there was no smooth progression of types of drug jar in England, and it is now necessary to return to the early 19th century, when we see the introduction of stoneware drug jars. These were made from clay and fusible stone, fired to a high temperature when partial vitrification made the body impervious to liquids. Salt was thrown into the kiln, and combined with the alumina and silica in the clay, producing a finely pitted, shiny glaze. The variation in colour between dark brown and light brown or grey was achieved by using a ferruginous dip. Although stoneware is known to have been made in England from about 1660, I can find no evidence of it being used to produce labelled drug jars before 1800. Many of these drug jars were decorated with the Hanoverian coat of arms, used until 1837 in relief. These moulds were still used well into the Victorian period, because of the expense of making new ones, but a few can be found with the Victorian coat of arms. Occasionally the Royal arms were flanked by other raised figures, for example lions or mounted knights.

Some very attractive sets of drug jars were made by artist potters at the Doulton factory in Lambeth, the impressed marks showing that they were made after 1891.

Plain stoneware jars with painted labels were used well into the 20th century, and ointments were still commonly being supplied in stoneware jars with paper labels in the 1950s.

Pill tiles[67]

Although this chapter is about drug jars, I feel that a brief mention should be made of the decorated tin-glazed earthenware tiles found in apothecaries' shops. These could be heart or shield-shaped, octagonal or (rarely) elliptical, and were frequently pierced with one or, more usually, two holes that could be used for suspending them. It has been suggested that they were used as signs to indicate the shop of an apothecary, and that the Society of Apothecaries gave them to apprentices upon obtaining the freedom of the Company, but there is no evidence to support either of these hypotheses. The abraded surface displayed by some tiles indicates that they were probably used for making pills and ointments, and were not merely ornamental.

Decoration

Both polychrome and blue and white tiles are known, many being decorated with variations of the arms of the Society of Apothecaries. In some examples Apollo is holding a bow in his right hand and an arrow in his left, instead of vice versa. Another inaccuracy is that sometimes the rhinoceros crest is surmounted by a tree (see, for example, Cat. 223). A number of tiles have the arms of the City of London below the Society's motto. Some tiles are dated and, of these, a number carry initials. An unusual polychrome one has the initials 'N B' and the date 1664, and is decorated with the arms of Charles II and the letters 'C R' (for Carolus Rex).[68] Even more unusual is a heart-shaped pictorial tile showing a man and dog mounting some steps towards a building.[69]

Later tiles made from lead-glazed earthenware were usually plain, although some were graduated to help divide the pill mass. Ones carrying the name of a manufacturer or wholesaler and/or coat of arms are rare.[70]

Conclusion

Nowadays we have little use for custom-made containers to hold drugs in the pharmacy, as they are kept in the containers in which they are received from the manufacturers or wholesalers, and the serried ranks of drug jars and shop rounds can no longer be seen. With their disappearance we also seem to have lost the characteristic smell, composed largely of herbs, spices, scented soap and perfume, that older readers will remember greeting them when they entered the shop. I still miss these things, and will always be grateful that I worked in the days when we dispensed medicines 'secundem artem'.

References and endnotes

1 Howard G E. *Early English Drug Jars*. London: The Medici Society, 1931.

2 Haslam J. *Medieval Pottery*. Princes Risborough: Shire Publications Ltd, 1984.

3 Rowe M, Trease G E. Thomas Baskerville, Elizabethan apothecary of Exeter. *Transactions of the British Society for the History of Pharmacy* 1970; 1(1): 3–28.

4 Charleston R J. The social background of English delftware. In: Lipski L L, Archer M, eds. *Dated English Delftware*. London: Philip Wilson Publishers Ltd, for Sotheby Publications, 1984: 9.

5 Burnby J. English apothecaries and probate entries: their use in pharmaceutical history. *Pharmaceutical Historian* 1997; 27(4): 53–58.

6 Garner F H, Archer M. *English Delftware*, 2nd edn. London: Faber and Faber, 1972: 2–3.

7 Savage G, Newman H. *An Illlustrated Dictionary of Ceramics*. London: Thames and Hudson, 1974: 291–292.

8 Britton F. *London Delftware*. London: Jonathon Horne, 1987: 19–22.

9 Britton F. *London Delftware*. London: Jonathon Horne, 1987: 103–104.

10 Wittop Koning D A. *Apothekerspotten uit de Nederlanden*. Haarle: Twist Productions, 1991: 28.

11 Drey R E A. *Apothecary Jars. Pharmaceutical Pottery and Porcelain in Europe and the East, 1150–1850*. London and Boston: Faber & Faber, 1978: 129–130.

12 Britton F. *London Delftware*. London: Jonathon Horne, 1987: 10.

13 Garner F H, Archer M. *English Delftware*, 2nd edn. London: Faber and Faber, 1972: 52–57.

14 Britton F. *English Delftware in the Bristol Collection*. London: Philip Wilson Publishers Ltd, for Sotheby Publications, 1982: 14.

15 Garner F H, Archer M. *English Delftware*, 2nd edn. London: Faber and Faber, 1972: 64–67 and illustration 121A. One of these plates is in the Glaisher Collection in the Fitzwilliam Museum, Cambridge, and the other in the Wilkinson Collection in the Thackray Medical Museum, Leeds.

16 Rackham B. *Catalogue of the Glaisher Collection of Pottery and Porcelain in the Fitzwilliam Museum, Cambridge*, Vol. 1, 1987, Woodbridge, Suffolk, by permission of Cambridge University Press, p. 212.

17 Wilkinson J F. Old English apothecary jars. *Proceedings of the Royal Society of Medicine* 1970; 63: 137–144.

18 Britton F. *English Delftware in the Bristol Collection*. London: Philip Wilson Publishers Ltd, for Sotheby Publications, 1982: 12.

19 Garner F H, Archer M. *English Delftware*, 2nd edn. London: Faber and Faber, 1972: 58–63.

20 Smith A. *The Illustrated Guide to Liverpool Herculaneum Pottery 1796–1840*. London: Barrie and Jenkins, 1970: 2.

21 Garner F H, Archer M. *English Delftware*, 2nd edn. London: Faber and Faber, 1972: 68–73.

22 Austin J C. *British Delft at Williamsburg*. Virginia and London: The Colonial Williamsburg Foundation in association with Jonathon Horne Publications, 1994: 15–16.

23 Wilkinson J. Apothecaries' jars. *The Antique Collector* 1974 (March); 51–53.

24 Howard G E. *Early English Drug Jars*. London: The Medici Society, 1931: 12.

25 Wilkinson J. Apothecaries' jars. *The Antique Collector* 1974 (March); 53.

26 Jackson W A. Is the man depicted on early English drug jars really smoking a pipe? *Pharmaceutical Journal* 2001; 267: 918–919.

27 Anderson W. *The Green Man*. London and San Francisco: HarperCollins, 1990.

28 Tugores M. Dutch gapers. *Pharmaceutical Journal* 1985; 235: 827–828.

29 Lipski L L, Archer M (eds). *Dated English Delftware. Tin-Glazed Earthenware 1600–1800*. London: Philip Wilson Publishers Ltd, for Sotheby Publications, 1984: 161, 164 (Nos. 724 and 739).

30 *Pharmaceutical Journal* 10 December 1977: 534.

31 Lothian A. The pipe-smoking man on 17th century English delft drug jars. *The Chemist and Druggist* 1955; 163: 568.

32 Howard G E. *Early English Drug Jars*. London: The Medici Society, 1931: 13–17.

33 Lothian A. Angels in the design of 17th century English delft drug jars. *Chemist and Druggist* 1955; 163: 734.

34 Wilkinson J F. Old English apothecary jars. *Proceedings of the Royal Society of Medicine* 1970; 63: 139–140.

35 Crellin J K. *Medical Ceramics. A Catalogue of the English and Dutch Collections in the Museum of the Wellcome Institute of the History of Medicine*, Vol. 1. London: Wellcome Institute of the History of Medicine, 1969: 21.

36 Lipski L L, Archer M (eds). *Dated English Delftware. Tin-Glazed Earthenware 1600–1800*. London: Philip Wilson Publishers Ltd, for Sotheby Publications, 1984: 369 (Colour plate IX and No. 1602).

37 Drey R A. A dated slipware drug jar. *Pharmaceutical Historian* 1975; 5(1): 1.

38 Letter from John Gash to C J Lucas, Horsham Museum, Ref. K109.

39 Humphries A. Personal Communication. Information from Jonathan Horne, July 2005.

40 Lipski L L, Archer M (eds). *Dated English Delftware. Tin-Glazed Earthenware 1600–1800*. London: Philip Wilson Publishers Ltd, for Sotheby Publications, 1984: 386 (No. 1662).

41 Wilkinson J F. Early English apothecaries' drug jars, Part 1. *Art and Antiques* Part 1 1981 (March); 44(6): 29.

42 Grigsby L B. *The Longridge Collection of English Slipware and Delftware, Vol. 2, Delftware*. London: Jonathon Horne Publications, 2000: 451.

43 Lothian A. Bird designs on English drug jars. *Chemist and Druggist* 1954 (June); 161: 672–677.

44 Lipski L L, Archer M (eds). *Dated English Delftware. Tin-Glazed Earthenware 1600–1800*. London: Philip Wilson Publishers Ltd, for Sotheby Publications, 1984: 379.

45 Lipski L L, Archer M (eds). *Dated English Delftware. Tin-Glazed Earthenware 1600–1800*. London: Philip Wilson Publishers Ltd, for Sotheby Publications, 1984: 384–385 (Nos. 1659 and 1659A).

46 Lipski L L, Archer M (eds). *Dated English Delftware. Tin-Glazed Earthenware 1600–1800*. London: Philip Wilson Publishers Ltd, for Sotheby Publications, 1984: 386–387 (Nos. 1666 and 1666A).

47 Wilkinson J F. Early English apothecaries' drug jars, Part 2. *Art and Antiques* 1981 (March); 44(20–26): 28.

48 Lothian A. Vessels for apothecaries. English delft drug jars. Reprinted from *The Connoisseur Year Book*, 1953, Nos. XXIX a and b, p. 5.

[49]Lothian A. Vessels for apothecaries. English delft drug jars. Reprinted from *The Connoisseur Year Book*, 1953, No. XXXIII, p. 6.

[50] Lipski L L, Archer M (eds). *Dated English Delftware. Tin-Glazed Earthenware 1600–1800*. London: Philip Wilson Publishers Ltd, for Sotheby Publications, 1984: 388–389 (Nos. 1669 and 1671).

[51] Lothian A. Bird designs on English drug jars. *Chemist and Druggist* 1954 (June); 161: 674.

[52] Lothian A. Cherub designs on English delft apothecary ware. *Chemist and Druggist* 1956 (June); 165: 608–613.

[53] Negus V. *Artistic Possessions at the Royal College of Surgeons of England*. Edinburgh and London: E & S Livingstone Ltd, 1967: 108–109.

[54] Lothian A. Vessels for apothecaries. English delft drug jars. Reprinted from *The Connoisseur Year Book*, 1953, No. XL, p. 7.

[55] Lipski L L, Archer M (eds). *Dated English Delftware. Tin-Glazed Earthenware 1600–1800*. London: Philip Wilson Publishers Ltd, for Sotheby Publications, 1984: 390 (No. 1673).

[56] Lipski L L, Archer M (eds). *Dated English Delftware. Tin-Glazed Earthenware 1600–1800*. London: Philip Wilson Publishers Ltd, for Sotheby Publications, 1984: 376 (No. 1630).

[57] Howard G E. *Early English Drug Jars*. London: The Medici Society, 1931: No. 34, Plate IX.

[58] Grigsby L B. *The Longridge Collection of English Slipware and Delftware, Vol. 2, Delftware*. London: Jonathon Horne Publications, 2000: 444–445.

[59] Rackham B. *Catalogue of the Glaisher Collection of Pottery and Porcelain in the Fitzwilliam Museum, Cambridge*, Vol. 2, 1987, Woodbridge, Suffolk, by permission of the Cambridge University Press, p. 83 (No. 1311).

[60]Hohler C. The badge of St James. In: Cox I, ed. *The Scallop*. London: The Shell Transport and Trading Company: 49–70.

[61] Lothian A. Saints on drug jars. *Chemist and Druggist* 1953; 159 (June): 598–603.

[62] Matthews L G. *Antiques of the Pharmacy*. London: G Bell and Sons, 1971: 5.

[63] Towner D. *Creamware*. London and Boston: Faber & Faber, 1978.

[64] Crellin J K. *Medical Ceramics. A Catalogue of the English and Dutch Collections in the Museum of the Wellcome Institute of the History of Medicine*, Vol. 1. London: Wellcome Institute of the History of Medicine, 1969: 114 and 121 (No. 21).

[65] Lothian Short A. Corbyn, Stacey & Co. – a note on their antiques. *Pharmaceutical Journal* 1967 (September): 211–212.

[66] Oswald A. *English Brown Stoneware 1670–1900*. London: Faber & Faber, 1982: 23.

[67] A fuller discussion of the shapes and decoration of pharmaceutical tiles can be found in Crellin J K. *Medical Ceramics. A Catalogue of the English and Dutch Collections in the Museum of the Wellcome Institute of the History of Medicine*, Vol. 1. London: Wellcome Institute of the History of Medicine, 1969: 143–150.

[68] Lipski L L, Archer M (eds). *Dated English Delftware. Tin-Glazed Earthenware 1600–1800*. London: Philip Wilson Publishers Ltd, for Sotheby Publications, 1984.

[69] *Pharmaceutical Journal* 1990 (28 July); 245: 125.

[70] Jackson W A, Antiques of Mander, Weaver and Co, Wolverhampton. *Pharmaceutical Historian* 1978; 8(3) (unpaginated).

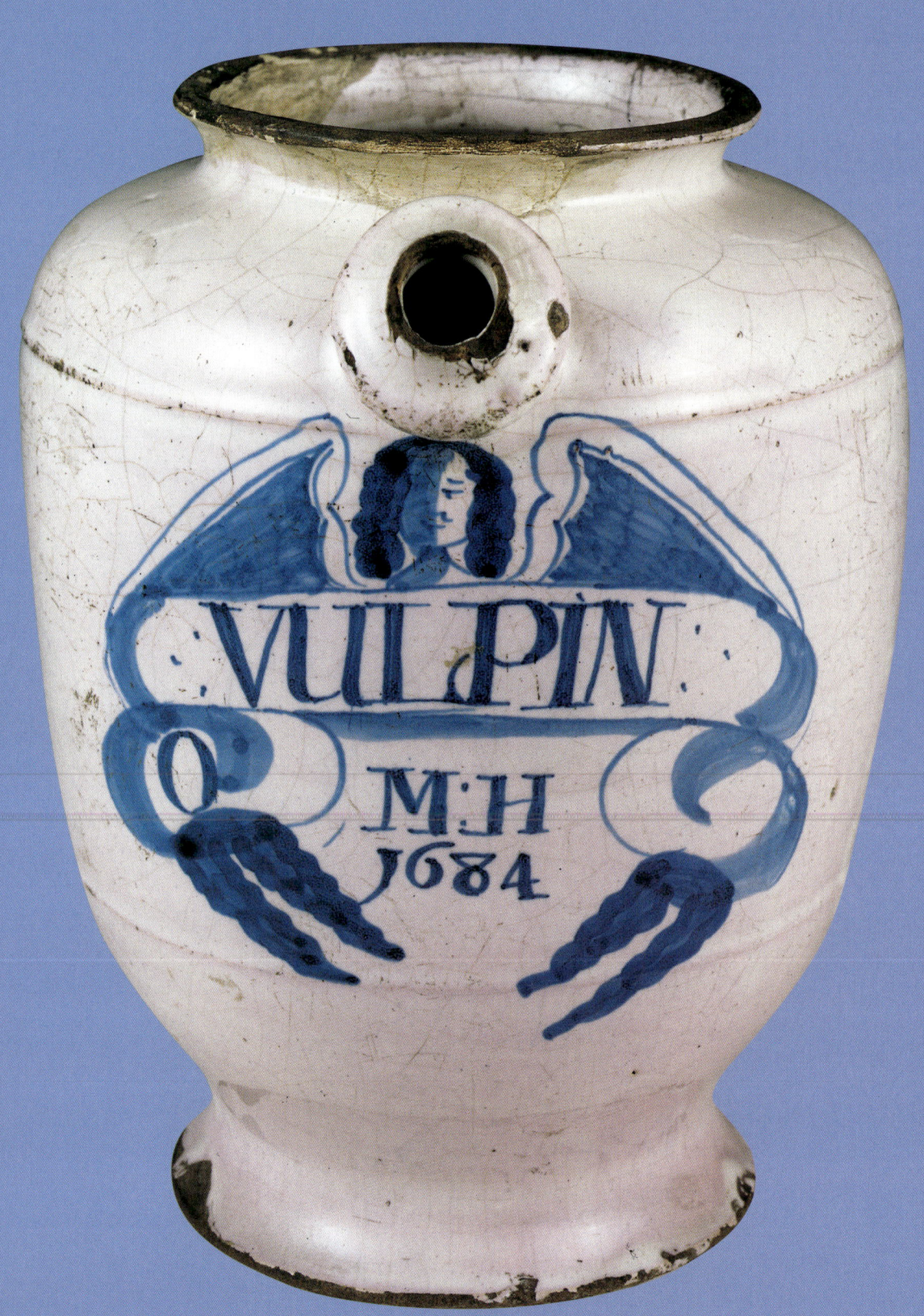

Catalogue

The catalogue has been arranged primarily by date and design. The overall structure is chronological, with the different designs placed together. Within each design type, the jars have been organised by date, and by group where it seems possible to draw conclusions. Of course, the jars were not made so that curators could order them neatly in a strict chronology and so there are inevitable overlaps and uncertainties.

The early cylindrical or albarello-shaped jars form the first section. In order to maintain groups according to acquisition and possible find dates and locations, some pots have been included that do not have tin glaze.

The objects that are not drug jars conclude the catalogue section. Delftware pill tiles, the Society's collection of barber's bowls, a porringer and a posset pot have been included.

Catalogue entries

Each catalogue entry consists of the following:

Simple name: e.g. Dry drug jar

Accession number: e.g. KCD/P1 (see below)

Description: A physical description of the object, its shape, colour and glaze.

Design: e.g. Pipe-smoking man

Inscription: Where relevant, quoted directly from what is shown on the object.

Wet drug jar depicting an angel with outspread wings, manufactured in London in 1684 (Cat. 86).

Meaning of inscription: In most cases this is an expansion of the Latin abbreviation (see below) and its English translation.

Contemporary account: This quotation aims to put into context the preparation that would have been stored in the jar (see below).

Date of manufacture: If a specific date is given, this is because it is inscribed on the jar. A date range suggests uncertainty. A date with c. (circa) means that the object compares closely with another example, which provides some certainty of a more specific date.

Place of manufacture: This is given as specifically as possible, but is often difficult to state accurately.

Dimensions: Each object's height and maximum width is given in millimetres.

Provenance: Details of how the Museum acquired the object, where known, and also information about previous owners where possible.

Condition: A brief note on the condition of the jar, under the broad terms poor, fair and good.

Comment: This section includes any additional information from a range of sources, including comparisons with objects in other collections, and detailed observations about design, shape or a jar's contents. Geoffrey Howard's comments on his own jars have been included whenever possible, even when, as in many cases, his suggestions have subsequently been questioned or disproved.

References: Publications where the item is illustrated or referred to. Full details for each publication are provided in the bibliography.

Accession numbers

In line with standard museum practice, each object has been assigned a unique accession number. The numbering system used at the Royal Pharmaceutical Society has changed once in its history. Robert Todd, the person in charge of the Museum's historical collections from 1969 to 1982, developed his own classification system for the entire collection. This generally consisted of a three-letter prefix, followed by a running number sequence. 'K' denotes a drug jar. 'KA' is a dated English dry drug jar, and 'KB' is a dated English wet drug jar. 'KC' is an undated English dry drug jar, and 'KD' is an undated English wet drug jar. The third letter in the prefix links to the jar's design. For example, 'D' is a pipe-smoking man design, and 'F' is fleur-de-lys.

More recently the Museum has adopted the widespread practice of forming the accession number from the year in which the object was acquired, and then sub-numbering each group of objects, and then each individual object. For example, 2002.60.1 is the first item in the sixtieth group of objects acquired in the year 2002.

Latin and abbreviations found on drug jars

The abbreviated Latin labels in decorative cartouches found on tin-glazed drug jars are characteristic of these objects. Translating these abbreviations is a task in itself, not made any easier by the sometimes inaccurate renditions of the abbreviations in question, the squashing in of certain letters when the artist appears to have run out of space, and the fashion of concealing some of the letters amongst the cartouche's decoration.

The abbreviation on each jar is translated and explained in each catalogue record. However, there are some general rules that help to read these labels, particularly relating to the type of preparation stored in the jar. Some of the most common in the Pharmaceutical Society's collection are as follows:

- B usually stands for *balsamum* (balsam).
- C may stand for *confectio* (confection), *conserva* (conserve) or *cortex* (bark).
- E is an abbreviation for *electuarium* (electuary) or *extractum* (extract).
- L refers to *lohoch* (lohoch) or *linimentum* (liniment).
- O stands for *oleum* (oil).
- P is usually for *pilulae* (pills).
- S for *syrupus* (syrup).
- T stands for *trochisici* (lozenges).
- Ther is short for *theriacum* (treacle).
- U is an abbreviation of *unguentum* (ointment). However, U is sometimes shown as a V, particularly on 17th century jars. Similarly, following a Roman styling, J is sometimes represented as I.

There is a useful summary of other features of drug jar labels in Drey R. *Apothecary Jars: Pharmaceutical Pottery and Porcelain in Europe and the East 1150–1850*. London and Boston: Faber & Faber, 1978, pp. 179–182.

Contemporary sources

In order to explain the labels on the jars and to put their intended contents in context, each catalogue entry includes a contemporary account of the preparation or one of the ingredients that would have been stored in the jar. The contemporary spelling, capital letters and italicisation have been kept in these quotations, even when spellings differ within a passage. The only amendment is that the long 's' has not been reproduced.

These contemporary insights have been taken from dispensatories or pharmacopoeias of the period.

Abbreviations and symbols found in recipes

The contemporary accounts included in each catalogue entry are primarily given in the form of a recipe or formula. As such they include standard Latin abbreviations and symbols for weights, used into the 20th century and beyond. For example, Roman numerals in lower case are used to indicate quantities – ii represents 2, iv represents 4. Other abbreviations include:

ana   of each

m.   *manipulus*, a handful

S.A.   *Secundum Artem*, meaning according to the skill of the apothecary or pharmacist. This is usually found at the end of a recipe, meaning use your skill to achieve the finished product.

ss   *semis, semissis*, a half

Apothecary weights

Apothecary weights were used in Europe for the measurement of pharmaceutical ingredients from the 1200s. Dispensing continued in the Apothecary system until 1 January 1971, when metric weights and measures were adopted. The basis of the Apothecary system was the grain.

One grain	gr.				
One scruple	Э	=	20 grains		
One drachm	ʒ	=	60 grains		
One ounce	℥	=	480 grains		
One pound	℔	=	12 ounces	=	5760 grains

Glossary

The medical terms used in the contemporary accounts in most catalogue entries are explained below. The spelling used in the accounts follows the 17th or 18th century original. For example, 'alexipharmick' or 'antiscorbutick' may be used. The spellings in the glossary are modern. The glossary does not include explanation of all of the many and varied ingredients used in the medicinal preparations. See the bibliography for suggestions of further reading on this subject.

Alexipharmic An antidote

Anodyne Analgesic, relieves pain, usually made with opium

Antidote Drug that counteracts or neutralises the effects of a poison or an unwanted condition

Antiscorbutic A treatment for scurvy

Antiseptic Drug that prevents 'sepsis' or putrefaction

Antispasmodic Preparation that reduces spasms

Antitussive Drug that alleviates or suppresses coughing

Aperient A mild laxative

Aromatic A plant or drug that gives off a fragrant smell

Astringent A substance that contracts tissues to stop blood flow or secretion of liquids. Used to reduce haemorrhage, diarrhoea, sweating. Externally, an astringent contracts broken or ulcerated skin

Basilicon An ointment, supposed to possess 'sovereign' qualities

Canary A sweet wine from the Canary Islands, similar to Madeira

Carminative A preparation that relieves flatulence, facilitates expulsion of gas from the intestines, most often prescribed for dyspepsia

Carus Profound sleep or insensibility

Cataplasm A poultice, usually with a water, rather than oil, base

Cathartic A purgative drug that prompts defecation

Cephalic Relating to the head

Cerate A hard ointment or paste, made by mixing lard or oil with wax or resin

Clyster Another term for an enema

Collyria An eyewash, a fluid or dry medication to apply to the eyes for inflammatory conditions

Conserve Flower or fruits of a single plant beaten into a uniform mass with sugar

Cordial A medicine that stimulates the heart

Decoction A liquid medicine that results from boiling a drug or medicinal plant to extract the water-soluble substances

Defluxion A flow or discharge from the eyes and nose, or a flow of humours from one part of the body to another in a particular disease

Detersive A preparation that is cleansing or scouring, either as a purge, or in the sense of removing corrupt matter from the body

Diaphoretic Drug that produces perspiration or sweating

Discutient A preparation that disperses morbid matter

Diuretic Drug that increases the flow of urine by stimulating the kidneys

Electuary A paste or lozenge made from powder mixed with honey, usually taken on the tip of a knife

Embrocation An ointment to rub into painful body parts, a liniment

Emetic A preparation that causes vomiting

Emmenagogue Promotes menstrual discharge, increases menstrual flow

Emollient Soothing or softening preparation, applied to skin

Emplaister Another term for a plaster or salve

Epatick Now 'hepatic'; relating to, or acting on the liver, good for the liver

Erysipela 'St Anthony's Fire', an acute streptococcal infection of the skin, resulting in fever, headache, vomiting and purple raised lesions, usually on the face

Expectorant Drug that promotes the secretion and rejection of mucus or other fluids from the lungs and windpipe. Used in pneumonia, catarrh, asthma

Fluxes Excessive blood flow, or excrement, or any other discharge

Fomentation Applying heat and moisture to the body to relieve pain and inflammation

Garagarism Another name for a gargle

Hydropic A treatment for dropsy, which cures the patient's thirst

Hysteric A preparation to treat uterine disorders

Incarn To promote healing

Infusion An extract obtained by soaking

Julep A sweet drink

Laxative Gentle cathartic, to stimulate the evacuation of faeces

Letharge White or red lead

Liniment External preparation to rub in for pain, stiffness or other muscle conditions

Lithontriptic A preparation that breaks up stones in the bladder

Lohoch Thick pectoral remedy, sucked from the end of a liquorice stick

Megrim Migraine, a severe headache

Mesue A figure in medieval medicine, possibly fictitious, to whom are ascribed various medical writings, including the Grabadia, one of the earliest collections of materia medica to be arranged in pharmacopoeical form

Mucilage A sticky preparation

Pectoral Medicine or a preparation for disorders of the chest or lungs

Purgative/purge Strong cathartic – prompting evacuation of the bowels

Quartan A fever or ague

Rheum Watery discharge from the nose or eyes

Rickets A disease caused by vitamin D deficiency, characterised by softening and consequent distortion of the bones

Stomachic Warms and strengthens the stomach, stimulates gastric activity

Tetters Eruption of the skin, caused by a wide range of complaints such as eczema, herpes, ringworm

Tonic Strengthens the body via the stomach, to increase circulation, digestion, muscular action, or sense of wellbeing

Theriac Literally 'treacle', an opium preparation with many other ingredients

Troche A lozenge

Unguent Ointment, plaster diluted with oil, to the consistency of stiff honey

Viscidities Sticky, glutinous substances

Vulnerary A preparation used to heal a wound

Catalogue contents

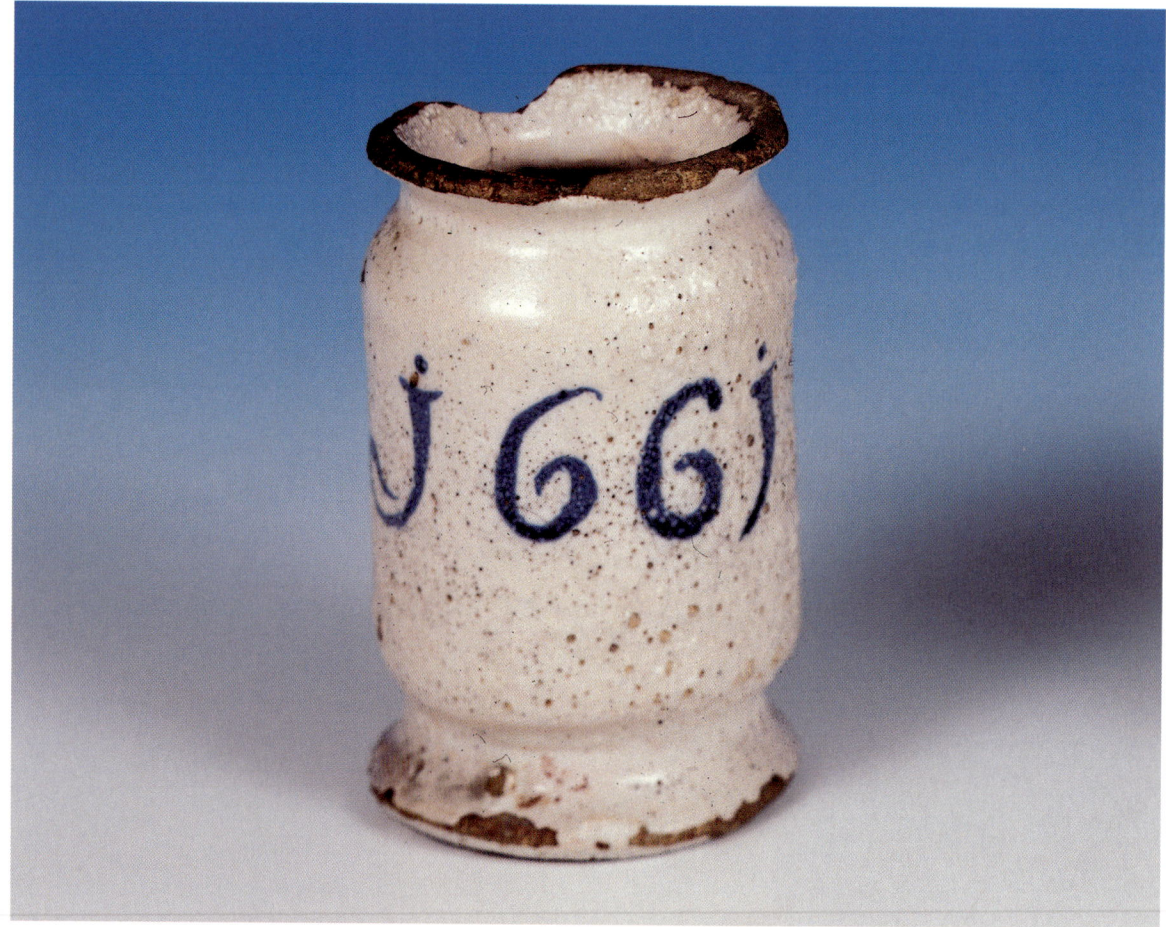

Dry drug jar (Cat.1)

ACCESSION NUMBER: KAA1
DESCRIPTION: Albarello shape, cream glaze with date in blue.
Neck everted with unglazed rim. Unglazed flat base.
INSCRIPTION: 1661
DATE OF MANUFACTURE: 1661
PLACE OF MANUFACTURE: London
DIMENSIONS: Height 60 mm, maximum width 38 mm
PROVENANCE: Bought in 1950
CONDITION: Good; large chips to rim, some loss of glaze on
body.

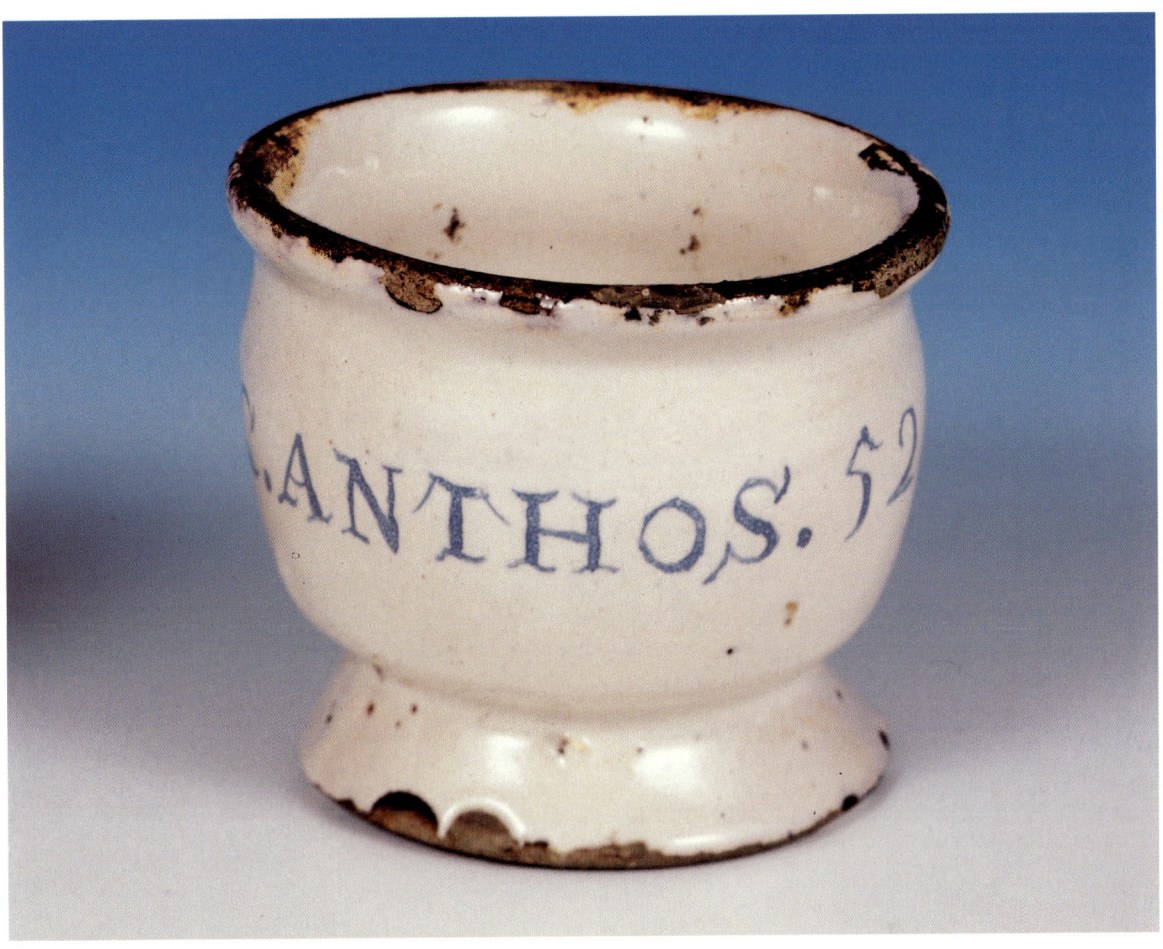

Dry drug jar (Cat.2)

ACCESSION NUMBER: KAA2

DESCRIPTION: Squat jar, tapering towards splayed base. White glaze with greyish tinge and design in blue, label panel straight. Neck everted with unglazed rim, glazed concave base with unglazed edge.

INSCRIPTION: 16 C.ANTHOS.52

MEANING OF INSCRIPTION: *Conserva anthos*, conserve of rosemary flowers

CONTEMPORARY ACCOUNT: "Our Garden Rosemary is so wel known, that I need not describe it. It Flowereth in *April* and *May* with us, and sometimes again in August... The flowers, and the Conserve made of them, is singular good to comfort the Heart, and to expel the contagion of the Pestilence..." (Culpeper, *The English Physician Enlarged*, 1655, pp. 319–320).

DATE OF MANUFACTURE: 1652

PLACE OF MANUFACTURE: London

DIMENSIONS: Height 53 mm, maximum width 68 mm

PROVENANCE: Bought in 1957, Howard Collection.

CONDITION: Good; glaze flaked on neck and base of rim.

COMMENT: It has been suspected that the inscription on this jar could be fake.

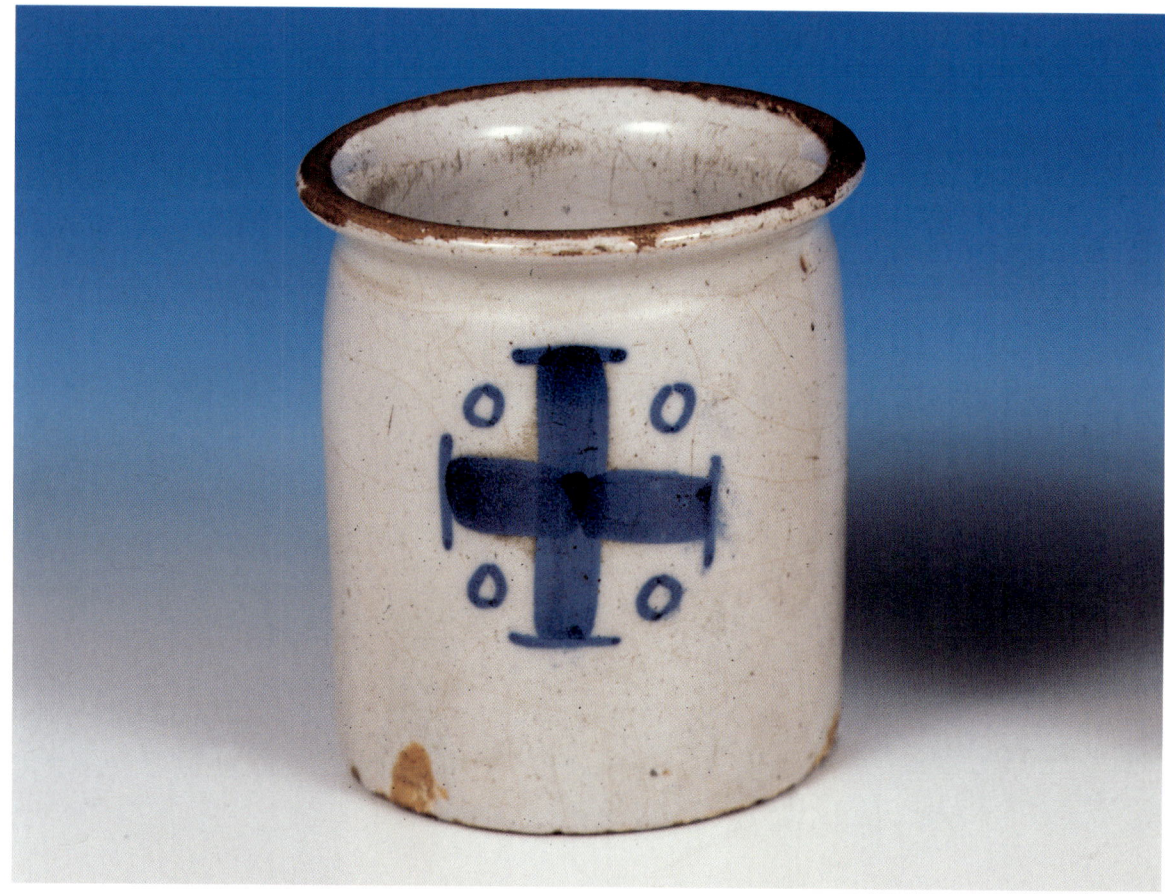

Dry drug jar (Cat.3)

ACCESSION NUMBER: KCA1

DESCRIPTION: Cylindrical jar. White glaze with pinkish tinge and design in blue. Neck everted with unglazed rim, concave unglazed base.

DESIGN: A cross, with four circles.

DATE OF MANUFACTURE: 1600–1800

PLACE OF MANUFACTURE: Possibly Mortlake, London

DIMENSIONS: Height 80 mm, maximum width 78 mm

PROVENANCE: Donated by Mr Hammond, date unknown.

CONDITION: Good; chips to rim, and larger loss of glaze at base.

COMMENT: Stephenson in Sloane *et al.* (2003) states that this design was common on both the base and the body of ointment pots found on the site of a pot house on Mortlake High Street.

REFERENCE: Sloane et al. *Early Modern Industry and Settlement.*

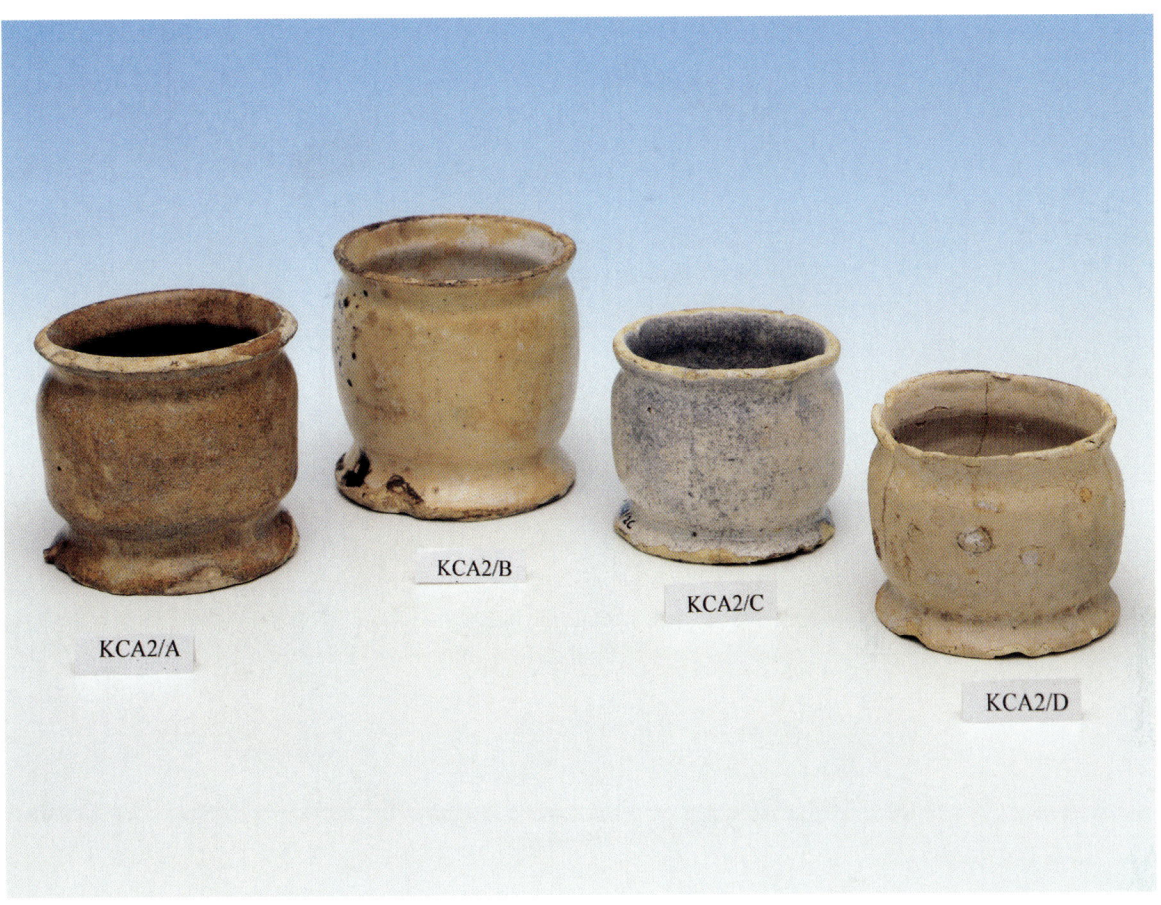

KCA2/B

KCA2/C

KCA2/A

KCA2/D

Dry drug jars (Cat.4–7)

The provenance of these jars is unclear. Museum records state that some jars were bought from "various" excavations. For example, in September 1961, the Museum purchased "An important collection of 34 Lambeth delft and other early unguent pots recovered from various London excavations in London circa 1926."

(Cat.4)

ACCESSION NUMBER: KCA2/A
DESCRIPTION: Squat jar, brown glaze. Neck everted with glazed rim.
DATE OF MANUFACTURE: 1570–1700
PLACE OF MANUFACTURE: London
DIMENSIONS: Height 62 mm, maximum width 73 mm
CONDITION: Good; very small chips.

(Cat.5)

ACCESSION NUMBER: KCA2/B
DESCRIPTION: Squat jar, white glaze with yellow tinge. Neck everted with glazed rim.
DATE OF MANUFACTURE: 1570-1700
PLACE OF MANUFACTURE: London

DIMENSIONS: Height 66 mm, maximum width 71 mm
CONDITION: Good; cracks to glaze, chips to rim and base

(Cat.6)

ACCESSION NUMBER: KCA2/C
DESCRIPTION: Squat jar, white glaze with grey tinge. Neck everted with unglazed rim.
DATE OF MANUFACTURE: 1570–1700
PLACE OF MANUFACTURE: London
DIMENSIONS: Height 51 mm, maximum width 64 mm
CONDITION: Good; chips to base and rim, addition of unglazed material on one side.

(Cat.7)

ACCESSION NUMBER: KCA2/D
DESCRIPTION: Squat jar, white glaze. Everted neck with unglazed rim.
DATE OF MANUFACTURE: 1570–1700
PLACE OF MANUFACTURE: London
DIMENSIONS: Height 51 mm, maximum width 63 mm
PROVENANCE: Label on base of jar reads 'Vandon St 31.8.27.' Assumed to be location and date of find. Vandon Street is close to Buckingham Palace.
CONDITION: Fair; many chips on base and rim

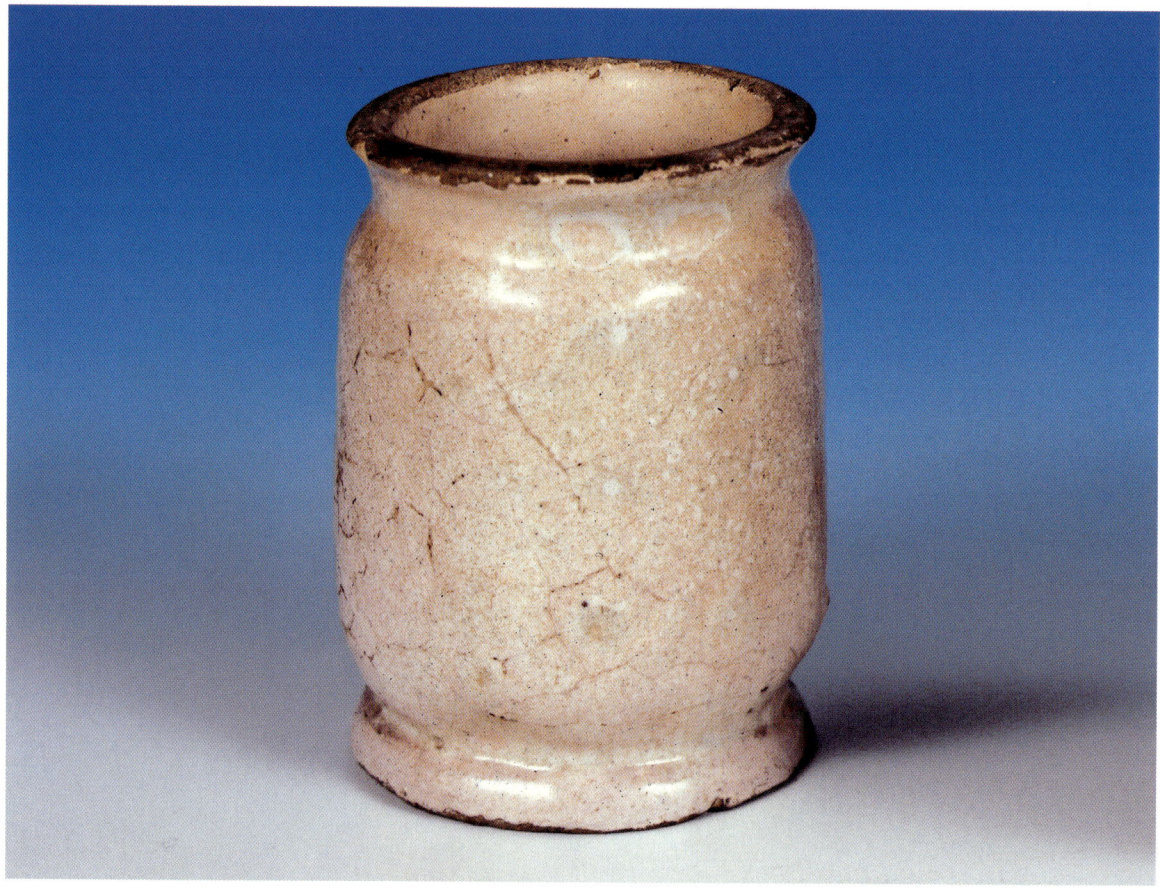

Dry drug jar (Cat.8)

ACCESSION NUMBER: KCA3
DESCRIPTION: Albarello-shaped jar with everted unglazed rim, white glaze.
DATE OF MANUFACTURE: 1600 - 1700
PLACE OF MANUFACTURE: London
DIMENSIONS: Height 75 mm, maximum width 60 mm
PROVENANCE: Has 'Gresham Street, Jan 26 1924' labelled on base of jar. Assumed to be location and date of find. Gresham Street is in the City of London.
CONDITION: Good; glaze crazed, some chips at rim and base.

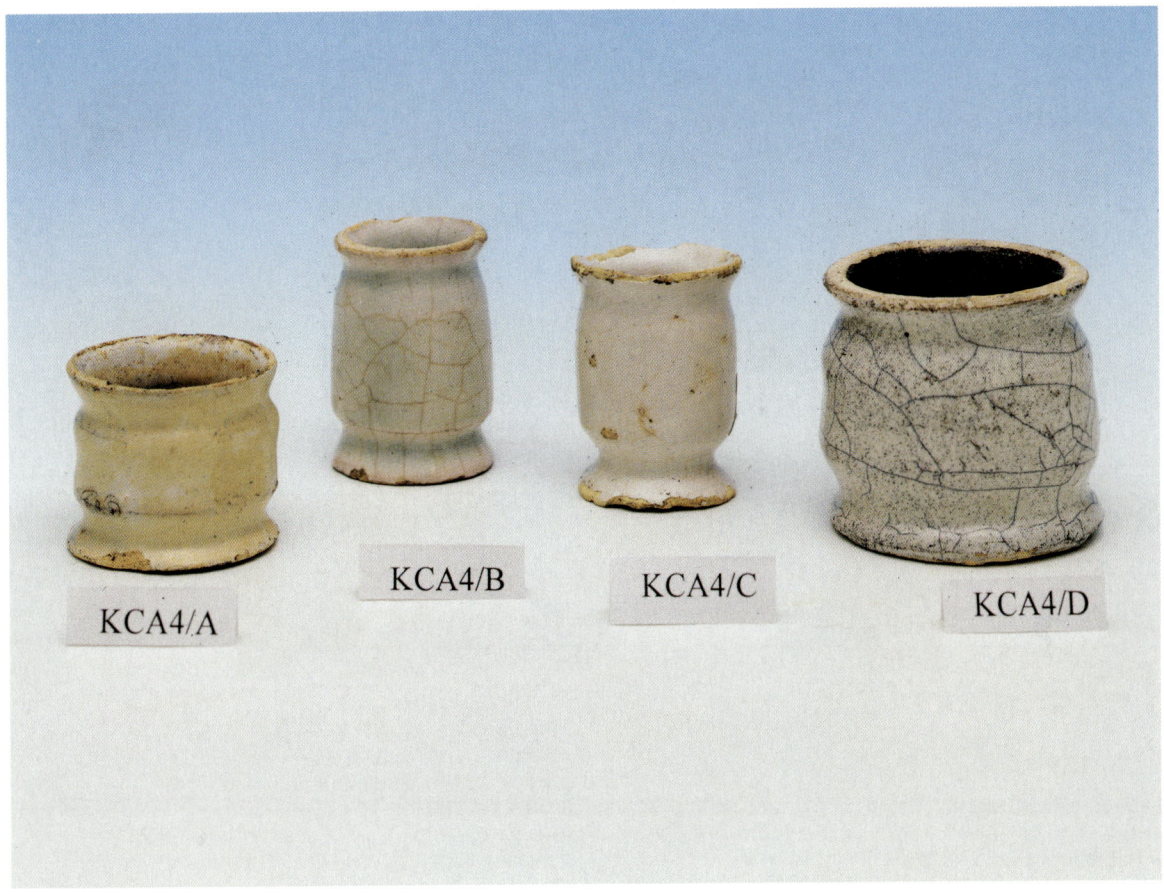

KCA4/A   KCA4/B   KCA4/C   KCA4/D

Dry drug jars (Cat.9–12)

The provenance of these jars is unclear. Museum records state that some jars were bought from "various" excavations. For example, in September 1961, the Museum purchased "An important collection of 34 Lambeth delft and other early unguent pots recovered from various London excavations in London circa 1926."

(Cat.9)
ACCESSION NUMBER: KCA4/A
DESCRIPTION: Squat jar, white glaze with yellow tinge. Everted neck with unglazed rim.
DATE OF MANUFACTURE: 1570–1700
PLACE OF MANUFACTURE: London
DIMENSIONS: Height 32 mm, maximum width 38 mm
CONDITION: Good; small chips and areas of glaze lost.

(Cat.10)
ACCESSION NUMBER: KCA4/B
DESCRIPTION: Albarello-shaped jar with white glaze, with blue and pink tinge. Everted neck with unglazed rim.
DATE OF MANUFACTURE: 1600-1700
PLACE OF MANUFACTURE: London

DIMENSIONS: Height 44 mm, maximum width 29 mm
PROVENANCE: Jar is labelled "730 Lambeth delft 17 C^Y L'DON 1935"
CONDITION: Fair; large chips to rim and some to base. Crazed glaze

(Cat.11)
ACCESSION NUMBER: KCA4/C
DESCRIPTION: Albarello-shaped jar, white glaze.
DATE OF MANUFACTURE: 1650–1700
PLACE OF MANUFACTURE: London
DIMENSIONS: Height 43 mm, maximum width 32 mm
PROVENANCE: Jar is labelled 'Wood St SW 19.3.28.' Assumed to be location and date of find.
CONDITION: Fair; chips to base and rim.

(Cat.12)
ACCESSION NUMBER: KCA4/D
DESCRIPTION: Squat jar with white glazed exterior and brown interior. Everted neck, unglazed rim.
DATE OF MANUFACTURE: 1650–1700
PLACE OF MANUFACTURE: London
DIMENSIONS: Height 46 mm, maximum width 49 mm
CONDITION: Good; very crazed glaze.

Early Jars

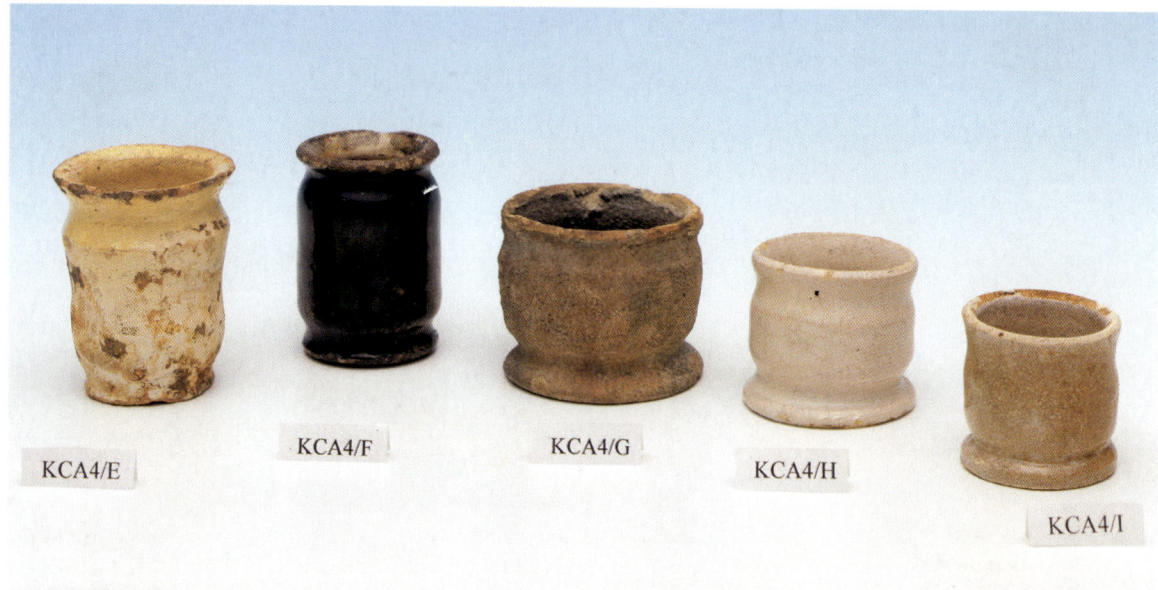

KCA4/E KCA4/F KCA4/G KCA4/H KCA4/I

Dry drug jars (Cat.13–17)

(Cat.13)

ACCESSION NUMBER: KCA4/E
DESCRIPTION: Albarello-shaped jar, white glaze with yellow tinge. Everted neck with glazed rim.
DATE OF MANUFACTURE: 1570-1700
PLACE OF MANUFACTURE: London
DIMENSIONS: Height 56 mm, maximum width 48 mm
PROVENANCE: Unclear. Museum records state that some of these jars were bought from "various" excavations. For example, in September 1961, the Museum purchased "An important collection of 34 Lambeth delft and other early unguent pots recovered from various London excavations in London circa 1926."
CONDITION: Fair; a large number of chips and loss of glaze.

(Cat.14)

ACCESSION NUMBER: KCA4/F
DESCRIPTION: Albarello-shaped jar, dark brown glaze with black. Everted neck with unglazed rim.
DATE OF MANUFACTURE: 1600–1650
PLACE OF MANUFACTURE: London
DIMENSIONS: Height 57 mm, maximum width 40 mm
PROVENANCE: Unclear. Museum records state that some of these jars were bought from "various" excavations. For example, in September 1961, the Museum purchased "An important collection of 34 Lambeth delft and other early unguent pots recovered from various London excavations in London circa 1926."
CONDITION: Good; chip from rim, and small chips at base.

(Cat.15)

ACCESSION NUMBER: KCA4/G
DESCRIPTION: Squat jar, unglazed, everted rim.
DATE OF MANUFACTURE: 1570–1700
PLACE OF MANUFACTURE: London
DIMENSIONS: Height 41 mm, maximum width 43 mm
PROVENANCE: Jar is labelled '845 Lambeth 17 CY J.D. Nottingham 1936' Assumed location and date of find.
CONDITION: Good; small chips to rim and base.

(Cat.16)

ACCESSION NUMBER: KCA4/H
DESCRIPTION: Squat jar, white glaze. Everted neck, glazed rim.
DATE OF MANUFACTURE: 1570–1700
PLACE OF MANUFACTURE: London
DIMENSIONS: Height 45 mm, maximum width 56 mm
PROVENANCE: Donated by Mrs J Thomas, Brocksom collection,1985
CONDITION: Good; chips to rim and base

(Cat.17)

ACCESSION NUMBER: KCA4/I
DESCRIPTION: Squat jar, light brown glaze. Everted neck with glazed rim.
DATE OF MANUFACTURE: 1606
PLACE OF MANUFACTURE: London
DIMENSIONS: Height 38 mm, maximum width 40 mm
PROVENANCE: Donated by Mrs J Thomas, Brocksom Collection, 1985. The base of the jar is labelled Seething Lane, which is assumed to be the location of find. This road is located in the City of London, close to the Tower of London. Incidentally, Samuel Pepys worked at the Navy Office on Seething Lane.
CONDITION: Good; some chips to rim.

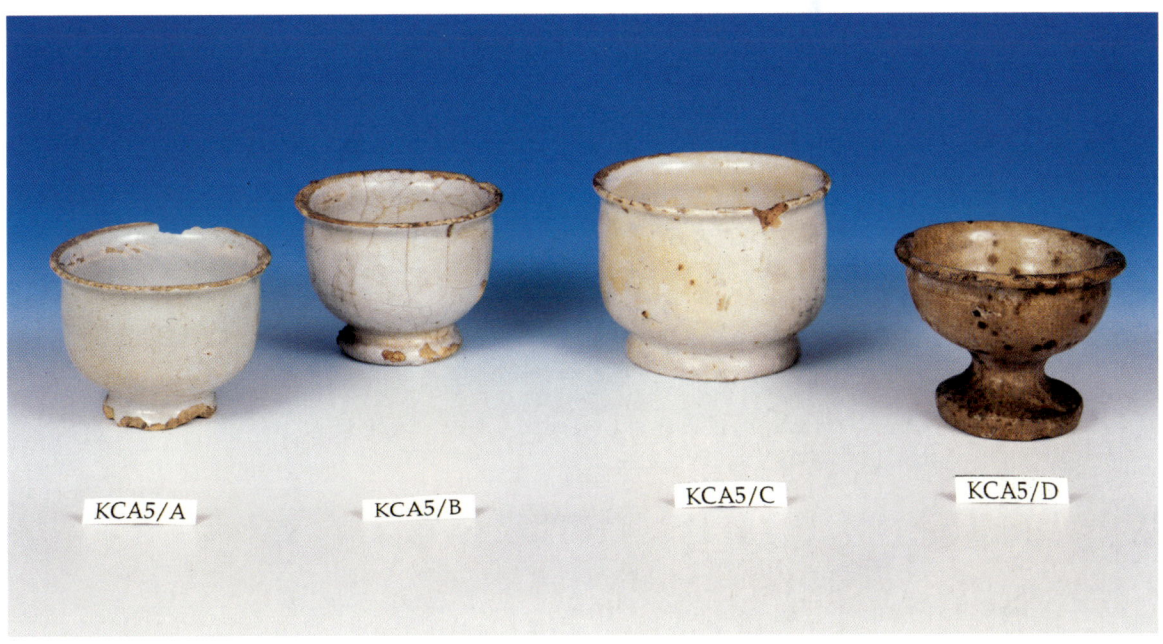

KCA5/A   KCA5/B   KCA5/C   KCA5/D

Dry drug jars (Cat.18–21)

(Cat.18)

ACCESSION NUMBER: KCA5/A

DESCRIPTION: Roughly cup-shaped jar, white glaze with blue tinge, unglazed rim.

DATE OF MANUFACTURE: 1570–1700

PLACE OF MANUFACTURE: London

DIMENSIONS: Height 57 mm, maximum width 82 mm

PROVENANCE: Donated by Mrs J Thomas, Brocksom collection, 1985

CONDITION: Fair; large chips to rim and base, loss of glaze on body.

(Cat.19)

ACCESSION NUMBER: KCA5/B

DESCRIPTION: Roughly cup-shaped jar, white glaze, unglazed rim.

DATE OF MANUFACTURE: 1570–1700

PLACE OF MANUFACTURE: London

DIMENSIONS: Height 58 mm, maximum width 83 mm

PROVENANCE: Jar labelled 'Wilton Rd Victoria 19.6.26' on base. Assumed location and date of find.

CONDITION: Fair; cracked glaze and chips

(Cat.20)

ACCESSION NUMBER: KCA5/C

DESCRIPTION: Roughly cup-shaped jar, white glaze, glazed rim.

DATE OF MANUFACTURE: 1750–1800

PLACE OF MANUFACTURE: London

DIMENSIONS: Height 64 mm, maximum width 91 mm

PROVENANCE: Unclear. Museum records state that some of these jars were bought from "various" excavations. For example, in September 1961, the Museum purchased "An important collection of 34 Lambeth delft and other early unguent pots recovered from various London excavations in London circa 1926 £50"

CONDITION: Good; large chip to rim, pitting to body.

(Cat.21)

ACCESSION NUMBER: KCA5/D

DESCRIPTION: Roughly cup-shaped jar on significant foot, brown glaze.

DATE OF MANUFACTURE: 1570–1700

PLACE OF MANUFACTURE: London

DIMENSIONS: Height 59 mm, maximum width 84 mm

PROVENANCE: Donated by Mrs J Thomas, Brocksom collection, 1985

CONDITION: Good; some loss of glaze.

Early Jars

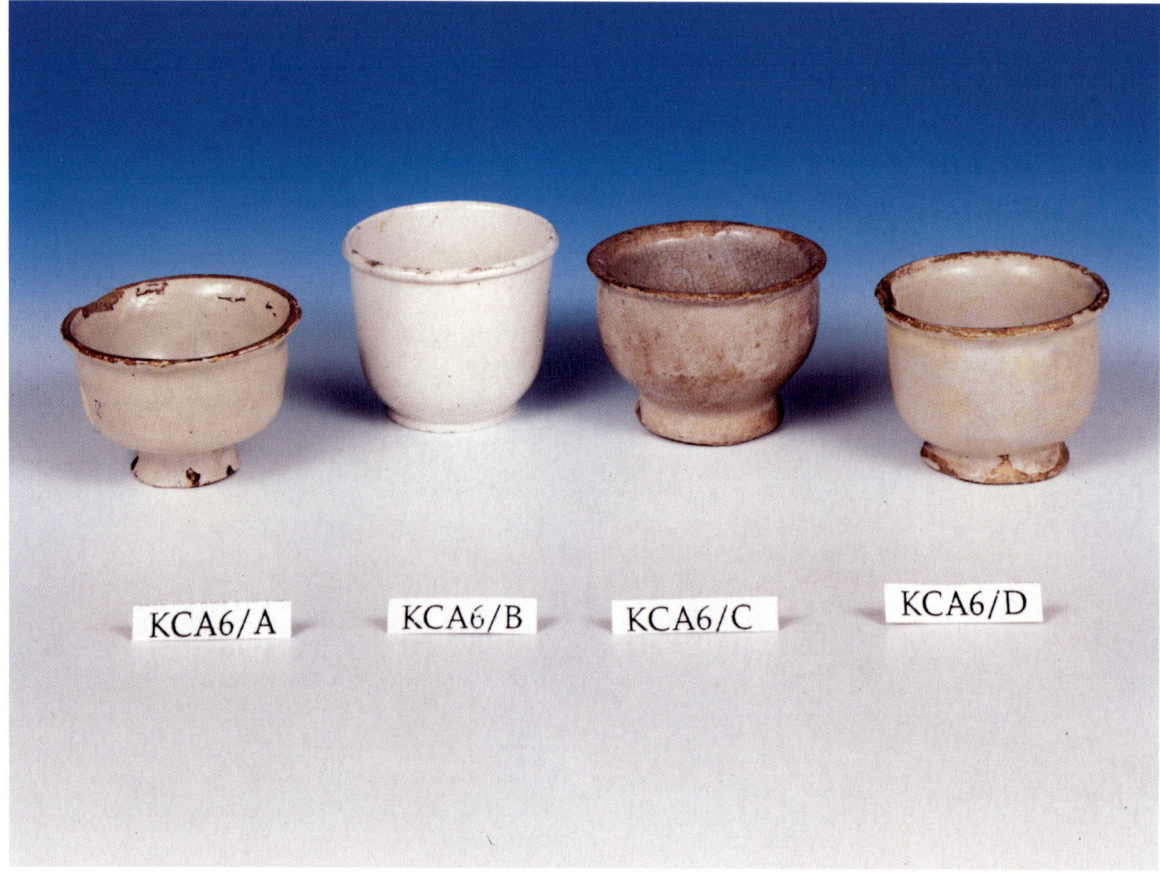

Dry drug jars (Cat.22–25)

The provenance of these jars is unclear. Museum records state that some jars were bought from "various" excavations. For example, in September 1961, the Museum purchased "An important collection of 34 Lambeth delft and other early unguent pots recovered from various London excavations in London circa 1926."

(Cat.22)
ACCESSION NUMBER: KCA6/A
DESCRIPTION: Roughly cup-shaped jar, white glaze, unglazed rim.
DATE OF MANUFACTURE: 1750-1800
PLACE OF MANUFACTURE: London
DIMENSIONS: Height 40 mm, maximum width 64 mm
CONDITION: Good, chips to rim and pedestal.

(Cat.23)
ACCESSION NUMBER: KCA6/B
DESCRIPTION: Cup-shaped jar, white glaze, glazed rim.
DATE OF MANUFACTURE: 1650–1800
PLACE OF MANUFACTURE: London
DIMENSIONS: Height 48 mm, maximum width 63 mm

PROVENANCE: Jar is labelled on base "Bernard St, Westminster [illegible].10.26". Assumed to be the location and date of the find.
CONDITION: Good, some small chips to rim.

(Cat.24)
ACCESSION NUMBER: KCA6/C
DESCRIPTION: Roughly cup-shaped jar, grey-brown glaze, unglazed rim.
DATE OF MANUFACTURE: 1570–1700
PLACE OF MANUFACTURE: London
DIMENSIONS: Height 46 mm, maximum width 68 mm
CONDITION: Good, some chips to base.

(Cat.25)
ACCESSION NUMBER: KCA6/D
DESCRIPTION: Roughly cup-shaped jar, white glaze, unglazed rim.
DATE OF MANUFACTURE: 1570–1700
PLACE OF MANUFACTURE: London
DIMENSIONS: Height 44 mm, maximum width 64 mm
CONDITION: Good, chips to rim and base.

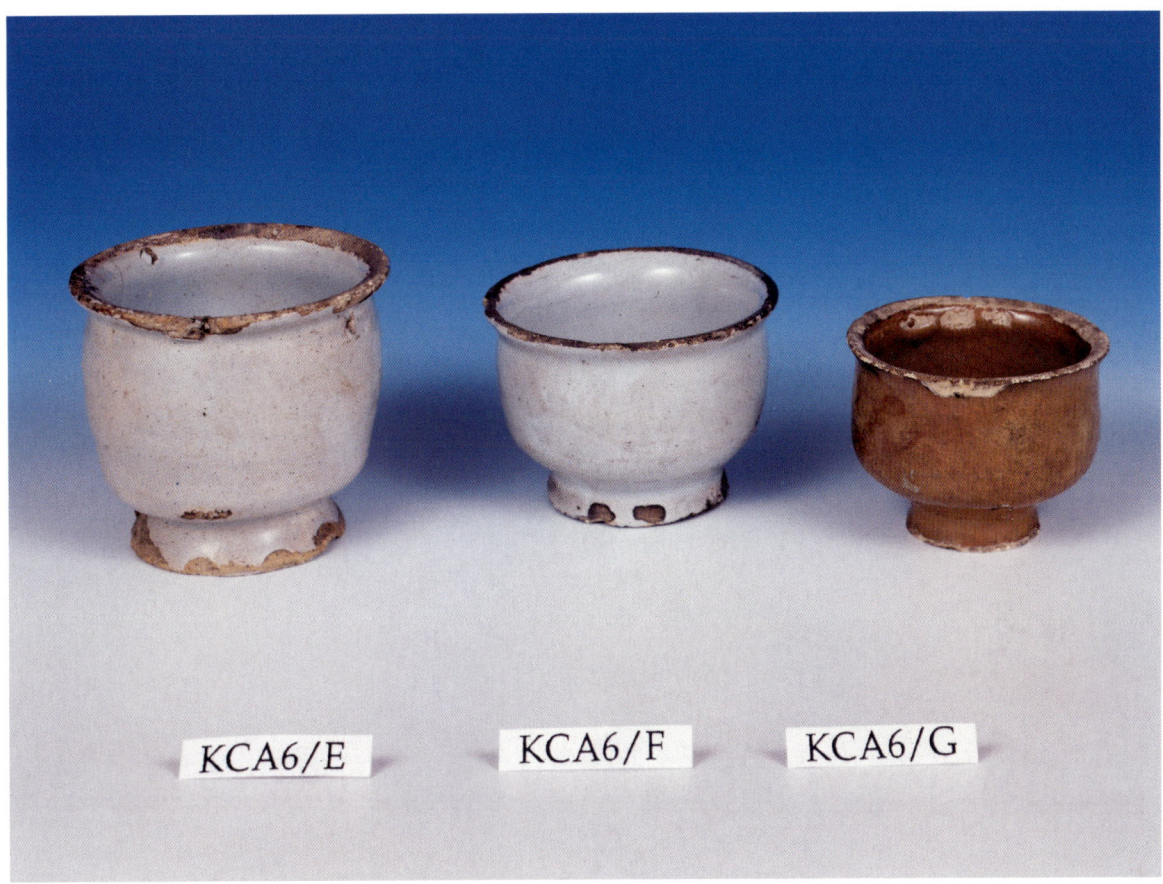

KCA6/E   KCA6/F   KCA6/G

Dry drug jars (Cat.26–28)

The provenance of these jars is unclear. Museum records state that some jars were bought from "various" excavations. For example, in September 1961, the Museum purchased "An important collection of 34 Lambeth delft and other early unguent pots recovered from various London excavations in London circa 1926."

(Cat.26)
ACCESSION NUMBER: KCA6/E
DESCRIPTION: Roughly cup-shaped jar, white glaze, unglazed rim.
DATE OF MANUFACTURE: 1570–1700
PLACE OF MANUFACTURE: London
DIMENSIONS: Height 61 mm, maximum width 75 mm
CONDITION: Good, chips to rim and base.

(cat.27)
ACCESSION NUMBER: KCA6/F
DESCRIPTION: Roughly cup-shaped jar, white glaze, unglazed rim.
DATE OF MANUFACTURE: 1700-1800
PLACE OF MANUFACTURE: London
DIMENSIONS: Height 47 mm, maximum width 71 mm
CONDITION: Good, chips to rim and base.

(Cat.28)
ACCESSION NUMBER: KCA6/G
DESCRIPTION: Roughly cup-shaped jar, brown glaze, unglazed rim.
DATE OF MANUFACTURE: 1570–1700
PLACE OF MANUFACTURE: London
DIMENSIONS: Height 43 mm, maximum width 70 mm
CONDITION: Good, chips to rim and base.

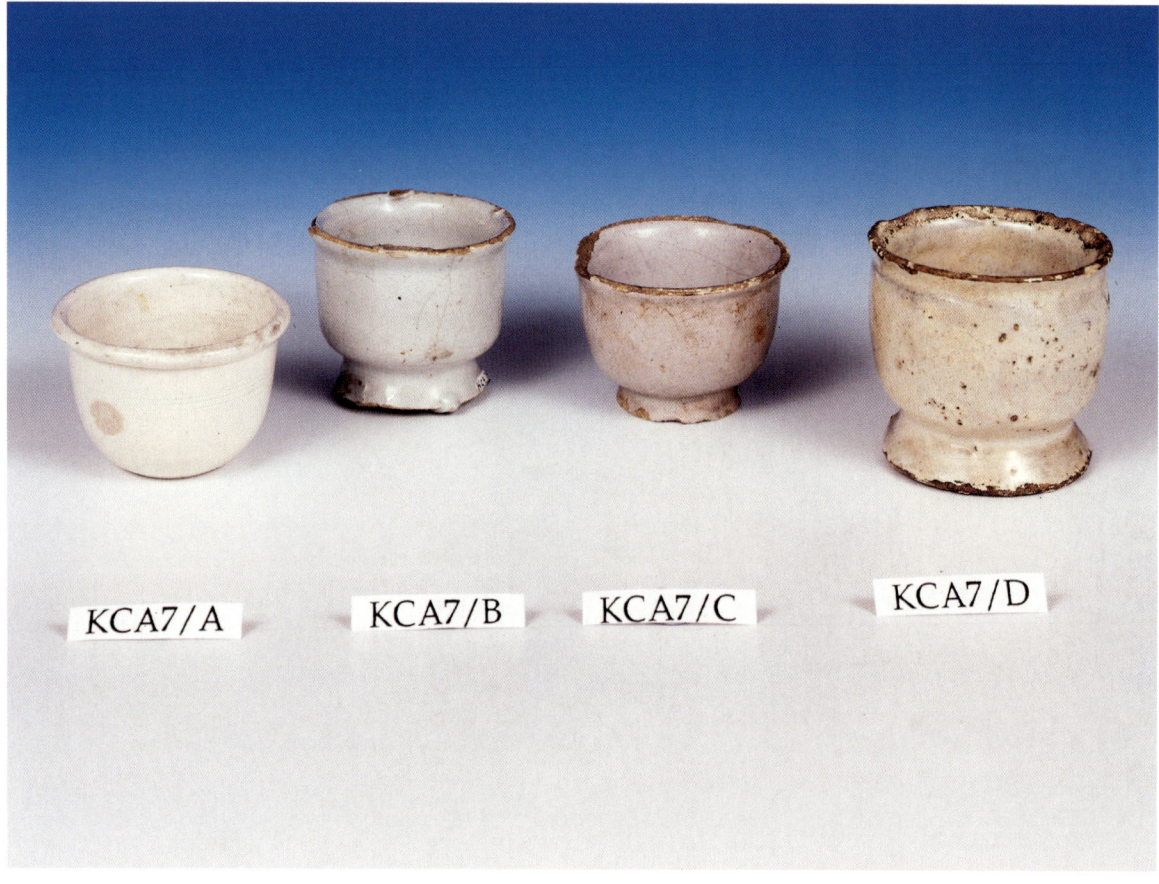

KCA7/A KCA7/B KCA7/C KCA7/D

Dry drug jars (Cat.29–32)

The provenance of these jars is unclear. Museum records state that some of these jars were bought from "various" excavations. For example, in September 1961, the Museum purchased "An important collection of 34 Lambeth delft and other early unguent pots recovered from various London excavations in London circa 1926."

(Cat.29)

ACCESSION NUMBER: KCA7/A
DESCRIPTION: Cup-shaped jar, white glaze, glazed rim.
DATE OF MANUFACTURE: 1700–1800
PLACE OF MANUFACTURE: London
DIMENSIONS: Height 35 mm, maximum width 60 mm
CONDITION: Good, chips to rim and base.

(Cat.30)

ACCESSION NUMBER: KCA7/B
DESCRIPTION: Roughly cup-shaped jar, white glaze, unglazed rim.
DATE OF MANUFACTURE: 1750–1800
PLACE OF MANUFACTURE: London
DIMENSIONS: Height 43 mm, maximum width 57 mm

PROVENANCE: A label on base of this jar reads '[illegible]/2/26'
CONDITION: Good, chips to rim and base, crazed glaze.

(Cat.31)

ACCESSION NUMBER: KCA7/C
DESCRIPTION: Roughly cup-shaped jar, white glaze, unglazed rim.
DATE OF MANUFACTURE: 1570–1700
PLACE OF MANUFACTURE: London
DIMENSIONS: Height 38 mm, maximum width 55 mm
CONDITION: Good, chips to rim and base.

(Cat.32)

ACCESSION NUMBER: KCA7/D
DESCRIPTION: Squat jar, white glaze, unglazed rim.
DATE OF MANUFACTURE: 1570–1700
PLACE OF MANUFACTURE: London
DIMENSIONS: Height 51 mm, maximum width 60 mm
PROVENANCE: Jar is labelled 'Vandon Street 31.8.27' Assumed to be location and date of find. Vandon Street is near Buckingham Palace.
CONDITION: Good, pitting to body

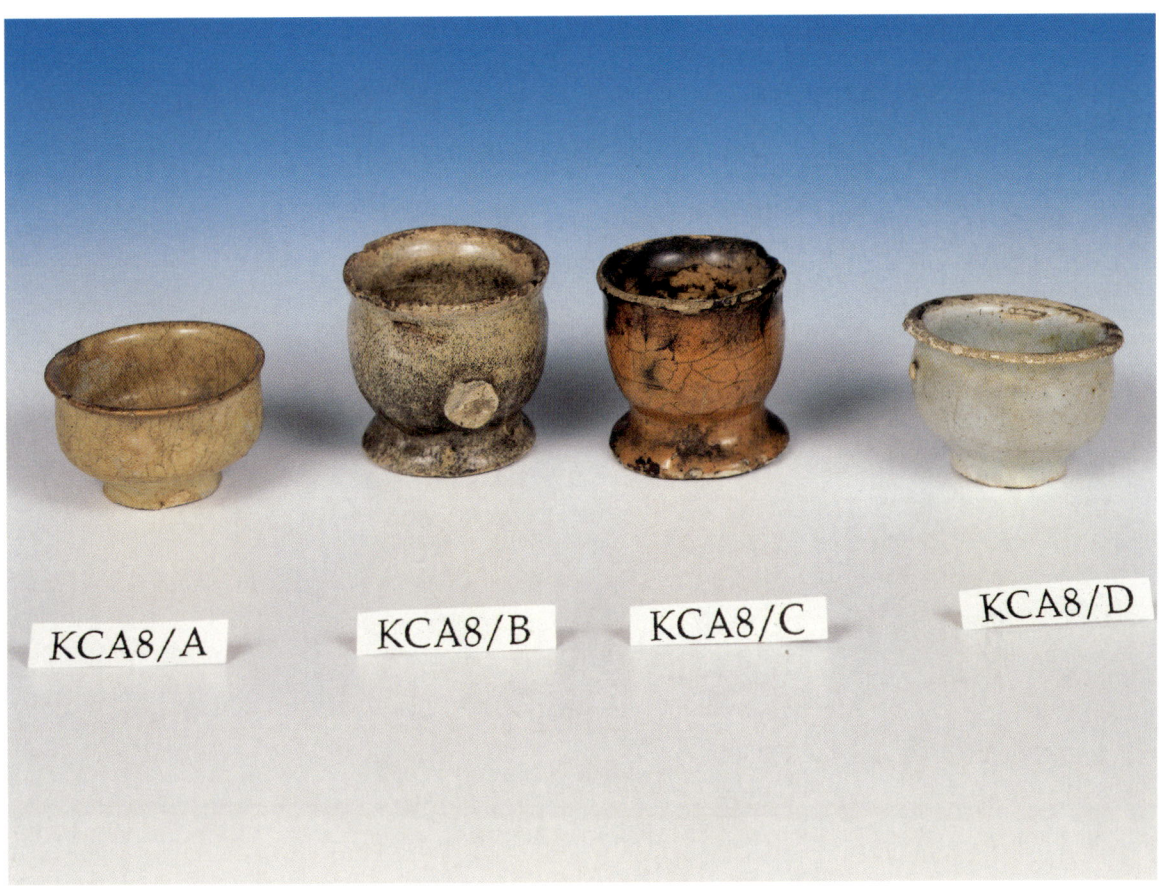

KCA8/A   KCA8/B   KCA8/C   KCA8/D

Dry drug jars (Cat.33-36)

The provenance of these jars is unclear. Museum records state that some of these jars were bought from "various" excavations. For example, in September 1961, the Museum purchased "An important collection of 34 Lambeth delft and other early unguent pots recovered from various London excavations in London circa 1926."

(Cat.33)

ACCESSION NUMBER: KCA8/A
DESCRIPTION: Roughly cup-shaped jar, brown glaze, glazed rim.
DATE OF MANUFACTURE: 1570-1700
PLACE OF MANUFACTURE: London
DIMENSIONS: Height 27 mm, maximum width 48 mm
PROVENANCE: Jar is labelled 'Vandon Street 31.8.27' Assumed to be location and date of find. Vandon Street is near Buckingham Palace.
CONDITION: Good, chip to base.

(Cat.34)

ACCESSION NUMBER: KCA8/B
DESCRIPTION: Squat jar, brown glaze, unglazed rim.
DATE OF MANUFACTURE: 1570-1700

PLACE OF MANUFACTURE: London
DIMENSIONS: Height 40 mm, maximum width 45 mm
PROVENANCE: Jar labelled on base 'Marsham S Westminr 10.2.28' Assumed to be location and date of find. Marsham Street is close to Westminster Abbey.
CONDITION: Fair, chips to rim, loss of glaze on body.

(Cat.35)

ACCESSION NUMBER: KCA8/C
DESCRIPTION: Squat jar, brown glaze, unglazed rim.
DATE OF MANUFACTURE: 1570-1700
PLACE OF MANUFACTURE: London
DIMENSIONS: Height 39 mm, maximum width 41 mm
CONDITION: Fair, some chips including large one to rim.

(Cat.36)

ACCESSION NUMBER: KCA8/D
DESCRIPTION: Roughly cup-shaped jar, grey glaze, unglazed rim.
DATE OF MANUFACTURE: 1750-1800
PLACE OF MANUFACTURE: London
DIMENSIONS: Height 30 mm, maximum width 47 mm
PROVENANCE: Jar labelled '[illegible] Westminster 5.7.27' Assumed to be location and date of find.
CONDITION: Good, some loss of glaze.

Early Jars

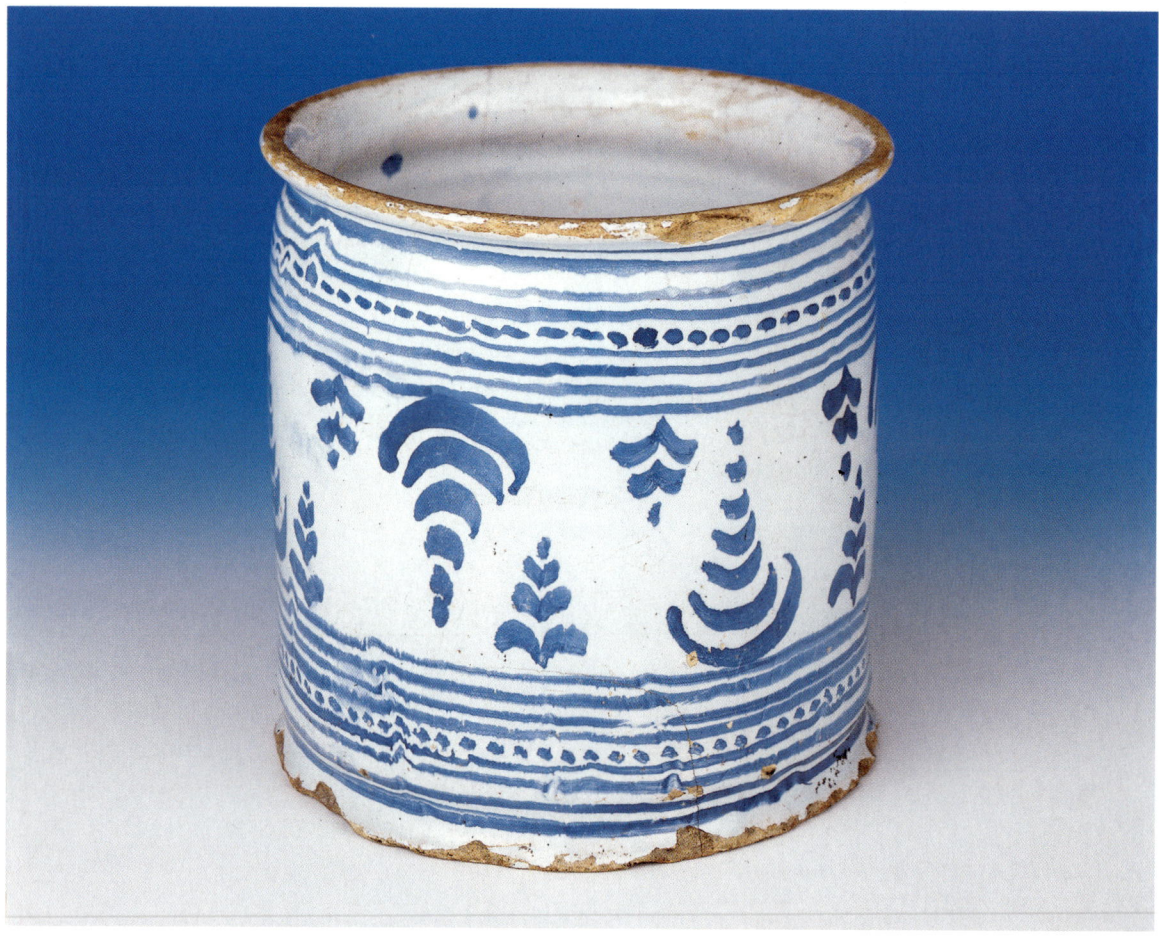

Dry drug jar (Cat.37)

ACCESSION NUMBER: KCB1
DESCRIPTION: Cylindrical, with slightly splayed base. Blue glaze with pinkish tinge and design in blue. Neck everted with unglazed rim, flat unglazed base.
DESIGN: Blue horizontal bands round neck and foot. Blue waist decoration.
DATE OF MANUFACTURE: 1570–1700
PLACE OF MANUFACTURE: London
DIMENSIONS: Height 185 mm, maximum width 185 mm
CONDITION: Fair; cracks descending from neck and ascending from base; neck and base rims chipped.

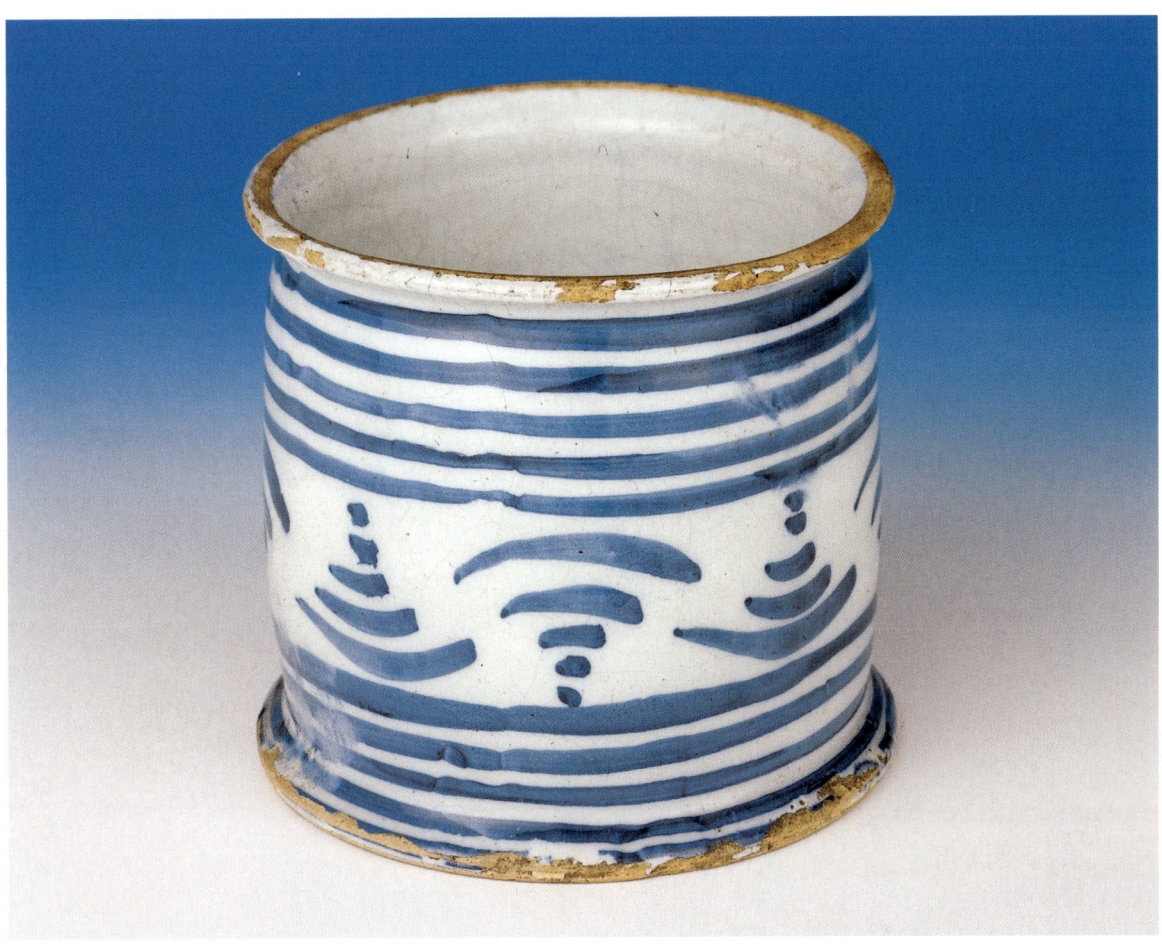

Dry drug jar (Cat.38)

ACCESSION NUMBER: KCB2
DESCRIPTION: Cylindrical, with slightly splayed base. Blue
glaze with pinkish tinge and design in blue. Neck everted with
unglazed rim, slightly concave unglazed base.
DESIGN: Blue horizontal bands round neck and foot. Blue waist
decoration.
DATE OF MANUFACTURE: 1570–1700
PLACE OF MANUFACTURE: London
DIMENSIONS: Height 140 mm, maximum width 165 mm
CONDITION: Good; base and neck rim chipped; glaze crazed
and flaked from neck and base rims.

Early Jars

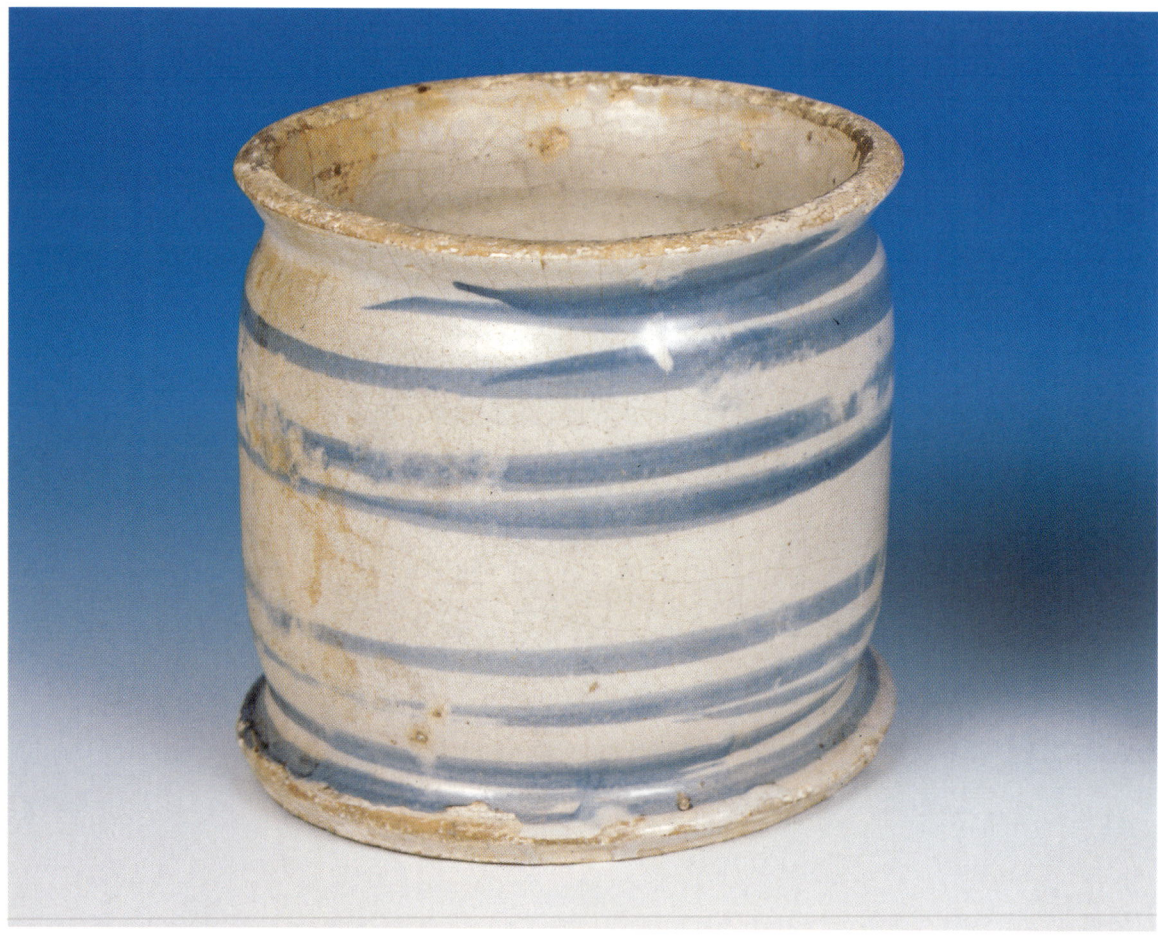

Dry drug jar (Cat.39)

ACCESSION NUMBER: KCB3/A
DESCRIPTION: Cylindrical jar with splayed base with blue
horizontal bands around neck and foot. No waist decoration.
Neck everted with unglazed rim, flat unglazed base.
DATE OF MANUFACTURE: 1570–1700
PLACE OF MANUFACTURE: London
DIMENSIONS: Height 96 mm, maximum width 119 mm
PROVENANCE: Jar labelled on base 'East India Hse, Regent St
[Libertys]'. Assumed to be location of find.
CONDITION: Good; small chips to base and rim, partial loss of
interior glaze.

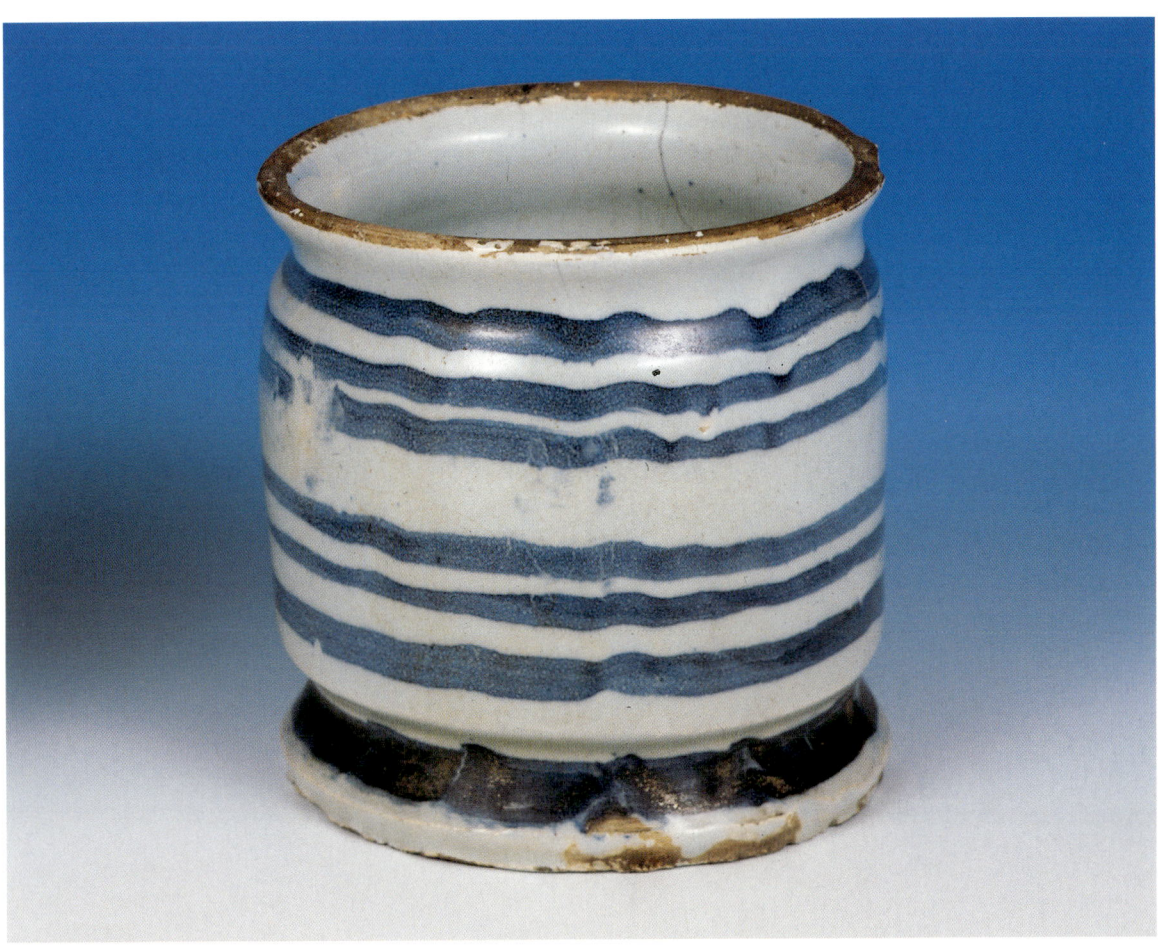

Dry drug jar (Cat.40)

ACCESSION NUMBER: KCB3/B
DESCRIPTION: Cylindrical jar with splayed base and blue horizontal bands around neck and foot. No waist decoration. Neck everted with unglazed rim, flat unglazed base.
DATE OF MANUFACTURE: 1570–1700
PLACE OF MANUFACTURE: London
DIMENSIONS: Height 86 mm, maximum width 94 mm
PROVENANCE: Donation, Hodgkin Collection, date unknown.
CONDITION: Good; chips to base and rim.

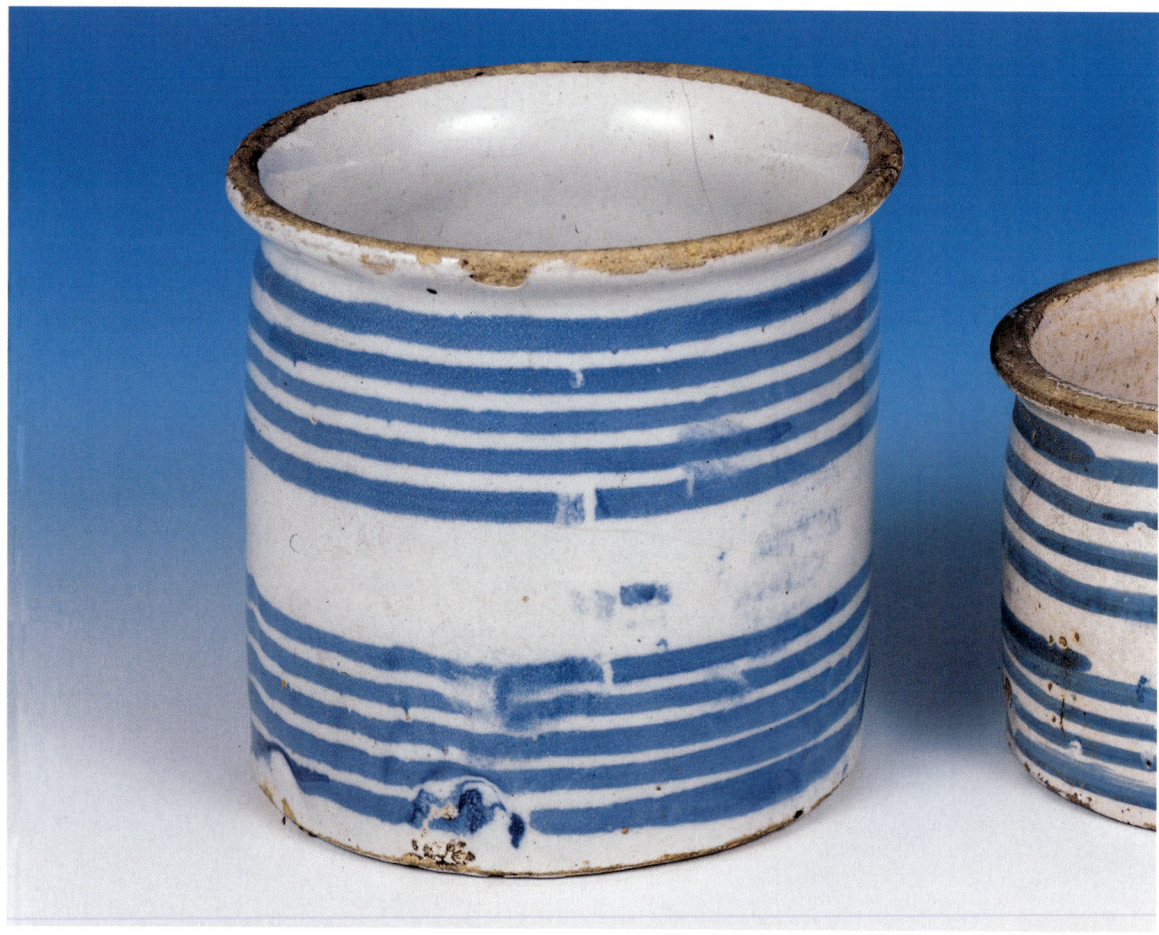

Dry drug jar (Cat.41)

ACCESSION NUMBER: KCB3/C
DESCRIPTION: Cylindrical jar with blue horizontal bands around neck and foot. No waist decoration. Neck everted with unglazed rim, flat unglazed base.
DATE OF MANUFACTURE: 1700–1800
PLACE OF MANUFACTURE: London
DIMENSIONS: Height 88 mm, maximum width 102 mm
PROVENANCE: Donated by Mrs J Thomas, Brocksom Collection, 1985.
CONDITION: Good; small chips at rim and base.

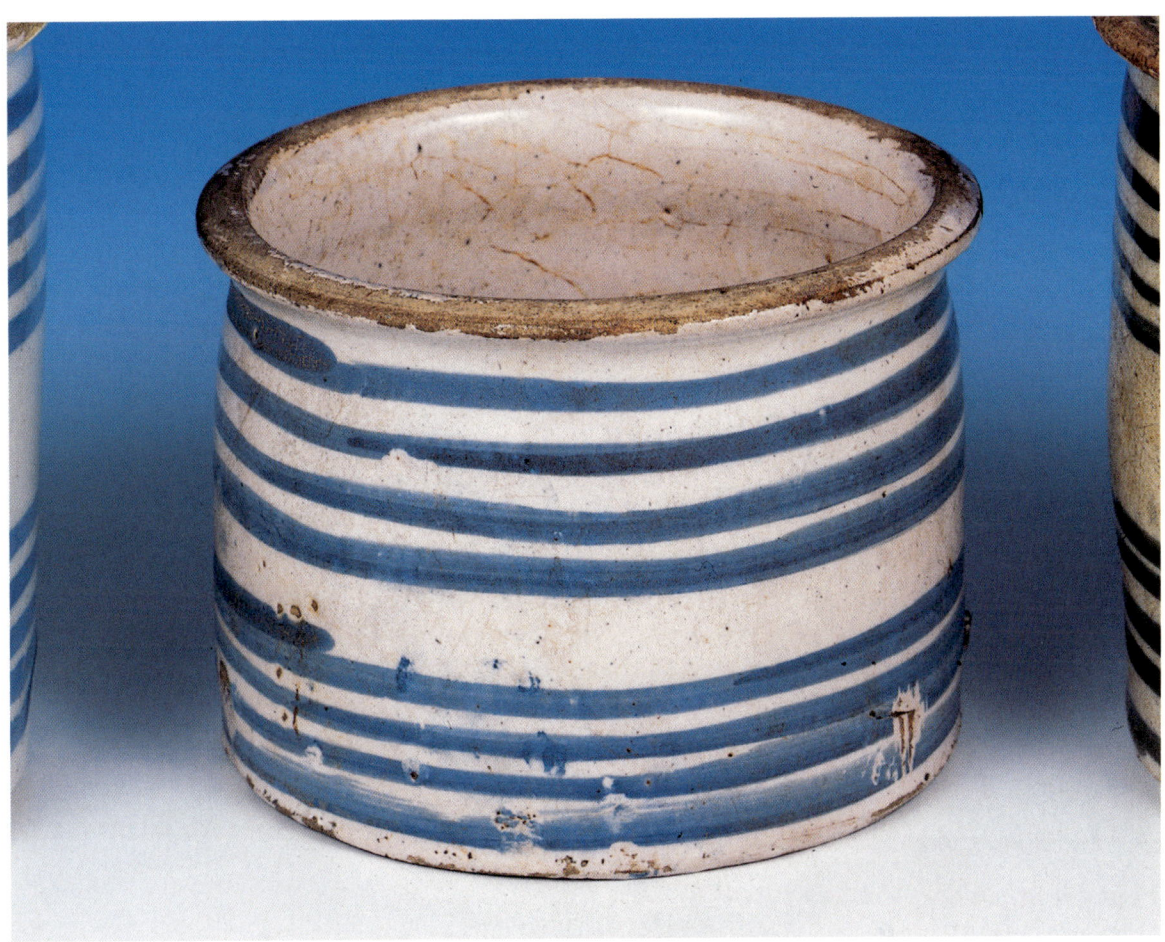

Dry drug jar (Cat.42)

ACCESSION NUMBER: KCB3/D

DESCRIPTION: Cylindrical jar with blue horizontal bands
around neck and foot. No waist decoration. Neck everted with
unglazed rim, flat unglazed base.

DATE OF MANUFACTURE: 1570–1700

PLACE OF MANUFACTURE: London

DIMENSIONS: Height 59 mm, maximum width 88 mm

PROVENANCE: Labelled 'Horseferry Road 17/2/33' on base.
Assumed to be location and date of find.

CONDITION: Good; some glaze loss and chips.

Early Jars

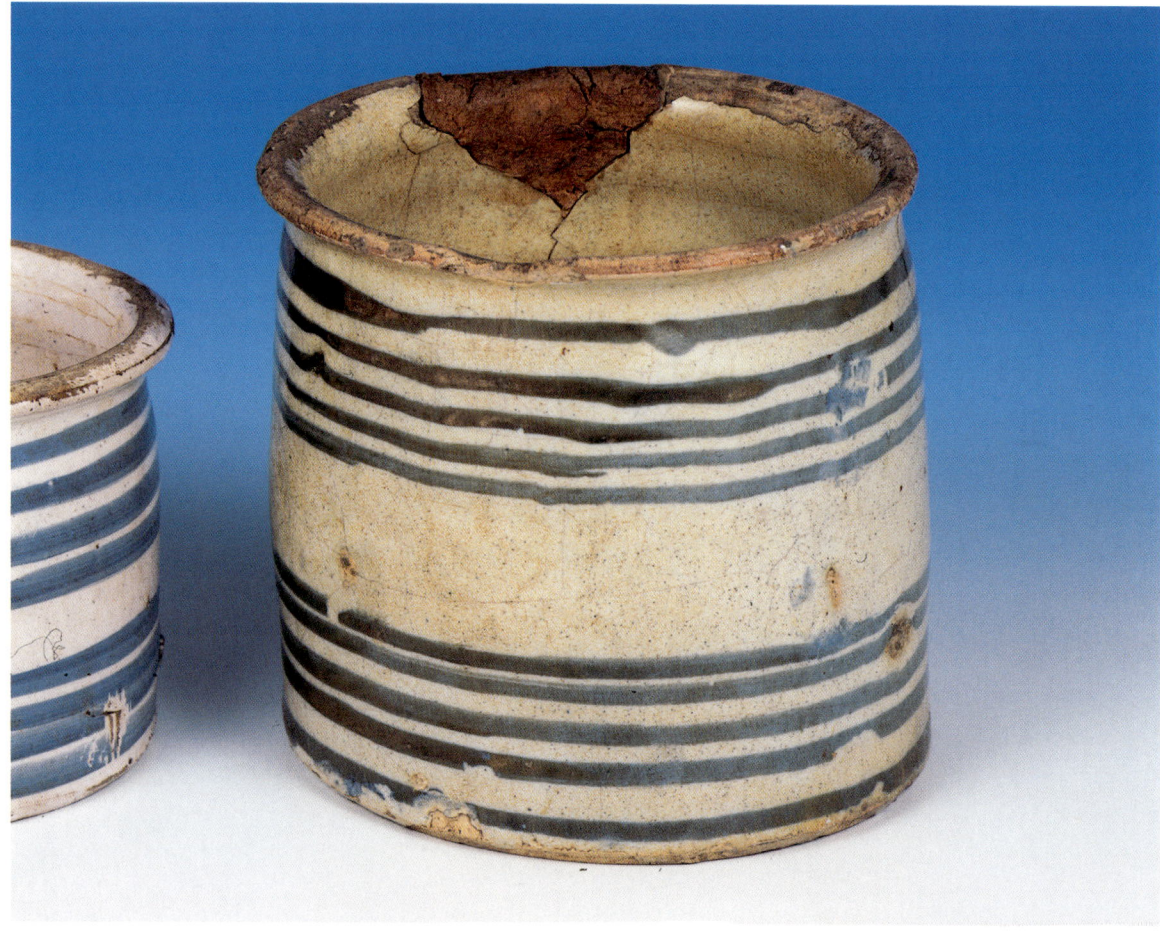

Dry drug jar (Cat.43)

ACCESSION NUMBER: KCB3/E
DESCRIPTION: Cylindrical jar with blue horizontal bands around neck and foot. No waist decoration. Neck everted with unglazed rim, flat unglazed base.
DATE OF MANUFACTURE: 1570–1700
PLACE OF MANUFACTURE: London
DIMENSIONS: Height 82 mm, maximum width 95 mm
CONDITION: Fair; some chips to base and rim, and glaze loss.

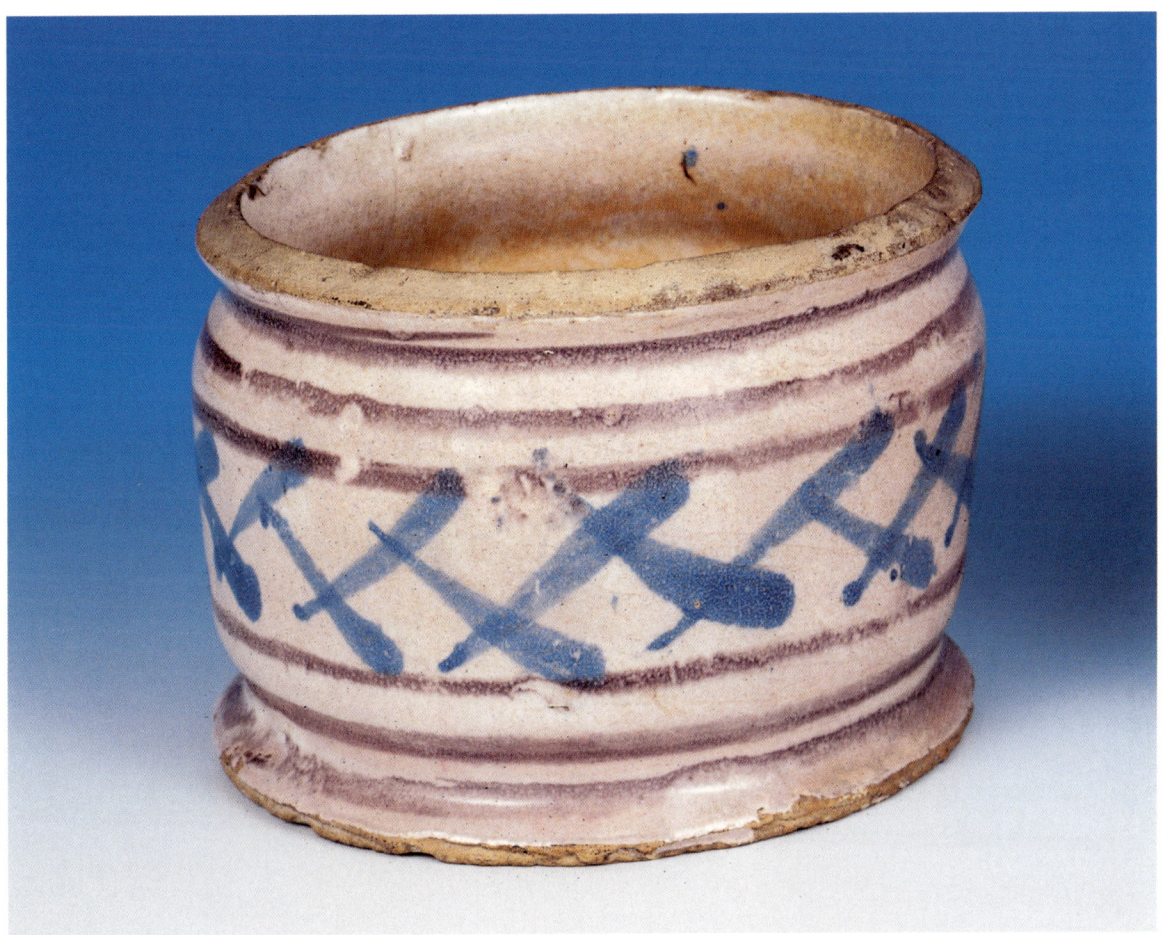

Dry drug jar (Cat.44)

ACCESSION NUMBER: KCB4/A
DESCRIPTION: Cylindrical jar with splayed base and mauve bands around neck and base. Blue waist decoration. Neck everted with unglazed rim, flat unglazed base.
DATE OF MANUFACTURE: 1570–1700
PLACE OF MANUFACTURE: London
DIMENSIONS: Height 32 mm, maximum width 39 mm
PROVENANCE: Unclear. Museum records state that some of these jars were bought from "various" excavations. For example, in September 1961, the Museum purchased "An important collection of 34 Lambeth delft and other early unguent pots recovered from various excavations in London circa 1926."
CONDITION: Good; small chips to base, rim and body.

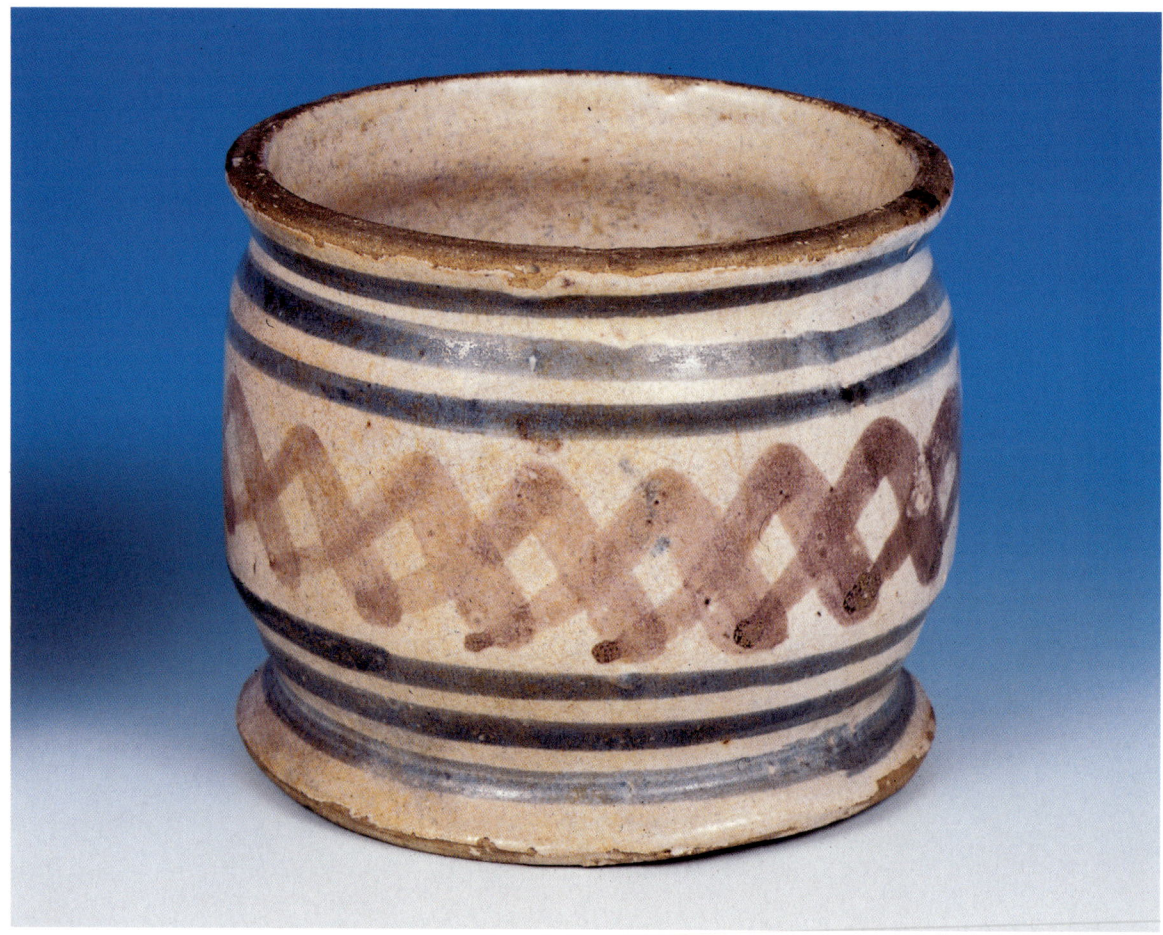

Dry drug jar (Cat.45)

ACCESSION NUMBER: KCB4/B

DESCRIPTION: Cylindrical jar with splayed base and blue bands around neck and base. Mauve waist decoration. Neck everted with unglazed rim, flat unglazed base.

DATE OF MANUFACTURE: 1570–1700

PLACE OF MANUFACTURE: London

DIMENSIONS: Height 90 mm, maximum width 119 mm

PROVENANCE: Jar is labelled 'S.Tel. Exchange 10/3/26' on base. Assumed to be location and date of find.

CONDITION: Good; slight chips.

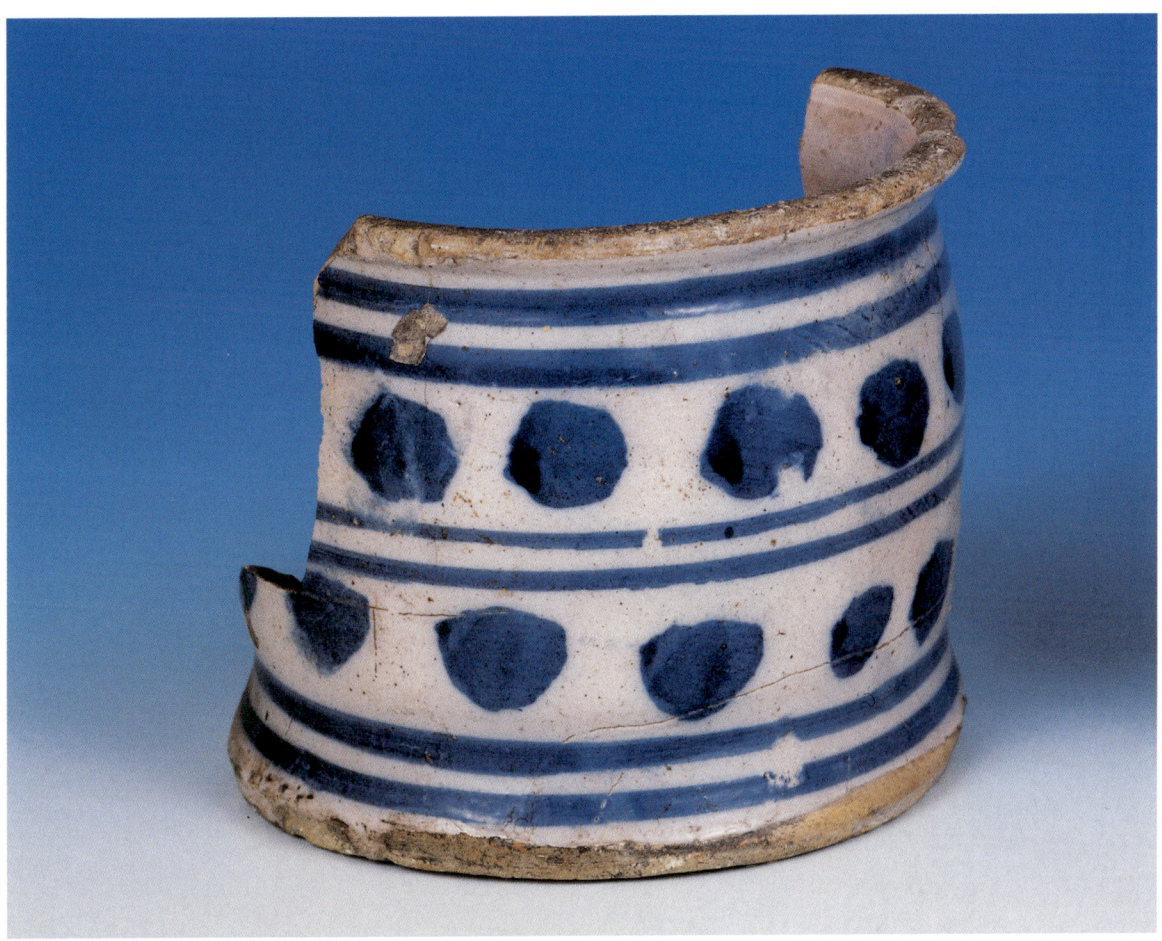

Dry drug jar (Cat.46)

ACCESSION NUMBER: KCB4/C
DESCRIPTION: Part of cylindrical jar with slightly splayed base and blue bands around neck, waist and base. Blue spots above and below waistline. Neck everted with unglazed rim, flat unglazed base.
DATE OF MANUFACTURE: 1650–1700
PLACE OF MANUFACTURE: London
DIMENSIONS: Height 92 mm, maximum width 113 mm
PROVENANCE: Jar is labelled on base 'Lower Regent St'. Assumed to be location of find.
CONDITION: Poor; chips, losses of glaze, scratches. Incomplete jar.

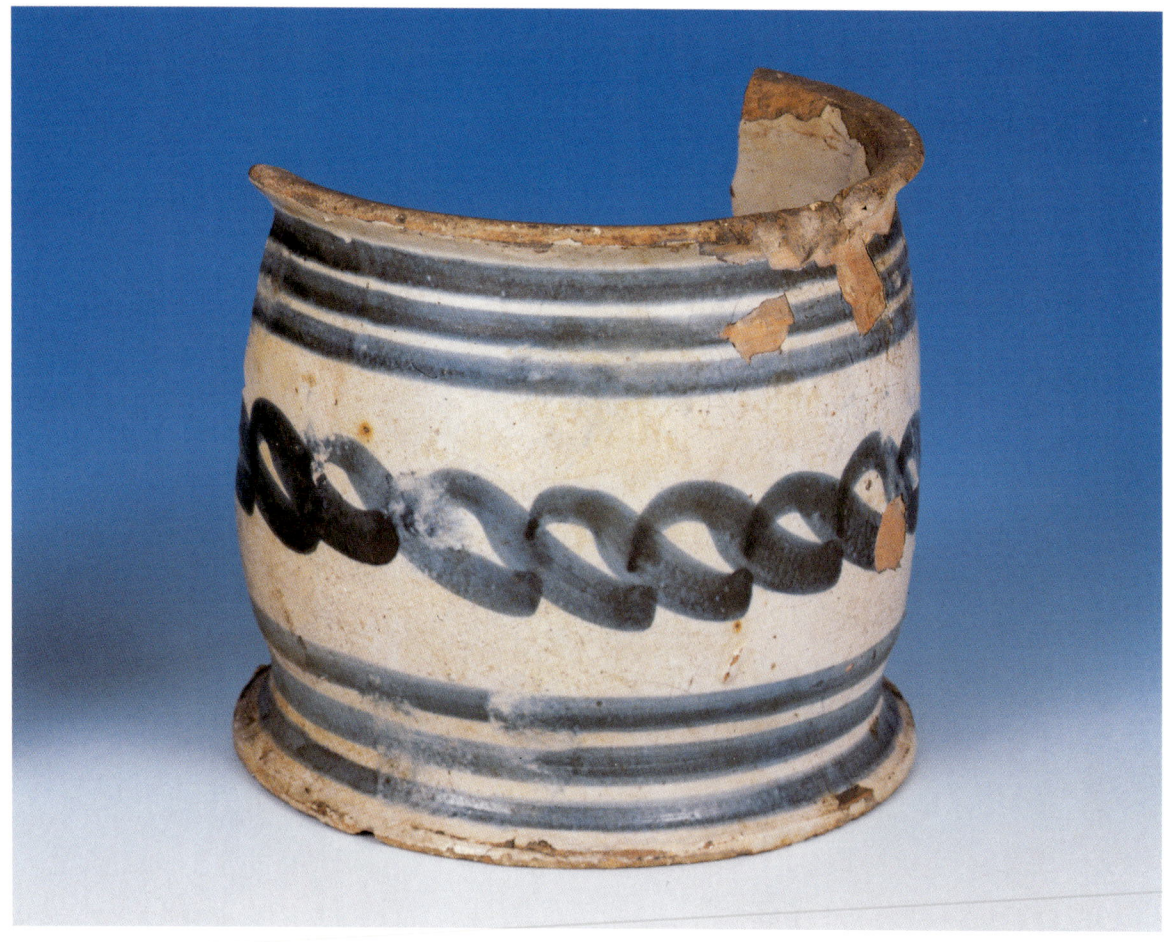

Dry drug jar (Cat.47)

ACCESSION NUMBER: KCB4/D
DESCRIPTION: Part of cylindrical jar with splayed base and blue bands around neck and base. Blue waist decoration. Neck everted with unglazed rim, flat unglazed base.
DATE OF MANUFACTURE: 1650–1700
PLACE OF MANUFACTURE: London
DIMENSIONS: Height 104 mm, maximum width 123 mm
PROVENANCE: Jar is labelled 'Lower Regent St 28/10/24' on base. Assumed to be location and date of find.
CONDITION: Poor; large losses of glaze and chips. Incomplete jar.

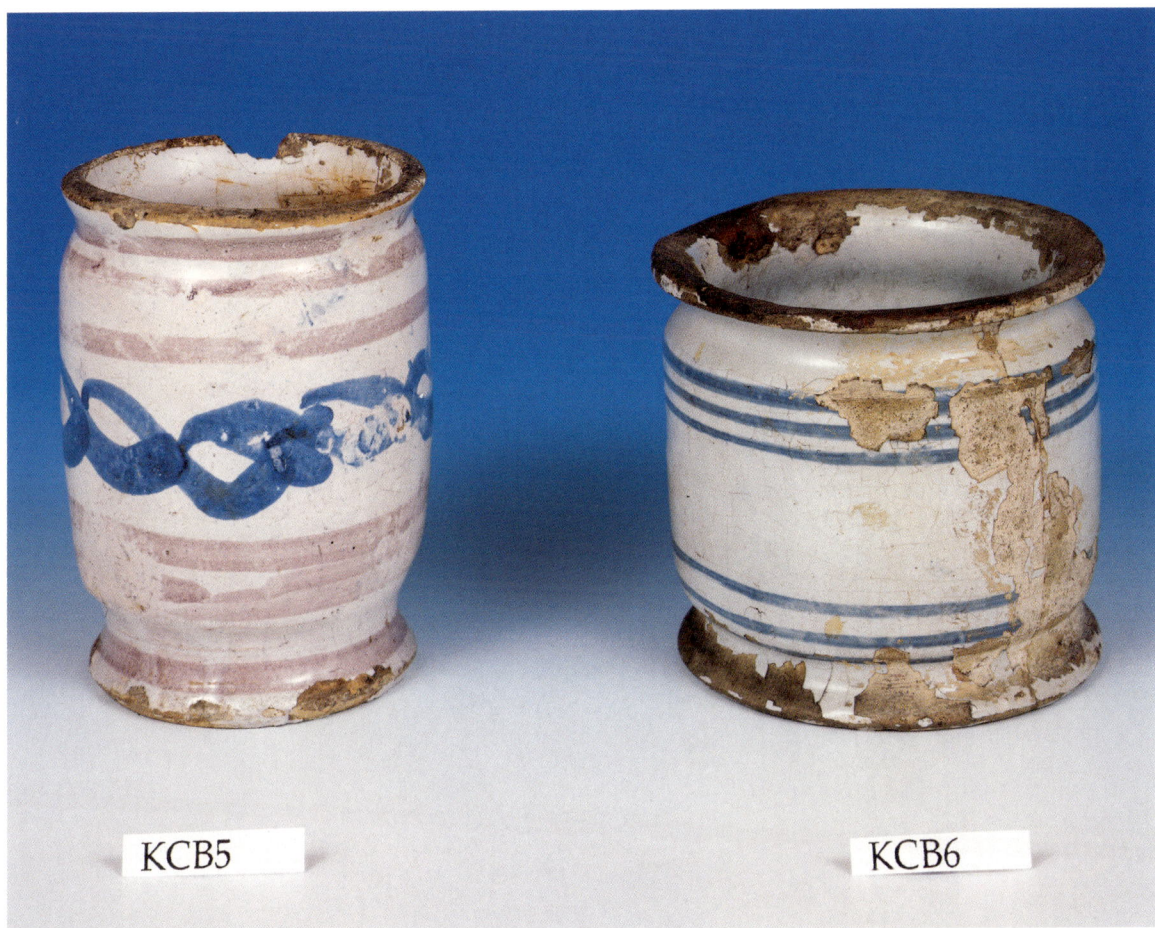

KCB5

KCB6

Dry drug jars

(Cat.48)

ACCESSION NUMBER: KCB5

DESCRIPTION: Cylindrical, with slightly splayed base. White glaze with greyish tinge and design in mauve and blue. Neck everted with unglazed rim, concave unglazed base.

DESIGN: Mauve horizontal bands round neck and foot. Blue waist decoration.

DATE OF MANUFACTURE: 1570–1700

PLACE OF MANUFACTURE: London

DIMENSIONS: Height 110 mm, maximum width 85 mm

PROVENANCE: Unclear. Museum records state that some of these jars were bought from "various" excavations. For example, in September 1961, the Museum purchased "An important collection of 34 Lambeth delft and other early unguent pots recovered from various excavations in London circa 1926."

CONDITION: Poor; neck chipped; cracks descending from neck; glaze flaked from neck and base rims.

(Cat.49)

ACCESSION NUMBER: KCB6

DESCRIPTION: Cylindrical, with slightly splayed base. Blue glaze and design in blue. Neck everted with unglazed rim, flat base. Labels on base: 'F.H. Garner No 264, L.L.L. No 112'.

DESIGN: Blue horizontal bands round neck and foot.

DATE OF MANUFACTURE: 1570–1700

PLACE OF MANUFACTURE: London

DIMENSIONS: Height 90 mm, maximum width 108 mm

PROVENANCE: Donated by Mrs J Thomas, Brocksom Collection, 1985.

COMMENT: L.L.L. refers to Louis L. Lipski.

CONDITION: Fair; significant loss of glaze.

Display jars

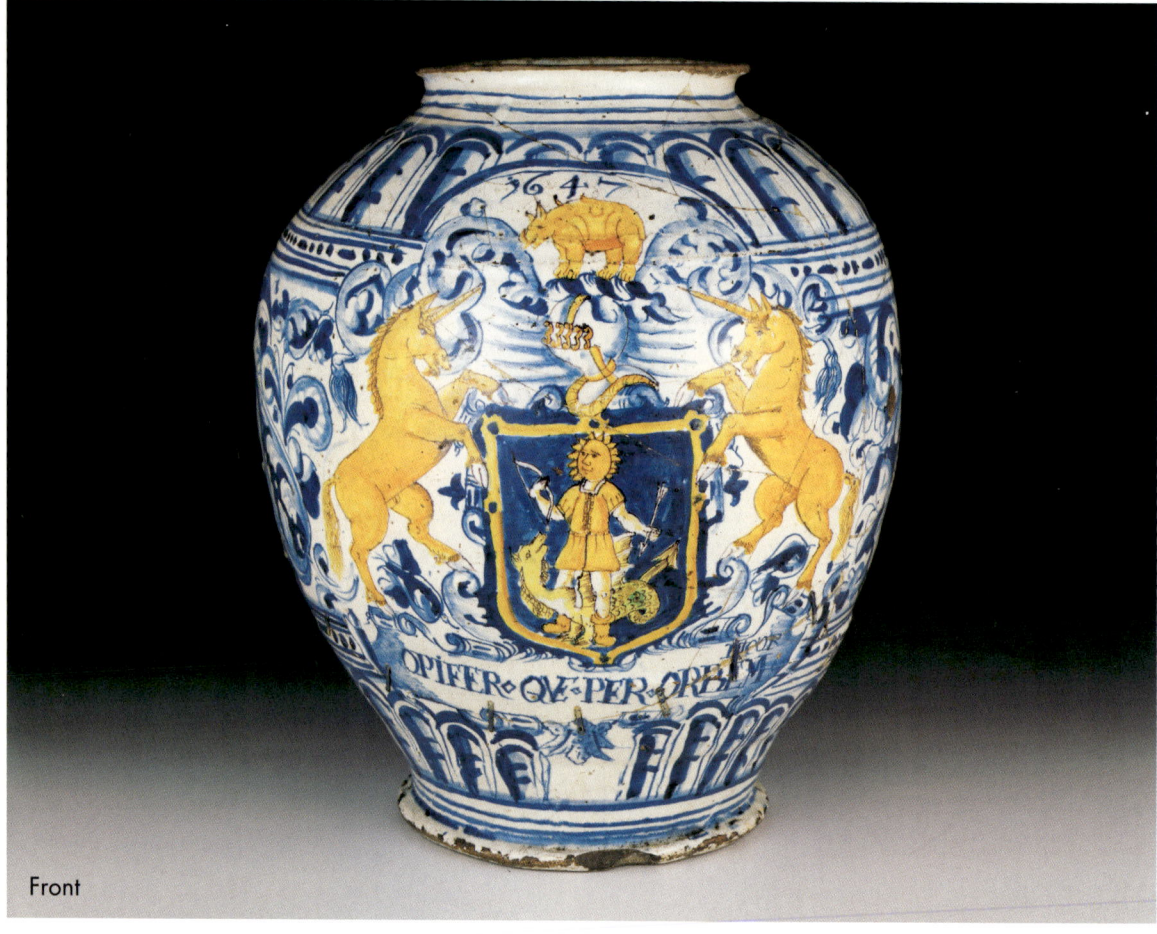

Front

Display jar (Cat.50)

ACCESSION NUMBER: KAC/P2

DESCRIPTION: Ovoid jar, tapering towards splayed base. White glaze with bluish tinge and design in brown, blue, green and yellow. Neck everted with unglazed rim, unglazed flat base.

DESIGN: Coat of arms of the Worshipful Society of Apothecaries, with leaf, pomegranate and flower design on reverse.

INSCRIPTION: OPIFER QUE PER ORBEM DICOR 1647

MEANING OF INSCRIPTION AND DESIGN: The Worshipful Society of Apothecaries is a livery company formed in 1617. The arms feature Apollo (the god of healing) killing the dragon of disease, supported by two unicorns (from King James's royal arms), and a rhinoceros as the crest (the powdered horn was believed to be medicinal). The motto, from the first book of Ovid's 'Metamorphoses', translates: "I am spoken of all over the world as one who brings help."

DATE OF MANUFACTURE: 1647

PLACE OF MANUFACTURE: Pickleherring, Rotherhithe or Montague Close potteries, Southwark, London

DIMENSIONS: Height 400 mm, maximum width 325 mm

PROVENANCE: Bought in 1953, London (Southwark).

CONDITION: Fair; has been repaired.

COMMENT: On 10 October 1953, Ernest Saville Peck wrote to Agnes Lothian. Peck had been contacted by Reverend H R Willimot of Langport in Somerset who was seeking his opinion about a large tin-glazed drug jar that he was planning to donate to a local museum. Peck sent a photograph of the jar in question to Agnes Lothian. She replied immediately: "This seems to be a very important 'find.' Can you not persuade him to leave it to the Society's Museum or give us the opportunity of acquiring it by purchase[?]." The evidence of Peck's powers of persuasion is obvious. Lothian wrote to Peck on 2 December 1953 saying that she had bought the jar for £100. He wrote back on 4 December saying that he was 'delighted'. The Establishment and Publications Committee also "congratulated the Librarian on this purchase".

This jar can boast two claims to fame: it is the earliest known dated English delftware drug jar, and it is also the earliest dated appearance of Apollo, the god of medicine, on an English drug jar. It is generally agreed that this jar was produced purely for display, rather than having any storage function. The

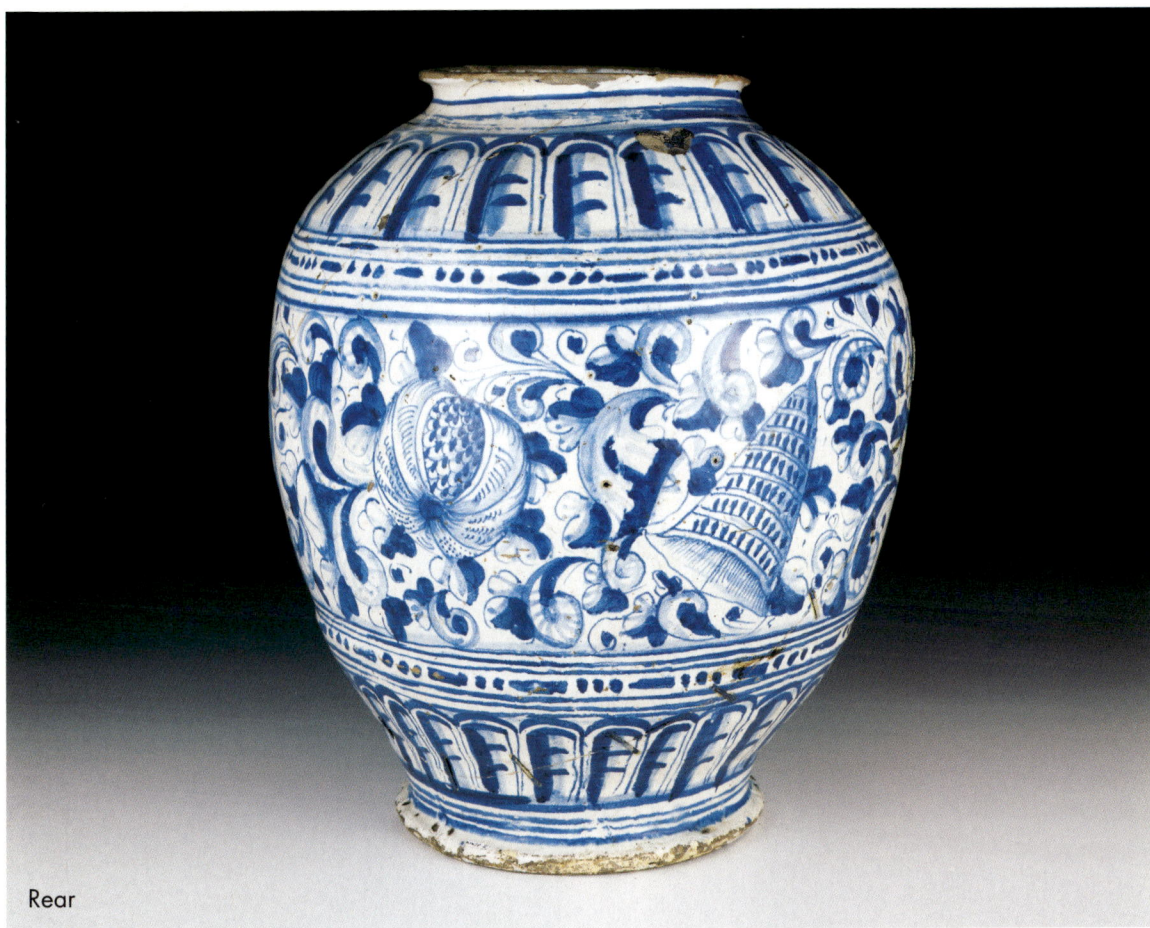

Rear

decoration declared proudly that the owner was a member of the Worshipful Society of Apothecaries.

The cartouche below the arms bearing the motto is a variant of the pipe-smoking man cartouche. Although it lacks the 'smoking' men, it has the same scrolls along the top and bottom edges, and the satyr-like head below the centre.

REFERENCES: Grigsby. The Longridge Collection of English Slipware and Delftware. Catalogue number D394.

Lipski and Archer, Dated English Delftware, No. 1592.

Lothian. Bird Designs p. 675.

Lothian. English Delftware in the Pharmaceutical Society's Collection. p. 1–2 and Plate 1.

Matthews. Antiques of the Pharmacy. Plate 26 and p. 4.

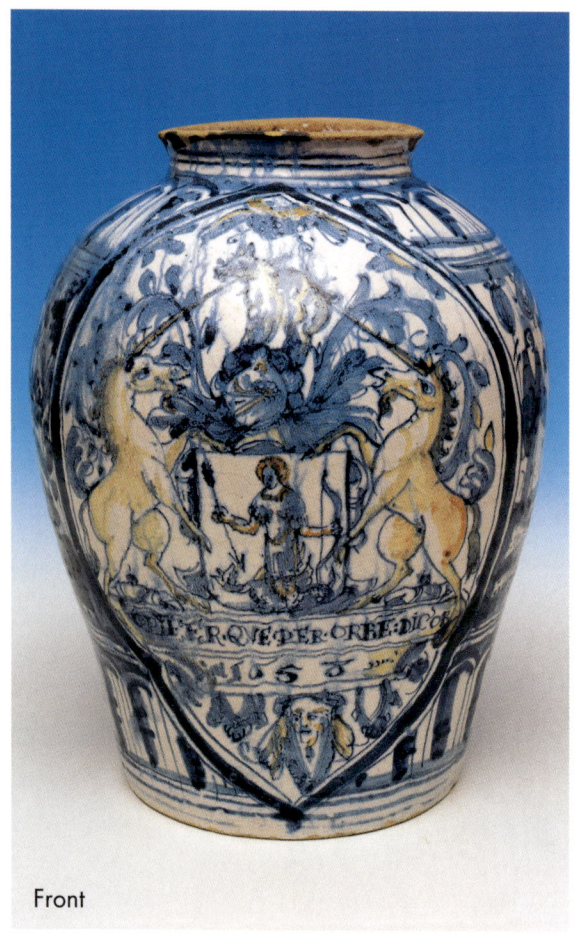

Front

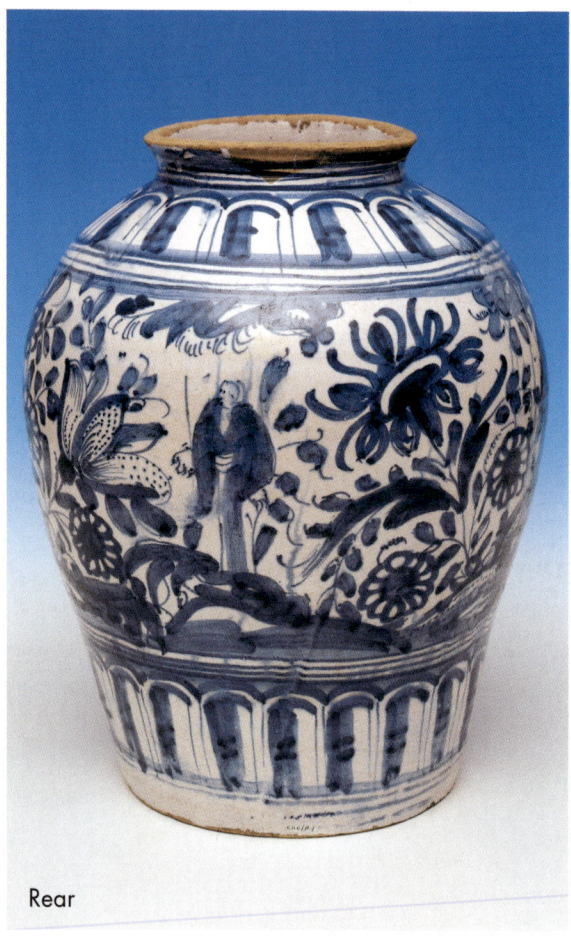

Rear

Display jar (Cat.51)

ACCESSION NUMBER: KAC/P1

DESCRIPTION: Ovoid jar, tapering slightly towards base. White glaze with design in blue and yellow. Neck slightly everted with unglazed rim, unglazed slightly concave base.

DESIGN: Arms of the Worshipful Society of Apothecaries on front. Chinese figures and flowers in blue on reverse.

INSCRIPTION: OPIFER.QVE.PER.ORBE:DICOR 1658

MEANING OF INSCRIPTION AND DESIGN: The Worshipful Society of Apothecaries is a livery company formed in 1617. The arms feature Apollo (the god of healing) killing the dragon of disease, supported by two unicorns (from King James's royal arms), and a rhinoceros as the crest (the powdered horn was believed to be medicinal). The motto, from the first book of Ovid's 'Metamorphoses', translates: "I am spoken of all over the world as one who brings help."

DATE OF MANUFACTURE: 1658

PLACE OF MANUFACTURE: Pickleherring, Rotherhithe or Montague Close potteries, Southwark, London

DIMENSIONS: Height 340 mm, maximum width 265 mm

PROVENANCE: Bought in 1957, Howard Collection.

CONDITION: Good; two holes in base; crack descending from neck; glaze flaked from rim of neck.

COMMENT: It is generally agreed that this jar was produced purely for display, rather than having any storage function. The decoration declared proudly that the owner was a member of the Worshipful Society of Apothecaries.

Howard notes the "finely modelled" head beneath the coat of arms, and proposes that it could be a portrait (p. 12). It certainly does not form part of the Apothecaries' coat of arms. However, the head does resemble in shape the bearded satyr-like face below the cartouche on the display jar KAC/P2 (Cat. 50), and also on many of the jars with the pipe-smoking man design.

REFERENCES: Howard, English Delftware Drug Jars, No. 7.

Lipski and Archer, Dated English Delftware, No. 1594.

Lothian, English Delftware in the Pharmaceutical Society's Collection. 1960, p. 2.

Lothian. The Armorial London Delft of the Worshipful Society of Apothecaries, p. 22 and 25.

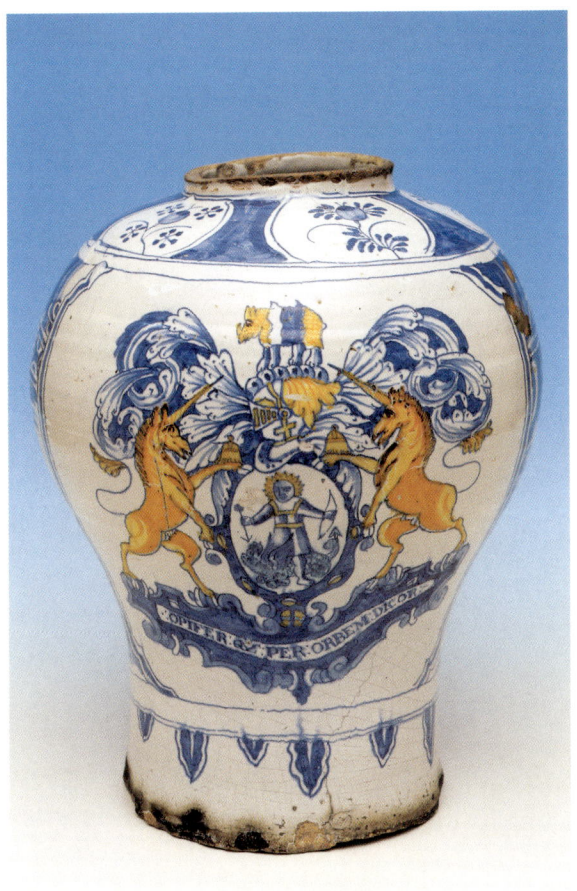

Front

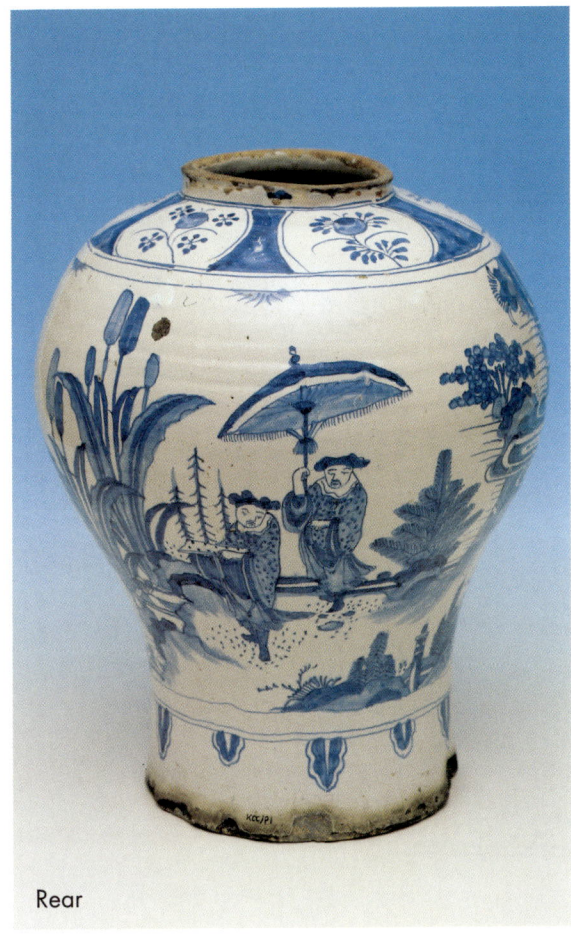

Rear

Display jar (Cat.52)

ACCESSION NUMBER: KCC/P1

DESCRIPTION: Bulbous jar, tapering towards base. White glaze with bluish tinge. Design in blue, yellow and green. Straight neck with unglazed rim, flat unglazed base.

DESIGN: Arms of the Worshipful Society of Apothecaries on front with Chinese figures, trees and a river scene on reverse.

INSCRIPTION: OPIFER:QVE:PER:ORBEM:DICOR:

MEANING OF INSCRIPTION AND DESIGN: The Worshipful Society of Apothecaries is a livery company formed in 1617. The arms feature Apollo (the god of healing) killing the dragon of disease, supported by two unicorns (from King James's royal arms), and a rhinoceros as the crest (the powdered horn was believed to be medicinal). The motto, from the first book of Ovid's 'Metamorphoses', translates: "I am spoken of all over the world as one who brings help."

The decoration on this jar is almost identical to, and certainly by the same hand as, that on seven polychrome and six blue and white pill tiles, including examples at the Society of Apothecaries, Colonial Williamsburg, and in the Longridge

Collection. The design on each even has the same slight tilt to the left.

DATE OF MANUFACTURE: 1650–1660

PLACE OF MANUFACTURE: Southwark, London

DIMENSIONS: Height 350 mm, maximum width 275 mm

PROVENANCE: Bought in 1957, Howard Collection. Originally from the Harland Collection, sold at Sotheby's 11/2/1931. See also KAE1 (Cat. 62) and KAG6 (Cat. 69).

CONDITION: Fair; large hole in base, base chipped, glaze flaked from body and rims of neck and base.

REFERENCES: Howard, English Delftware Drug Jars, No. 7A.

Lothian. The Armorial London Delft of the Worshipful Society of Apothecaries, p. 22 and 24.

Lothian. English Delftware in the Pharmaceutical Society's Collection. Reprinted, p. 2.

Pipe-smoking man

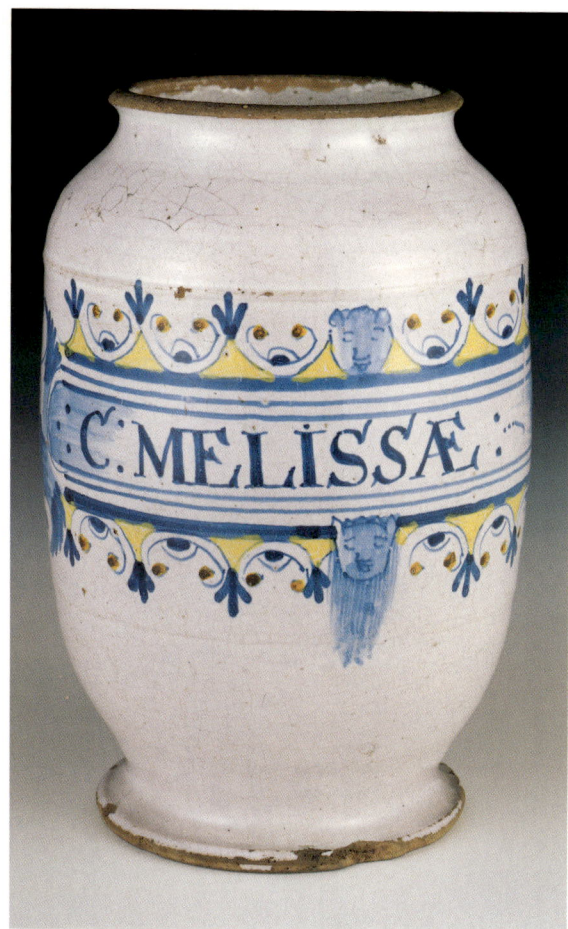

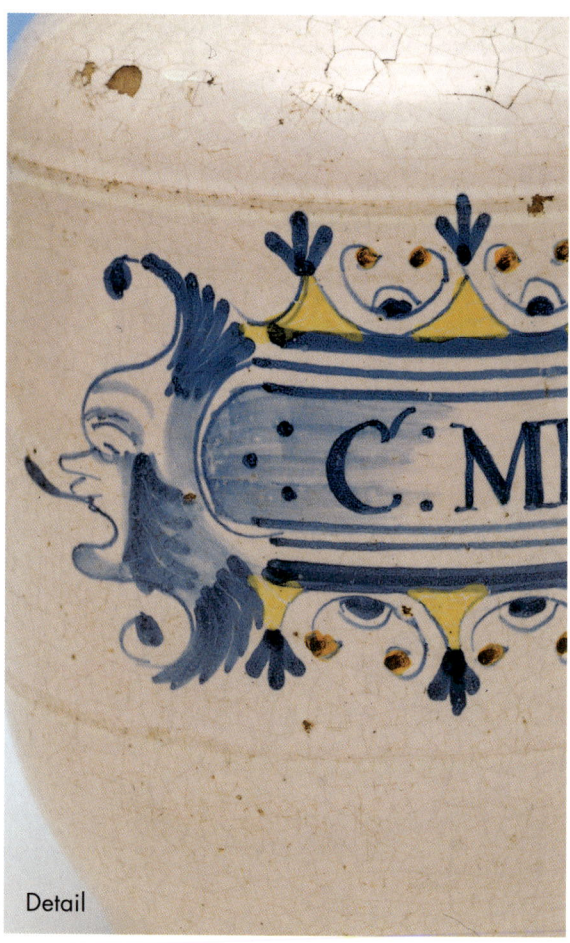

Detail

Dry drug jar (Cat.53)

ACCESSION NUMBER: KCD/P1

DESCRIPTION: Ovoid jar with splayed base and with two narrow ridges encircling bowl, one below the neck and the other above the foot. White glaze with pronounced pink tinge and design in blue, yellow and orange. Label panel straight, framed in two thin even lines and thicker (outer) third line. Neck ridged with unglazed rim, concave unglazed base.

DESIGN: Pipe-smoking man.

INSCRIPTION: C:MELISSAE:

MEANING OF INSCRIPTION: *Conserva melissae*, conserve of balm (*Melissa officinalis*)

CONTEMPORARY ACCOUNT: "It flowers in *July*. This Herb is very well known in our Gardens. It is of a fine Cordial Flavour; but it is so weak, that in most medicinal Forms it is lost, and 'tis hard even to dry it with its Natural Scent... It is a good Cordial, and makes an agreeable Ingredient in many *Alexipharmick* Waters. Any other *Forms* it is not fit for." (J. Quincy, *A Compleat English Dispensatory*, 1718, pp. 162–163)

DATE OF MANUFACTURE: c. 1645–1655

PLACE OF MANUFACTURE: London

CONDITION: Good; glaze crazed with chip off shoulder, base chipped in several places.

COMMENT: Howard claims that this is the earliest example of a polychrome drug jar (p. 12). The design is the same as a goblet in the Colonial Williamsburg Collection (catalogue ref. 81) dated 1655, and the cartouche border is the same design as a mug in the same collection (catalogue ref. 80), dated 1645.

DIMENSIONS: Height 210 mm, maximum width 143 mm

PROVENANCE: Bought in 1957, Howard Collection.

REFERENCES: Austin, British Delft at Williamsburg, p. 100, Nos. 80 and 81.

Howard, English Delftware Drug Jars, No. 4.

Lothian. English Delftware in the Pharmaceutical Society's Collection. p. 3 and Plates 4a and 4b.

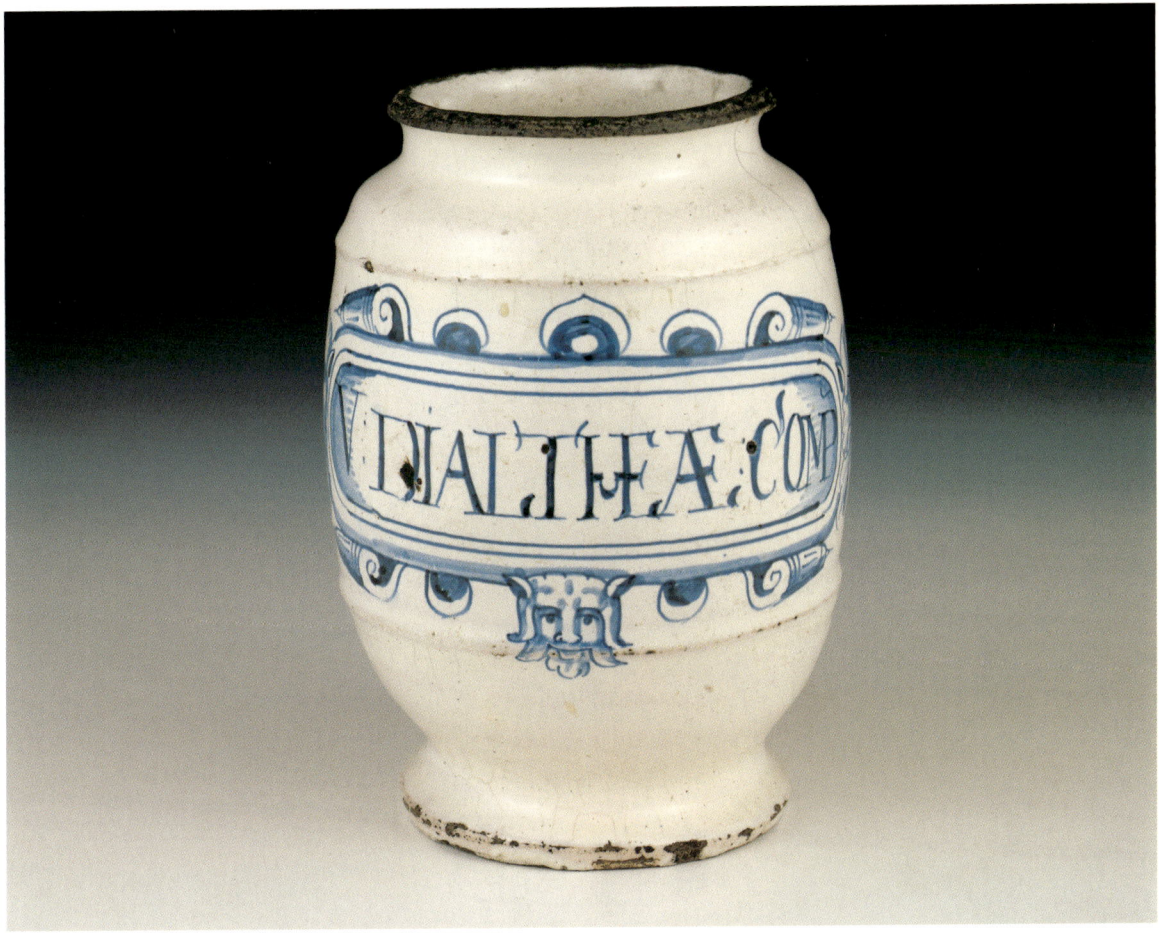

Dry drug jar (Cat.54)

ACCESSION NUMBER: KCD2

DESCRIPTION: Ovoid jar with splayed base and with two narrow ridges encircling bowl, one below the neck and the other above the foot. White glaze with pinkish tinge and design in blue. Label panel straight, framed in two thin even lines and thicker (outer) third line. Neck everted with unglazed rim, slightly concave unglazed base.

DESIGN: Pipe-smoking man.

INSCRIPTION: V:DIALTHEAE:COMP

MEANING OF INSCRIPTION: *Unguentum dialtheae compositium*, compound ointment made with marshmallow (*Althaea officinalis*)

CONTEMPORARY ACCOUNT: "Take the thick Mucilage made with Marshmallow-Roots, and Foenugreek and Linseed, ana ℔ ii. Oil of Olives ℔ iv. Wax ℔ i. Resin ℔ ss. Turpentine ʒ ii. Mix S.A."

"…This is reckon'd Emollient and Suppurative, and for such purposes is much used in extemporaneous Liniments and Cataplasms. By its Warmth, join'd with a relaxing Property, in such Forms, it greatly helps to rarefy the inclos'd Humours, and dispose them either for Transpiration or Revulsion, but most commonly for Maturation i.e. ripening into Matter: So as to render them fit for Discharge, either by Incision or Caustick." (J. Quincy, *A Compleat English Dispensatory*, 1718, p. 454)

DATE OF MANUFACTURE: c. 1650

PLACE OF MANUFACTURE: Probably Rotherhithe Pottery, Southwark, London.

DIMENSIONS: Height 190 mm, maximum width 143 mm

PROVENANCE: Bought in 1954 from the collection of Mrs Robert Sargeant.

CONDITION: Good; fine cracks descending from neck, glaze crazed, some pitting.

COMMENT: A fragment of a jar excavated by the Museum of London Archaeology Service at Rotherhithe appears to have been decorated by the same hand (MOLAS PW89, 1060 'LINIM [ARCAEI]').

REFERENCES: Archer. Delftware. p. 391.

Lothian. English Delftware in the Pharmaceutical Society's Collection. p. 2, Plate 3a.

Pipe-smoking man

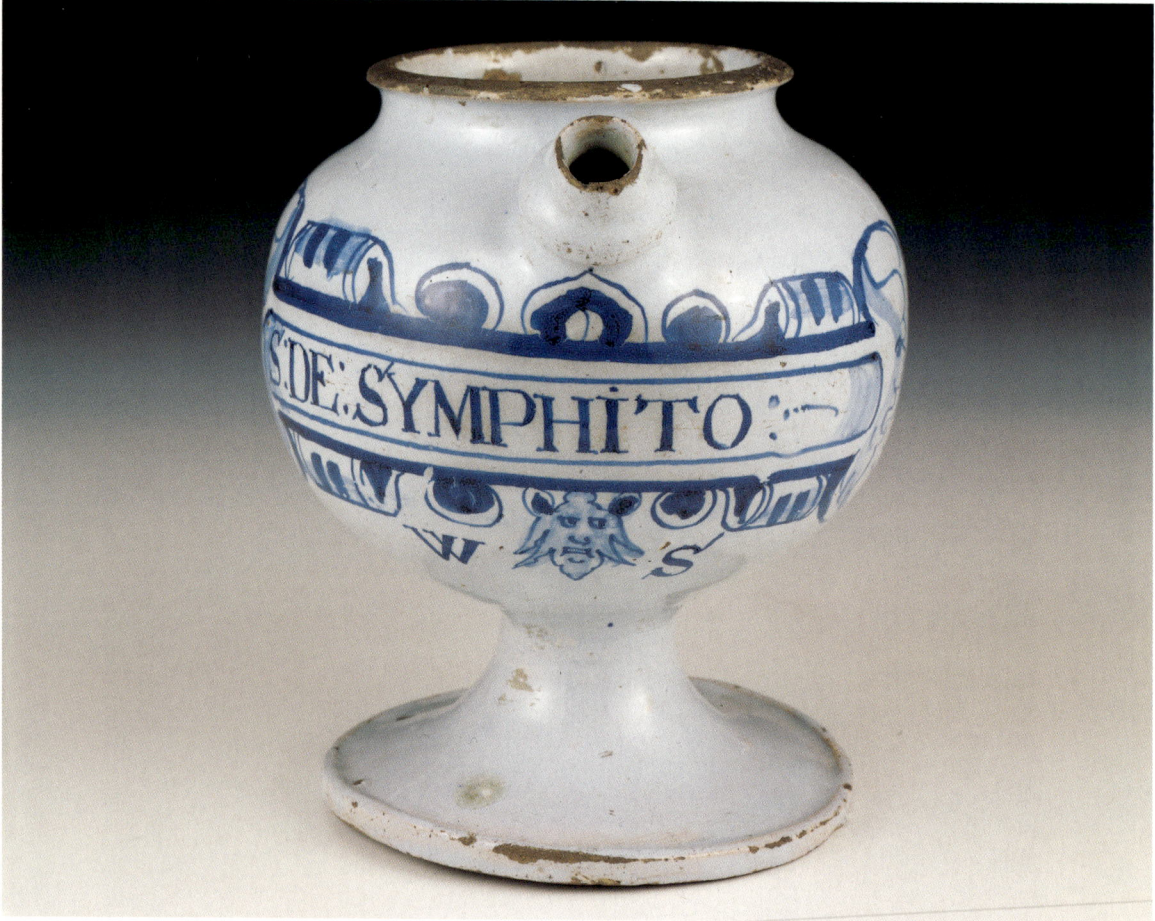

Wet drug jar (Cat.57)

ACCESSION NUMBER: KDD3

DESCRIPTION: Bulbous jar on spreading foot, with spout and fluted strap-like looped handle. White glaze with bluish tinge and design in blue. Label panel straight, framed in even outline with thicker outer line. Neck everted with unglazed rim, flanged spout, ridged, hollowed and unglazed base.

DESIGN: Pipe-smoking man.

INSCRIPTION: S:DE:SYMPHITO WS

MEANING OF INSCRIPTION: *Syrupus de symphito*, syrup of comfrey (*Symphytum officinale*). 'W.S. are the initials of the apothecary who commissioned the jar.

CONTEMPORARY ACCOUNT: "'Take the Roots and Leaves of the greater and lesser Comfrey, ana m.iii. fresh red Roses, Leaves of Betony, Plantain, Pimpernel, Knot-Grass, Scabious, and Colts-Foot, ana m.ii. Bruise them and press out their Juice; to each Pound of which put ℔ i. of Sugar, and boil up to a Syrup.'

"Ingredients of this Intention, which is to agglutinate, are the most improper of any for this Form; for that adhesive Property in which such Virtues reside, is spoil'd by the Interposition of Sugar, whose Parts are rigid and very detersive. For this reason, notwithstanding this Syrup is sometimes required, it is good for nothing." (J. Quincy, *A Compleat English Dispensatory*, 1718, p. 381)

DATE OF MANUFACTURE: 1650–1670

PLACE OF MANUFACTURE: Probably Southwark, London.

DIMENSIONS: Height 170 mm, maximum width 145 mm

PROVENANCE: Bequest, Saville Peck, 1955.

CONDITION: Good; glaze crazed and flaked on handle and rim of base.

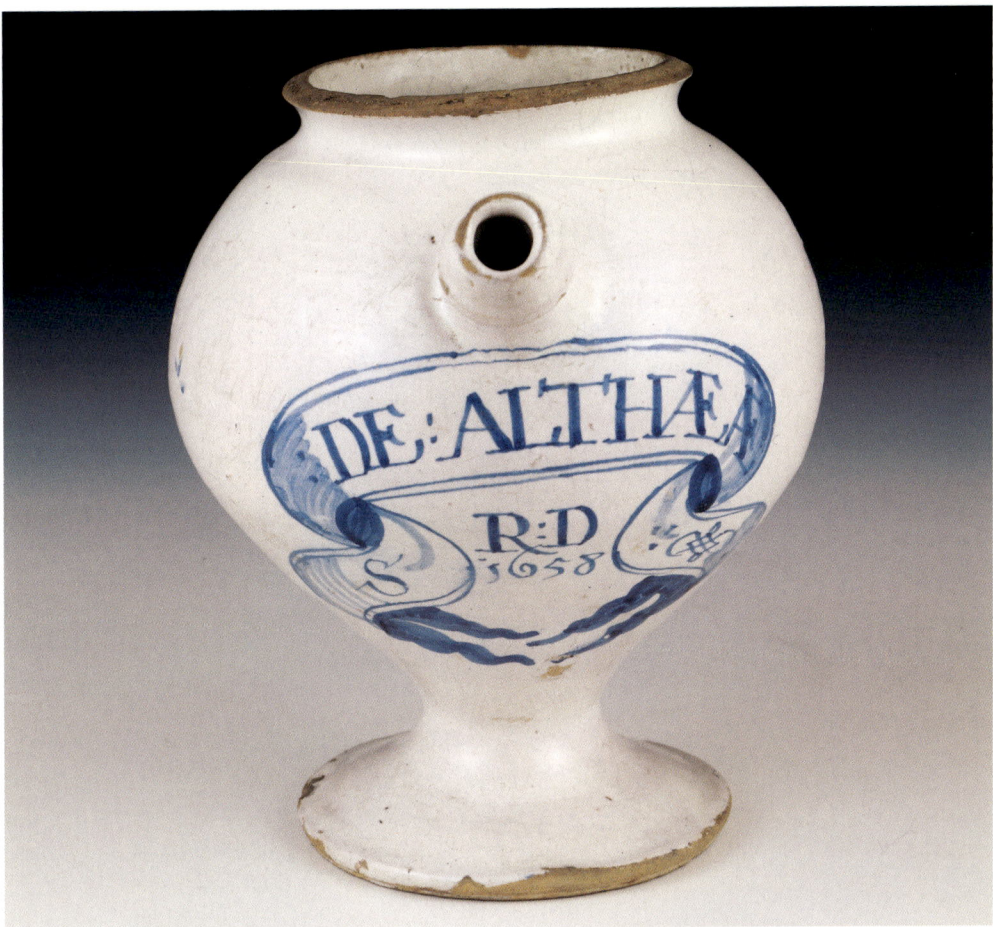

Wet drug jar (Cat.58)

ACCESSION NUMBER: KBE1

DESCRIPTION: Bulbous jar on spreading foot, with spout and (broken) handle. White glaze with pinkish tinge and design in blue. Label panel curved slightly upwards, framed in two thin even lines. Neck everted with unglazed rim, flanged spout, flat unglazed base.

DESIGN: Ribbon cartouche.

INSCRIPTION: S:DE:ALTHAEAE R:D1658

MEANING OF INSCRIPTION: *Syrupus de althaea*, syrup of marshmallow (*Althaea officinalis*). 'R.D.' are the initials of apothecary who commissioned the jar.

CONTEMPORARY ACCOUNT: "Take Marsh-Mallow Roots ℥ ii. of Grass, Asparagus, Liquorise, Roots and Raisins ston'd, ana ℥ ss. leaves of Marsh-Mallows, common Mallows, Pellitory of the Wall, Pimpernel, Saxifrage, Plantain, white and black Maiden-hair, ana m.i. red Chiches ℥ i. the four greater and lesser cold Seeds, ana ℥ iii. Boil them in a Sufficient quantity of Water, strain the Liquor out hard and boil it up when clarify'd into a Syrup, with ℔ iiiss. of white Sugar."

(J. Quincy, *A Compleat English Dispensatory*, 1718, p. 394)

DATE OF MANUFACTURE: 1658

PLACE OF MANUFACTURE: Possibly Pickleherring Pottery, Southwark, London.

DIMENSIONS: Height 185 mm, maximum width 165 mm

PROVENANCE: Bought in 1957, Howard Collection.

CONDITION: Good; base chipped, glaze crazed and flaked on body (1 cm at base of scroll) and rims of spout, neck and base, fragments of broken handle remaining.

COMMENT: Howard states that this is the earliest example of this design. He also suggests that it is by the same artist as KAG11 (Cat. 68) (p. 13). However, this seems unlikely as the A and R are formed differently.

REFERENCES: Howard, English Delftware Drug Jars, No. 6.

Lipski and Archer, Dated English Delftware, No. 1597.

Lothian, Agnes. Vessels for Apothecaries. 1953, p. 1 and Plate No. XI.

Lothian. Seventeenth Century English History Reflected in Pharmaceutical Antiques, pp. 7–8.

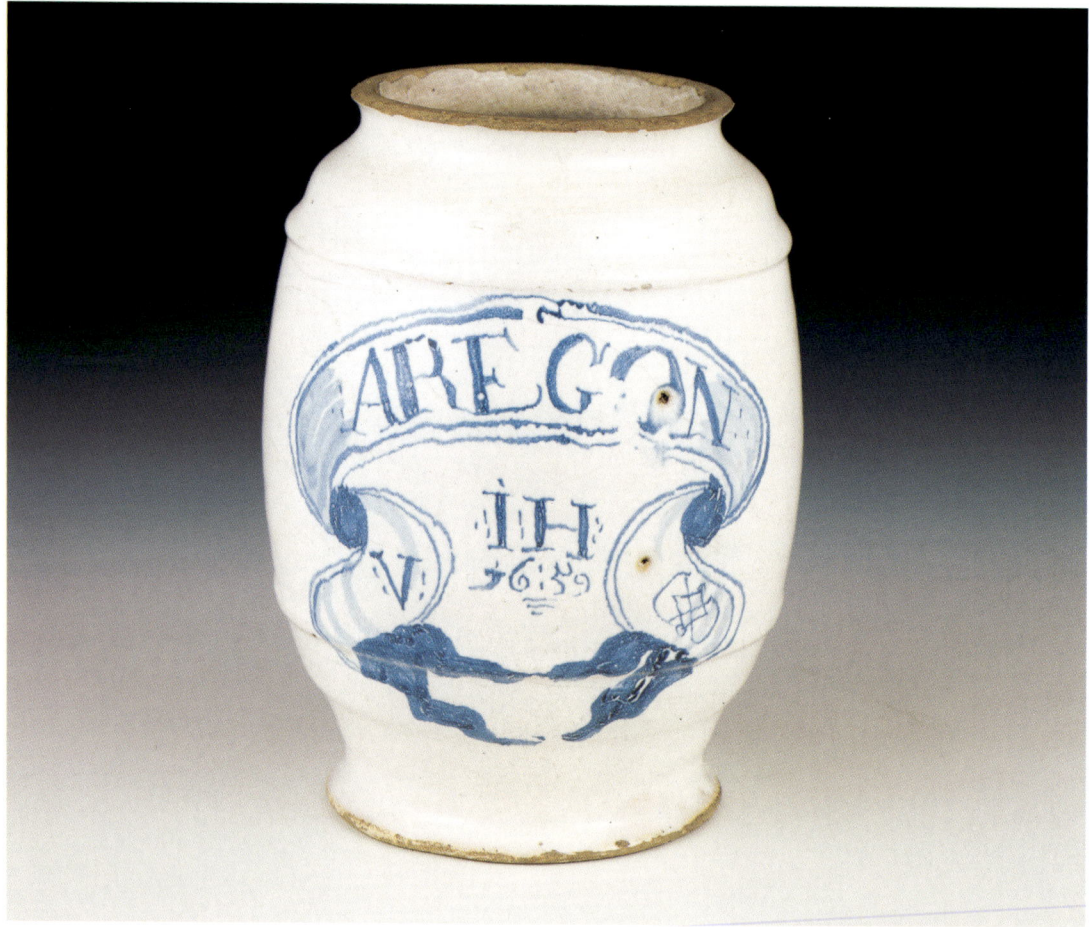

Dry drug jar (Cat.59)

ACCESSION NUMBER: KAE2

DESCRIPTION: Barrel-shaped jar, with splayed base and two narrow ridges encircling bowl, one below the neck and the other below the label. White glaze with pinkish tinge and design in blue. Label panel curved slightly upwards framed in two thin lines. Neck everted with unglazed rim, slightly concave unglazed base.

DESIGN: Ribbon cartouche.

INSCRIPTION: V:AREGON: (part of 'O' missing) I:H 16:59

MEANING OF INSCRIPTION: *Unguentum aregon*, aregon ointment. 'I:H' are the initials of the apothecary who commissioned the jar.

CONTEMPORARY ACCOUNT: Aregon ointment is described by Salmon in his New London Dispensatory, 1678, as a 'helpful' ointment. Its ingredients included tops of rosemary, marjoram, thyme, rue, roots of aron, wild cucumbers, bay leaves, sage, savin, bryony root, fleabaine, and laurel. However, Culpeper wrote: "It mightily digestive and maketh thin, and that not without some purging quality; and is very comodius against cold afflictions of the body but especially of the sinnews, convulsions, falling sickness, pains of the joynts, and great guts; I cannot much commend it, unless I should commend it for its length and tediousness" (N. Culpeper, *Pharmacopoeia Londinensis*, 1653, p. 168).

DATE OF MANUFACTURE: 1659

PLACE OF MANUFACTURE: Probably Southwark, London.

DIMENSIONS: Height 190 mm, maximum width 145 mm

PROVENANCE: Bought in 1957, Howard Collection.

CONDITION: Good; three fine cracks encircling bowl and one ascending from base, base chipped, glaze pitted and flaked from neck and base rims.

REFERENCES: Lipski and Archer, Dated English Delftware, No. 1598.

Lothian. Angels p. 732.

Lothian. English Delftware in the Pharmaceutical Society's Collection. p. 3 and Plate 3b.

Ribbon cartouche

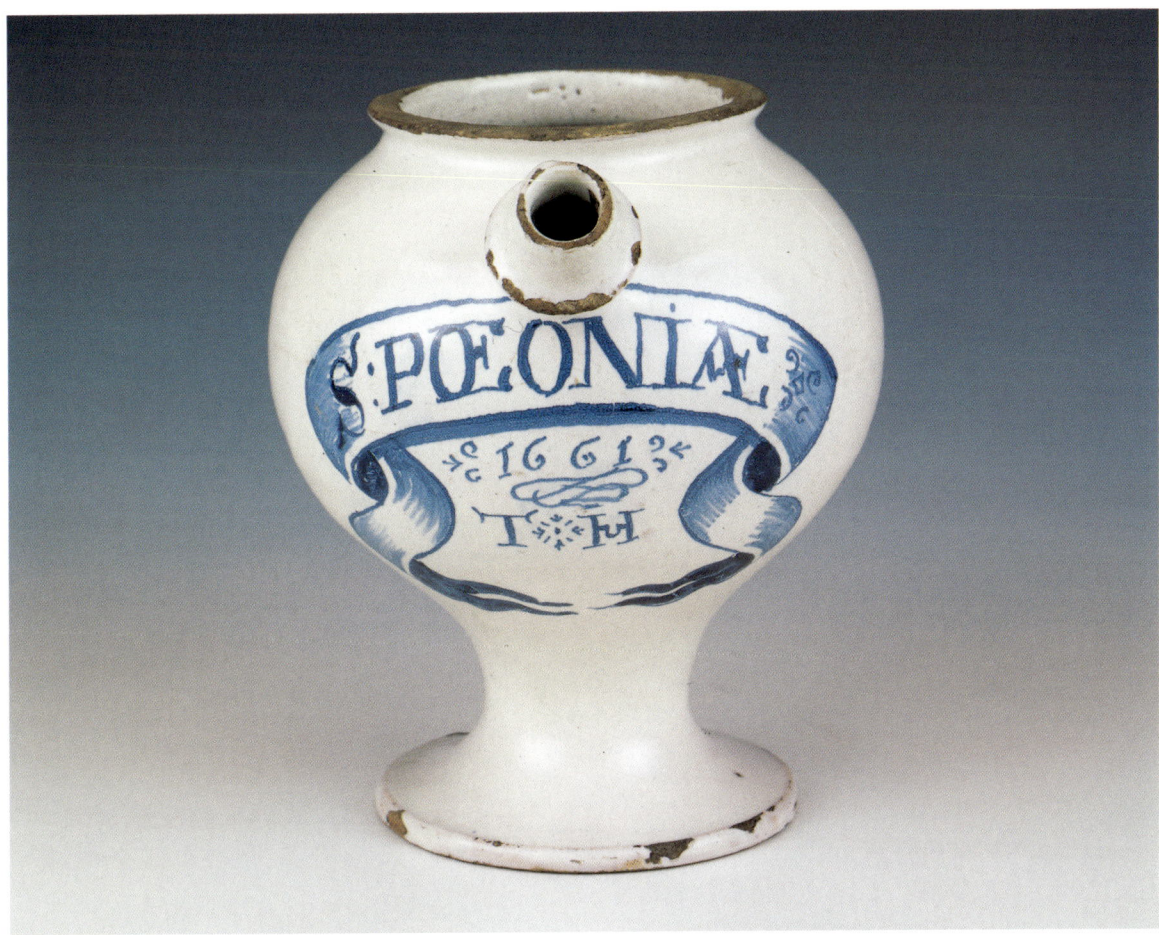

Wet drug jar (Cat.60)

ACCESSION NUMBER: KBE2

DESCRIPTION: Bulbous jar on spreading foot, with spout and fluted strap-like looped handle. White glaze with pinkish tinge and design in blue. Label panel curved slightly upwards with even outline. Neck everted with unglazed rim, flanged spout, hollowed unglazed base.

DESIGN: Ribbon cartouche.

INSCRIPTION: S:POEONIE 1661 TH

MEANING OF INSCRIPTION: *Syrupus paeoniae*, syrup of peonies (*Paeonia officinalis*). 'TH' are the initials of the apothecary who commissioned the jar.

CONTEMPORARY ACCOUNT: "'Take Roots of fresh Pioney, male and female, ana ℥ iss. Infused in White-Wine; of Contrayerva ℥ ss. Bastard-Lovage ℥ vi. Elks-Hoof ℥ i. Rosemary with the Flowers m.i. Betony, Origanum, Hyssop, Ground-Pine, and Rue ana ℥ iii. Wood of Aloes, Cloves and the lesser Cardamoms, ana ℥ ii. Ginger and Spikenard, ana ℥ ii. Staechas and Nutmegs, ana ℥ iiss. Water of Pioney-Root ℔ vi. Digest them together some hours, and boil to ℔ iv. To the straining add ℔

ivss. of Sugar, and make into a Syrup.' This is much prescribed in extemporaneous Forms, either to sweeten Liquors, or to give due Consistence, in all nervous Intentions; but very little good can be expected from it." (J. Quincy, *A Compleat English Dispensatory*, 1718, p. 379)

DATE OF MANUFACTURE: 1661

PLACE OF MANUFACTURE: Possibly Rotherhithe Pottery, Southwark, London.

DIMENSIONS: Height 190 mm, maximum width 170 mm

PROVENANCE: Bought in 1957, Howard Collection.

CONDITION: Good; 3.5 cm chip in base, glaze flaked on handle and spout, and neck and base rims.

REFERENCE: Lipski and Archer, Dated English Delftware, No. 1601.

Ribbon cartouche

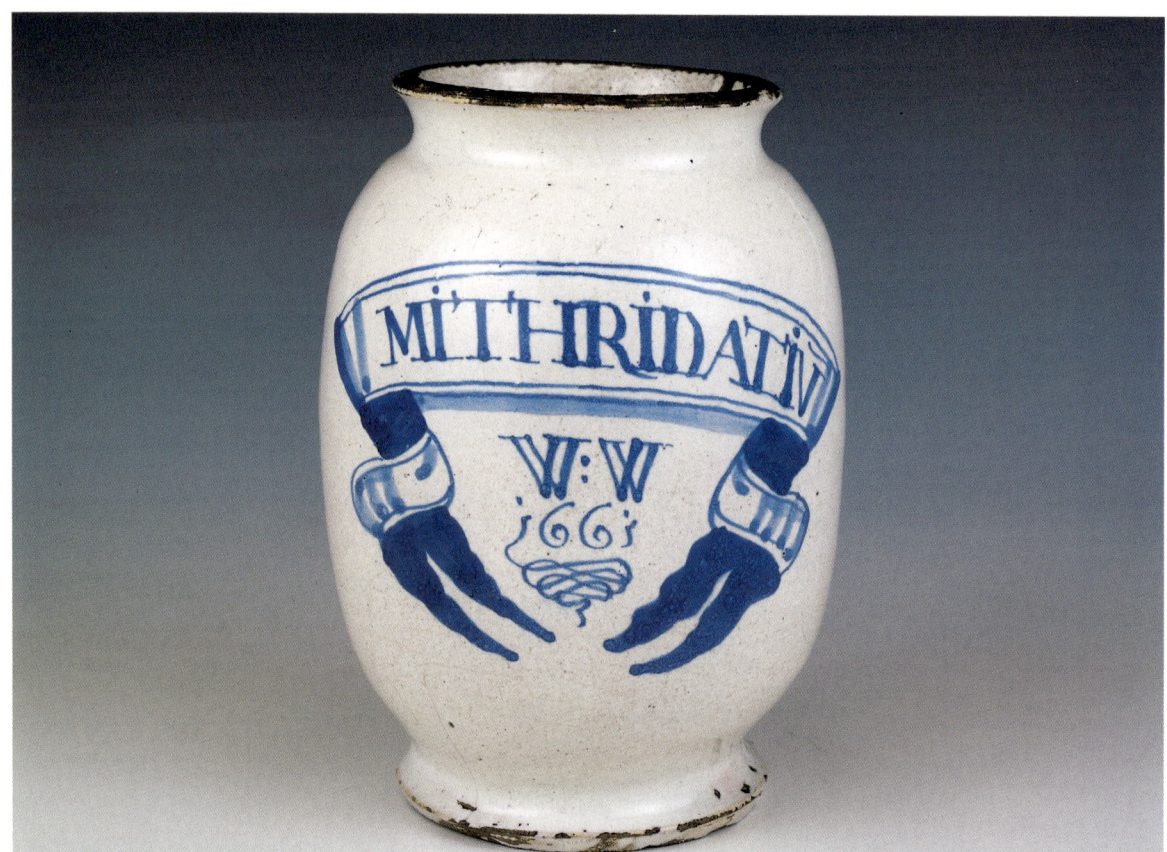

Dry drug jar (Cat.61)

ACCESSION NUMBER: KAE3

DESCRIPTION: Ovoid jar with splayed base. White glaze with pinkish tinge and design in blue. Label panel curved slightly upwards, framed in two thin lines. Neck everted with unglazed rim, very slightly concave, unglazed base.

DESIGN: Ribbon cartouche.

INSCRIPTION: MITHRIDATIV W:W 1661

MEANING OF INSCRIPTION: *Electuarium Mithridatium*, Mithridates' electuary. One of several forms of theriac (treacle) still popular in the 17th century as a universal antidote against poisons and infectious diseases. The name Mithridate is derived from Mithridates VI, king of Pontus (132–63 BC), who was believed to have rendered himself immune to poisoning by the constant use of antidotes. 'W:W' are the initials of the apothecary who commissioned the jar.

CONTEMPORARY ACCOUNT: "Take of Arabian Myrrh, Saffron, Agaric, Ginger, Cinnamon, Spikenard, Frankincense, and Seeds of Treacle-Mustard, ana ʒ x. of the Seeds of Hartwort, Opobalsamum, or in its stead, expressed Oil of Nutmegs, Sweet-Rush, Arabian Stoechas, the true Costus, Galbanum, Cyprus Turpentine, Long Pepper, Castor, Juice of Hypocistis, Styrax,

Opoanax, and Indian Leaf, or in its stead Mace, ana ʒ i. of Cassia Bark, Polymountain, white Pepper, Scordium, Seeds of wild Carrot, Carpobalsam, or Cubebs, Troches of Cypheos, and Bdellium, ana ʒ vii. of Spikenard cleansed, Gum Arabic, Macedonian Parsley Seed, Opium, the lesser Cardamoms, Fennel Seeds, Gentian Root, red Rose Flowers, and Dittany of Crete, ana ʒ v. of Aniseeds, Asarum, Acorus or Calamus Aromaticus, Orrice, the greater Valerian, and Sagapenum, ana ʒ iii. of Meum Root, Acacia, Stinks, and the tops of St. John's Wort, ana ʒ iiss. of the best Canary, enough to dissolve the Gums and Juices, which will take up about ʒ xxvi. of clarify'd Honey as much as the Weight of all the Ingredients, except the Wine; and make into an Electuary, S.A." (J. Quincy, *A Compleat English Dispensatory*, 1718, pp. 431–432)

DATE OF MANUFACTURE: 1661

PLACE OF MANUFACTURE: London

DIMENSIONS: Height 185 mm, maximum width 145 mm

PROVENANCE: Bought in 1957, Howard Collection.

CONDITION: Good; crack ascending from base, glaze crazed and flaked from rim of base.

REFERENCES: 'The Queen', Vol III, May 1907, Fig. 3, then in the collection of Mr B. Butler of Reading.

Lipski and Archer, Dated English Delftware, No. 1603 (and 1614 in error).

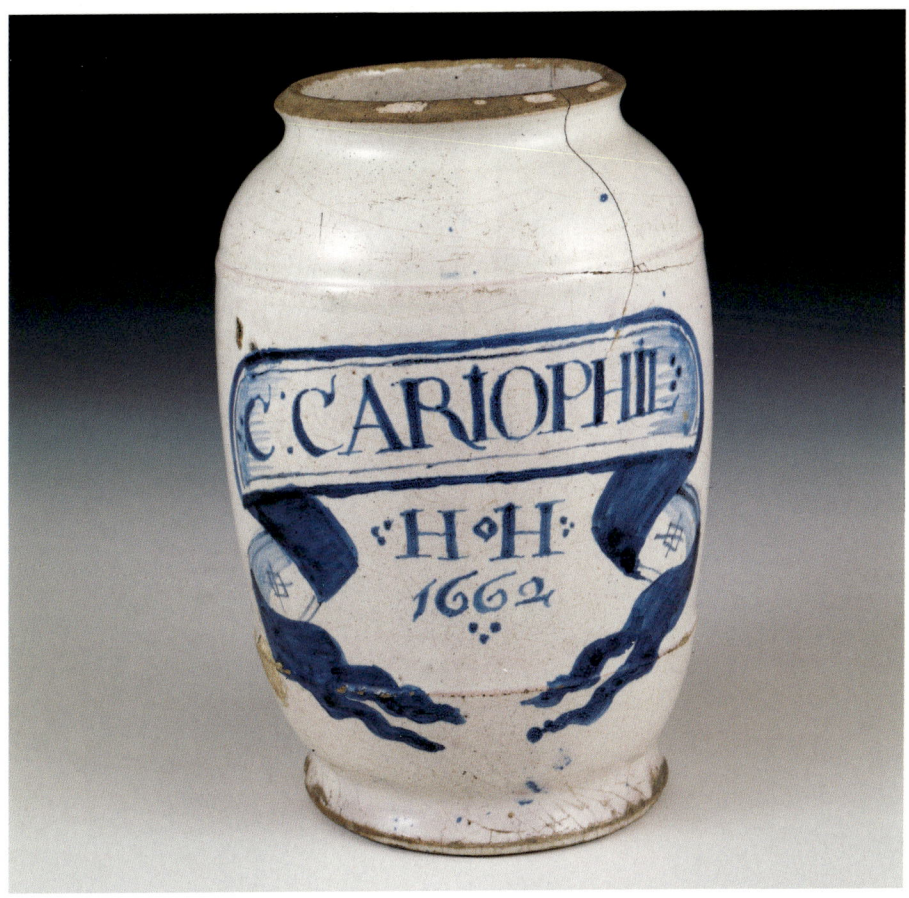

Dry drug jar (Cat.62)

ACCESSION NUMBER: KAE1

DESCRIPTION: Ovoid jar tapering slightly towards splayed base, with two narrow ridges encircling bowl, one below the neck and the other below the label. White glaze with pinkish tinge and design in blue. Label panel curved slightly upwards, framed in thin line and thicker outer line. Neck everted with unglazed rim, unglazed flat base.

DESIGN: Ribbon cartouche.

INSCRIPTION: C:CARIOPHIL: H H 1662

MEANING OF INSCRIPTION: *Conserva cariophyllus*, conserve of clove gillyflowers (*Dianthus caryophyllus*). 'H H' are the initials of the apothecary who commissioned the jar.

CONTEMPORARY ACCOUNT: "Clove Gillyflowers; call'd also very commonly, Flores Tunica… They blow in June. They are a fine Aromatick, and very grateful to Smell and Taste. They have place in the Syrup made of them, and most Cephalic and Cordial Juleps. There is also a Conserve made of them, but it is hardly ever used." (J. Quincy, *A Compleat English Dispensatory*, 1718, p. 81)

DATE OF MANUFACTURE: 1662

PLACE OF MANUFACTURE: London

DIMENSIONS: Height 190 mm, maximum width 135 mm

PROVENANCE: Bought in 1957, Howard Collection. Previously Harland Collection, sold as a part lot (18), 11/2/1931, with KAG6 (Cat. 69).

CONDITION: Fair; two cracks descending from neck, 2 cm of glaze flaked from bowl, at base of left end of scroll; glaze crazed and flaked on rim of base.

COMMENT: Howard suggested that this jar was by the same hand as KBE1 (Cat. 58) (p. 14). However, although the H is quite similar, the A and R are formed differently and the ornaments are different. He also notes the "cyphers" on the cartouche "lozenges", and links these to other jars including KBG3 (Cat. 72), KAG11 (Cat. 68), KAG6 (Cat. 69) and KDG10 (Cat. 105). Grigsby notes that this jar is from a set (p. 450), with other jars in the Longridge Collection, the Wilkinson Collection, the Glaisher Collection (Fitzwilliam Museum), and the Greg Collection (Manchester City Art Gallery).

REFERENCES: Grigsby. The Longridge Collection of English Slipware and Delftware. Catalogue number D450.

　　Howard, G. E. English Delftware Drug Jars, No. 11.

　　Lipski and Archer, Dated English Delftware, No. 1605B.

Fleur-de-lys

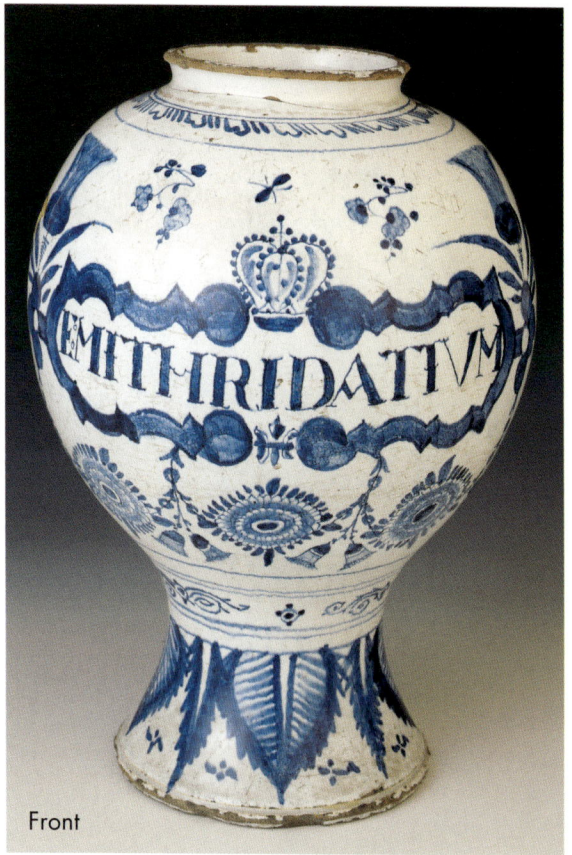

Front

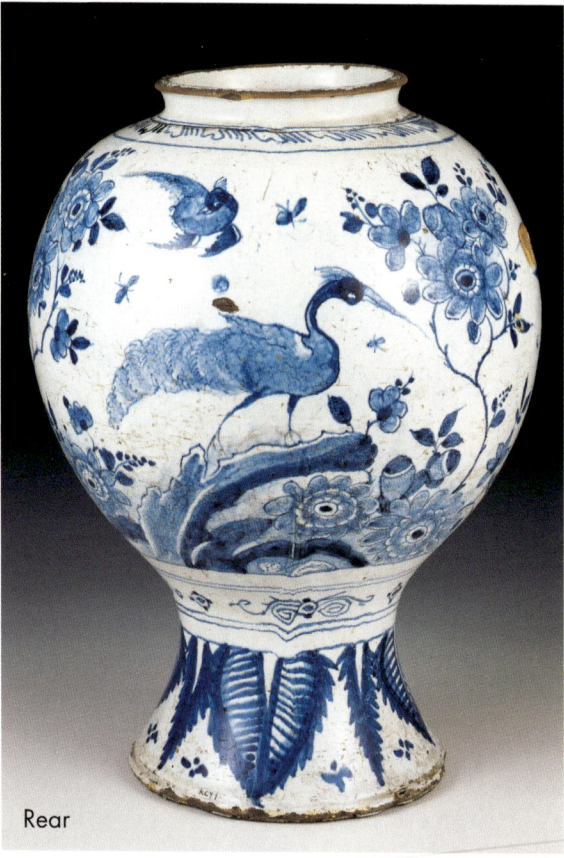

Rear

Dry drug jar (Cat.63)

ACCESSION NUMBER: KCY1

DESCRIPTION: Bulbous jar, tapering to broad slightly spreading foot. White glaze with bluish tinge and design in blue. Label panel straight, with very thick wavy strap-work frame. Neck everted, with unglazed rim, flat unglazed base.

DESIGN: Fleur-de-lys with crown, and Chinese style decoration of birds, insects, flowers and foliage on reverse.

INSCRIPTION: E:MITHRIDATIVM

MEANING OF INSCRIPTION: *Electuarium Mithridatium*, Mithridates' electuary. One of several forms of theriac (treacle) still popular in the 17th century as a universal antidote against poisons and infectious diseases. The name Mithridate is derived from Mithridates VI, king of Pontus (132–63 BC), who was believed to have rendered himself immune to poisoning by the constant use of antidotes.

CONTEMPORARY ACCOUNT: "Take of Arabian Myrrh, Saffron, Agaric, Ginger, Cinnamon, Spikenard, Frankincense, and Seeds of Treacle-Mustard, ana ʒ x. of the Seeds of Hartwort, Opobalsamum, or in its stead, expressed Oil of Nutmegs, Sweet-Rush, Arabian Stoechas, the true Costus, Galbanum, Cyprus Turpentine, Long Pepper, Castor, Juice of Hypocistis, Styrax, Opoanax, and Indian Leaf, or in its stead Mace, ana ʒ i. of Cassia

Bark, Polymountain, white Pepper, Scordium, Seeds of wild Carrot, Carpobalsam, or Cubebs, Troches of Cypheos, and Bdellium, ana ʒ vii. of Spikenard cleansed, Gum Arabic, Macedonian Parsley Seed, Opium, the lesser Cardamoms, Fennel Seeds, Gentian Root, red Rose Flowers, and Dittany of Crete, ana (ʒ) v. of Aniseeds, Asarum, Acorus or Calamus Aromaticus, Orrice, the greater Valerian, and Sagapenum, ana ʒ iii. of Meum Root, Acacia, Stinks, and the tops of St. John's Wort, ana ʒ iiss. of the best Canary, enough to dissolve the Gums and Juices, which will take up about ʒ xxvi. of clarify'd Honey as much as the Weight of all the Ingredients, except the Wine; and make into an Electuary, S.A." (J. Quincy, *A Compleat English Dispensatory*, 1718, pp. 431–432)

DATE OF MANUFACTURE: 1700–1720

PLACE OF MANUFACTURE: Lambeth, London, or possibly Bristol.

DIMENSIONS: Height 330 mm, maximum width 248 mm

PROVENANCE: Donation, J. W. Cooper, 1955.

CONDITION: Good; large chip off glaze (top left of label panel), crack below neck, base and neck rims chipped.

COMMENT: There is a pair to this jar (E: DIASCORDIVM, retaining its domed lid with tall bulbous knop), in a private collection in Scotland.

REFERENCE: An English Delft Mithridatium Jar, The Pharmaceutical Journal, 174, February 5, 1955.

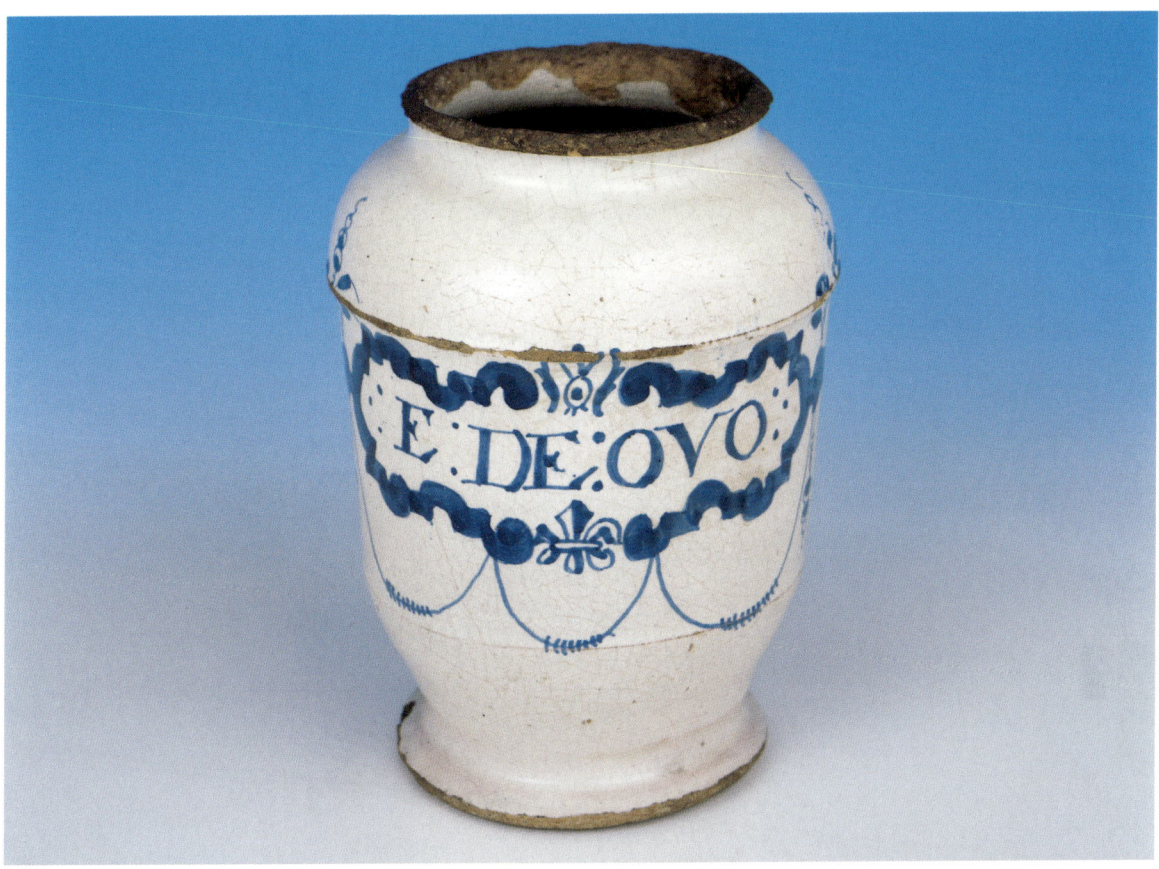

Dry drug jar (Cat.64)

ACCESSION NUMBER: KCF1

DESCRIPTION: Ovoid jar, tapering slightly towards splayed base, with two narrow ridges encircling bowl; one below label and the other below the neck. White glaze with pinkish tinge and design in blue. Label panel straight with wavy strap-work frame. Neck everted with unglazed rim, slightly concave unglazed base.

DESIGN: Fleur-de-lys.

INSCRIPTION: E:DE:OVO:

MEANING OF INSCRIPTION: *Electuarium de ovo*, electuary of egg

CONTEMPORARY ACCOUNT: "'Take a new-laid Egg, and thro a hole made in the Shell, draw out the White: then thrust in as much Saffron to the Yolk, as the Shell will hold, and roast them together until they are brought into a dry Substance so as to powder, taking care that it be in a Heat not great enough to burn the Saffron black. Powder this mixture with its equal weight of white Mustard-Seed; Roots of white Dittany or Fraxinel, and Tormentils, ana ℥ ii. Myrrh, Raspings of Harts-horn, and Butter-Bur Root, ana ℥ i. Roots of Angelica, Burnet, Juniper Berries, Zedoary and Camphor, ana ℥ ss. Mix all together with their weight of Venice Treacle, by help of a sufficient quantity of Syrup of Lemons, into an Electuary.'

There are a few trifling things in this Composition, but all together it makes an admirable Alexipharmick." (J. Quincy, *A Compleat English Dispensatory*, 1718, p. 407)

DATE OF MANUFACTURE: c. 1670

PLACE OF MANUFACTURE: London

DIMENSIONS: Height 175 mm, maximum width 140 mm

PROVENANCE: Bequest, Saville Peck, 1955. Formerly from Prior Collection.

CONDITION: Good; glaze crazed and flaked from body and neck and base rims.

REFERENCES: Grigsby. The Longridge Collection of English Slipware and Delftware. Catalogue number D402.

Lothian. English Delftware in the Pharmaceutical Society's Collection. p. 4 and Plate 7a.

Walker. Ancient pharmacy jars: p. 251, number 1.

Fleur-de-lys

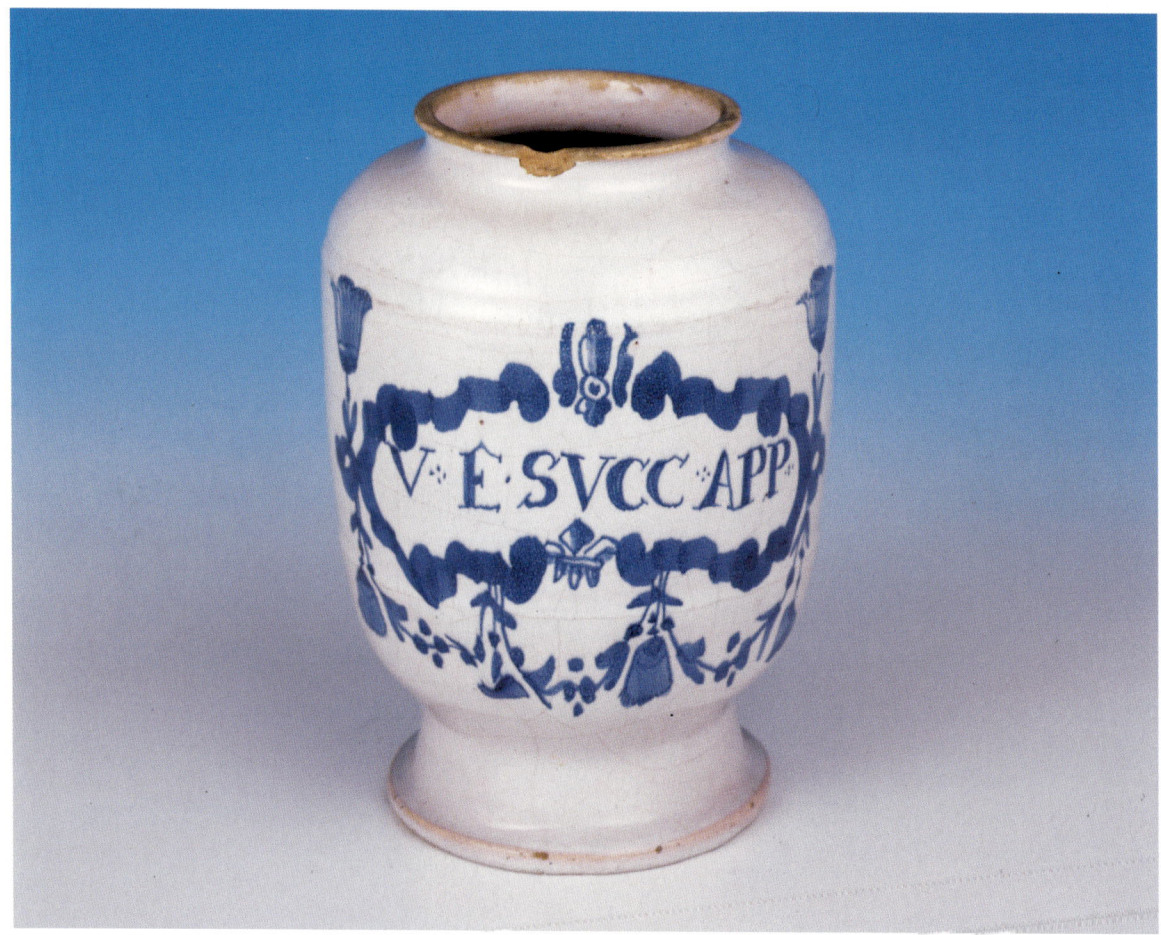

Dry drug jar (Cat.65)

ACCESSION NUMBER: KCF2

DESCRIPTION: Ovoid jar, tapering slightly towards splayed base, with two narrow ridges encircling bowl, one below the neck and the other below the label. White glaze with pinkish tinge. Slightly concave unglazed base.

DESIGN: Fleur-de-lys.

INSCRIPTION: V E SVCC APP

MEANING OF INSCRIPTION: *Unguentum e succis aperitivis primum*, ointment of aperient juice

CONTEMPORARY ACCOUNT: "Take of the juyce of Smallage, Endive, Mints, Wormwood, Common Parsly, Valerian, of each three ounces; oyl of Wormwood and Mints, of each half a pound; yellow Wax three ounces: mix them together over the fire, and make of them an Oyntment. Sometimes is added also the pouders of Calamus Aromaticus, Spicknard, of each one drachm; a little oyl of Cappers."

"It opens stoppages of the stomach and spleen, easeth the Rickets, the breast and sides being anointed with it." (Culpeper, *Pharmacopoeia Londoniensis or the London Dispensatory*, 1653, p. 171)

DATE OF MANUFACTURE: 1670–1690

PLACE OF MANUFACTURE: London

DIMENSIONS: Height 175 mm, maximum width 135 mm

PROVENANCE: Bought in 1957, Howard Collection.

CONDITION: Good; four chips on rim of neck, glaze crazed and flaked from rim of base.

COMMENT: Howard remarks on the "peculiarly distinctive border", more characteristic of 18th century jars. He dates this jar earlier because of its similarity to a jar in the Fitzwilliam Museum, Cambridge (Glaisher Collection) dated 1669. However the jar in the Glaisher Collection is of a slightly different design.

REFERENCES: Howard. English Delftware Drug Jars, p. 15 and No. 10.

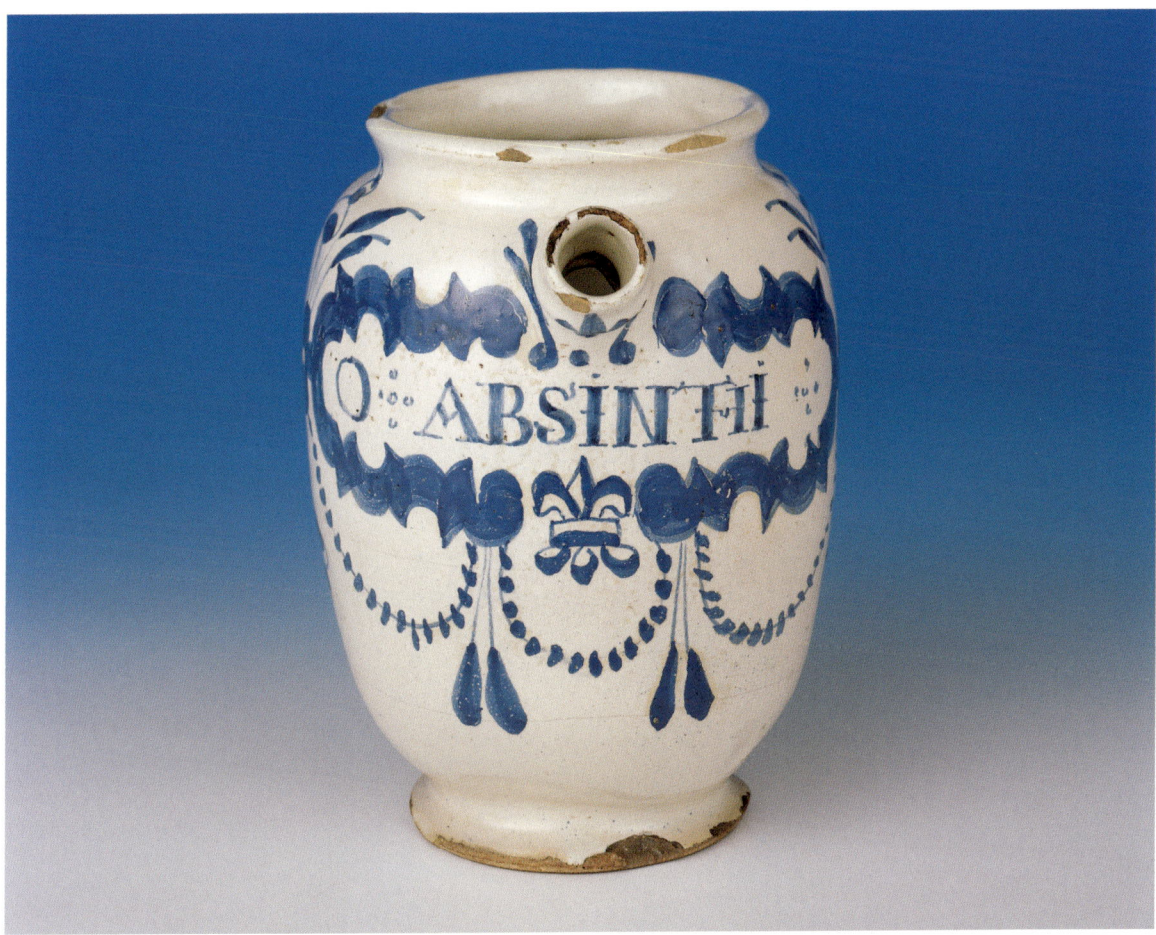

Wet drug jar (Cat.66)

ACCESSION NUMBER: KDF1
DESCRIPTION: Ovoid jar, tapering slightly towards splayed base, with spout and (broken) handle. White glaze with pinkish tinge and design in blue. Label panel straight with wavy strap-work frame. Neck ridged with glazed rim, spout with small flange, slightly concave, unglazed base.
DESIGN: Fleur-de-lys.
INSCRIPTION: O ABSINTHI
MEANING OF INSCRIPTION: *Oleum absinthii*, oil of wormwood (*Artemisia absinthum*)
CONTEMPORARY ACCOUNT: "This is very fetid and nauseous, as are all which are drawn from Plants of a tough, gummy, or balsamick Texture, as those of Box, Savine, &c. and therefore it is not much, or hardly at all in internal Prescription: but it is frequently order'd on Emplaisters against Worms in Children, which are to be apply'd to the Belly; for its penetrating Nauseousness is reckon'd so far to get thorow the Pores as to disturb those ugly Inhabitants, and promote their Ejectment. Some make also the Oil of Roman Wormwood; but this is a Plant which affords its Oil with so much difficulty, and in such small quantities, that it is hardly worth drawing, both on account of its Unpleasantness and its Scarcity, and therefore is little us'd." (J. Quincy, *A Compleat English Dispensatory*, 1718, p. 368)
DATE OF MANUFACTURE: c. 1680–1700
PLACE OF MANUFACTURE: Possibly Brislington/Bristol.
DIMENSIONS: Height 185 mm, maximum width 145 mm
PROVENANCE: Bequest, Saville Peck, 1955.
CONDITION: Fair; several cracks encircling bowl, fragments of handle remaining, base chipped, glaze crazed and flaked from spout and rims of neck and base.

Fleur-de-lys

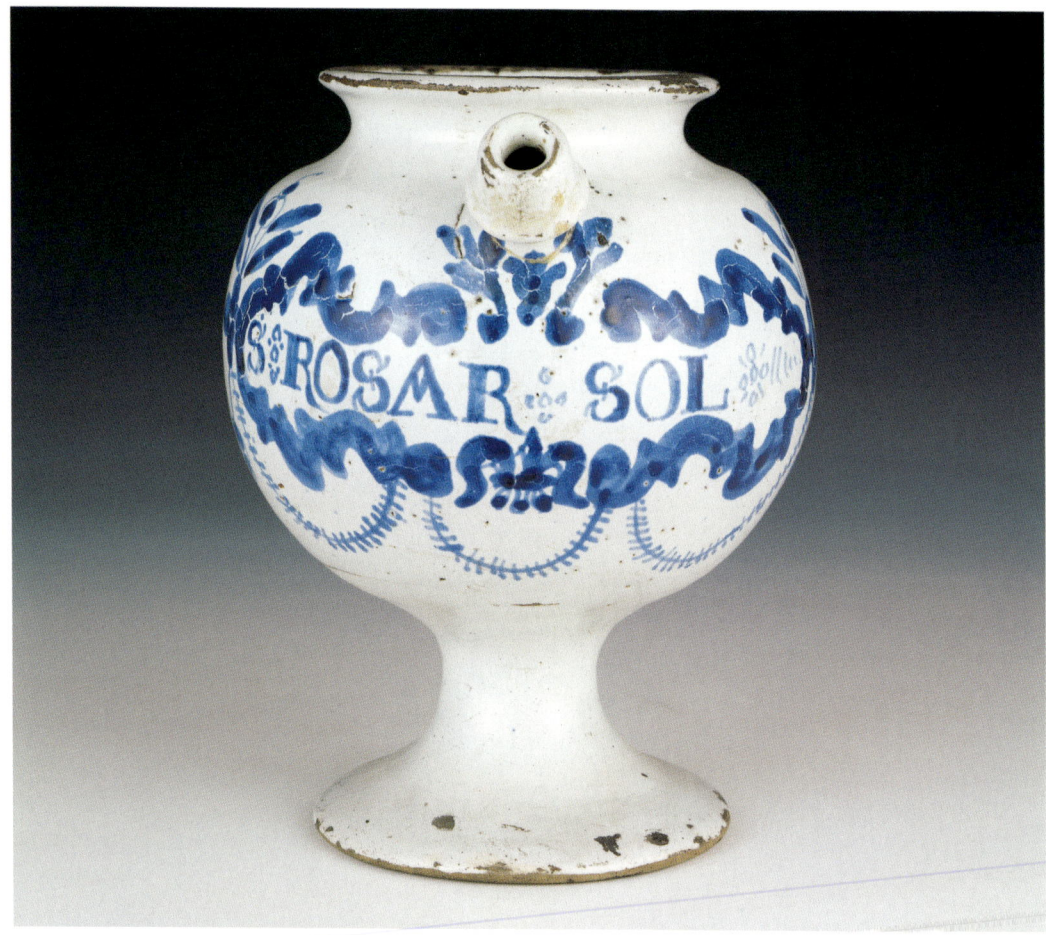

Wet drug jar (Cat. 67)

ACCESSION NUMBER: KDY3

DESCRIPTION: Bulbous jar on spreading foot, with spout and fluted strap-like looped handle. White glaze with pinkish tinge and design in blue. Label panel straight with wavy strap-work frame. Neck everted with flat unglazed rim, flanged spout, hollowed and glazed base with unglazed edge.

DESIGN: Fleur-de-lys.

INSCRIPTION: S ROSAR SOL

MEANING OF INSCRIPTION: *Syrupus rosarum solutivus*, solutive syrup of roses

CONTEMPORARY ACCOUNT: Quincy compares this recipe with syrup of damask roses. "These two differ only in the former [Damask Roses] being made with the express'd Juice of the Flowers lb vi. to lb iv. of Sugar) and the latter [Solutive] from a strong Infusion of the Flowers. The latter of which is much the best, and is conveniently made with the Residuum after Distillation of the Water, as has been already hinted. It is a stronger Purge than that of Rhubarb; and ʒ i. to a Child, ʒ ii. to a Man, is the Dose." (J. Quincy, *A Compleat English*

Dispensatory, 1718, p. 380)

DATE OF MANUFACTURE: 1700–1730

PLACE OF MANUFACTURE: London

DIMENSIONS: Height 200 mm, maximum width 165 mm

PROVENANCE: Bequest, Saville Peck, 1955.

CONDITION: Fair; one large crack and two small cracks encircling bowl, spout glued, glaze flaked from neck, spout, handle and base.

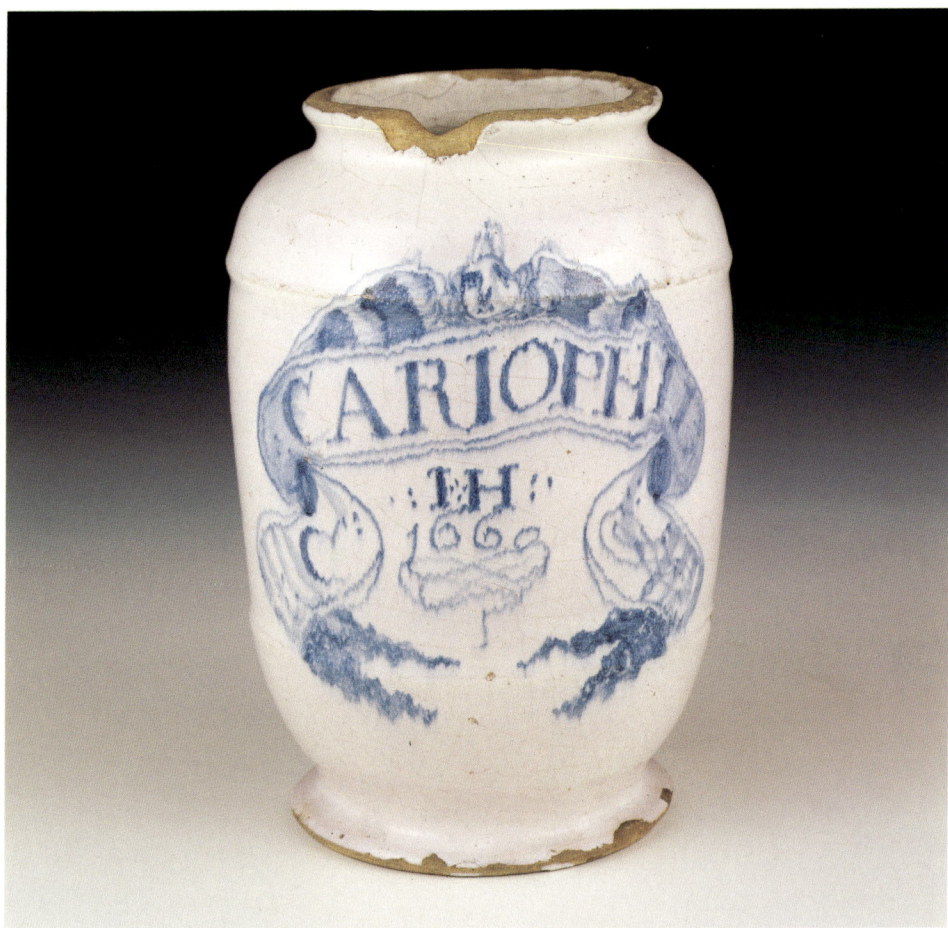

Dry drug jar (Cat.68)

ACCESSION NUMBER: KAG11

DESCRIPTION: Ovoid jar, tapering slightly towards splayed base, with two narrow ridges encircling bowl, one below the neck the other below the label. White glaze with pinkish tinge and design in blue. Label panel crooked and sloping upwards framed in two lines. Neck everted with unglazed rim, slightly concave unglazed base.

DESIGN: Angel with outspread wings.

INSCRIPTION: C CARIOPHIL I H 1660

MEANING OF INSCRIPTION: *Conserva cariophyllus*, conserve of clove gillyflowers (*Dianthus caryophyllus*). 'I H' are the initials of the apothecary who commissioned the jar.

CONTEMPORARY ACCOUNT: "CARIOPHYLLI HORTENSES, *Clove Gillyflowers*; call'd also very commonly, *Flores Tunica*... They blow in *June*. They are a fine *Aromatick*, and very grateful to *Smell* and *Taste*. They have place in the Syrup made of them, and most Cephalic and Cordial *Juleps*. There is also a *Conserve* made of them, but it is hardly ever used." (J. Quincy, *A Compleat English Dispensatory*,

1718, p. 81)

DATE OF MANUFACTURE: 1660

PLACE OF MANUFACTURE: London

DIMENSIONS: Height 200 mm, maximum width 140 mm

PROVENANCE: Bought in 1957, Howard Collection.

CONDITION: Fair; 3 cm chip from neck rim, crack ascending from base and encircling bowl, three portions of glaze peeling from bowl below lower ridge, glaze flaked from neck and base rims.

COMMENT: Howard notes the "cypher" on the right-hand "lozenge" of the cartouche, and links this to other jars including KBG3 (Cat. 72), KAG6 (Cat. 69), KAE1 (Cat. 62) and KDG10 (Cat. 105). He comments that the angel appears to have two "horns" on its head, and has "scanty locks", a Puritanical fashion (p. 13). He also states that this jar is the earliest appearance of the angel with outspread wings design. However, there is a jar dated 1659 in the Wellcome Collection at the Science Museum (ref: 1985-1903).

REFERENCES: Howard, English Delftware Drug Jars, No. 8.

Angel with outspread wings

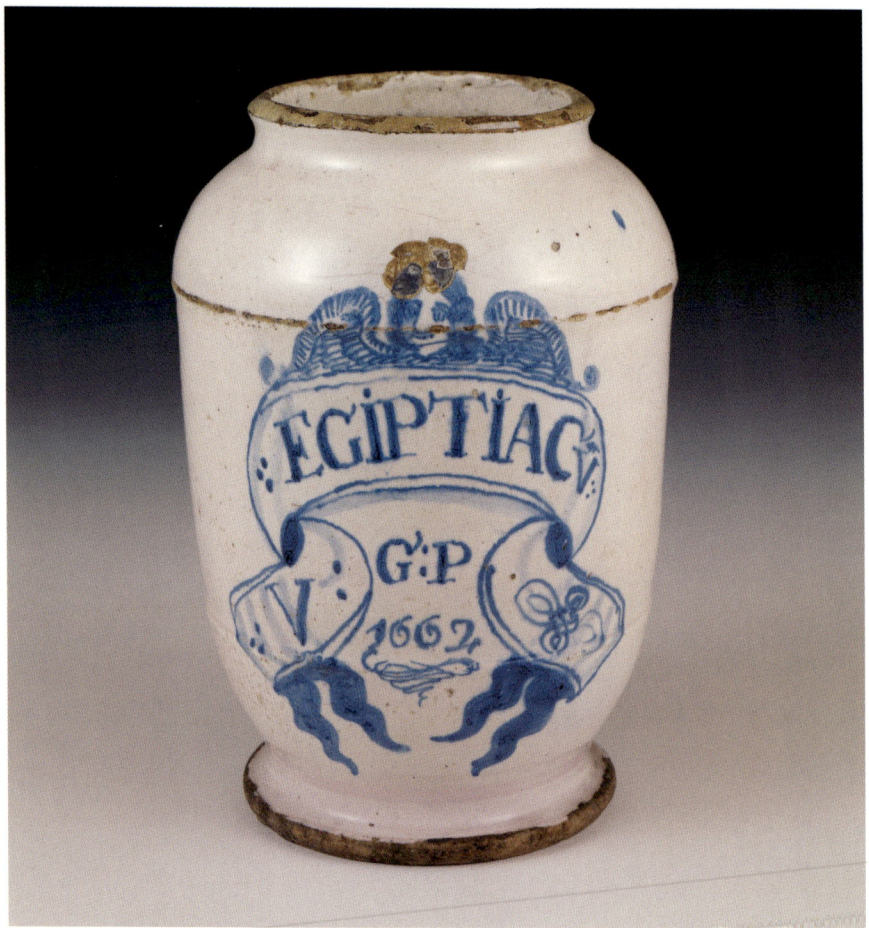

Dry drug jar (Cat.69)

ACCESSION NUMBER: KAG6
DESCRIPTION: Ovoid jar, tapering slightly towards splayed base, with two narrow ridges encircling bowl, one below the neck and the other above the base. White glaze with pinkish tinge and design in blue. Label panel curved slightly upwards with even outline. Neck ridged with partly glazed rim, slightly concave unglazed base.
DESIGN: Angel with outspread wings.
INSCRIPTION: V : EGIPTIACV: G:P 1662
MEANING OF INSCRIPTION: *Unguentum Egiptiacum*, Egyptian ointment. Verdigris ointment is mentioned in the ancient Egyptian papyrus, Ebers, which dates from 2500 BC. 'G:P' are the initials of the apothecary who commissioned the jar.
CONTEMPORARY ACCOUNT: "'Take Verdigrease in fine Powder ʒ v. Honey ʒ xiv. Vinegar ʒ vii. Boil all together till it is of a deep red, and as thick as Honey.'

"This is a Prescription of *Mesue*, *Fabricus Hildanus*, in a Discourse concerning a Gangrene and Mortification, gives this Medicine an extraordinary Recommendation, for deterging or eating off rotten Flesh, and cleansing to admiration foul Ulcers.

This is of great Use to destroy those cankerous Erosions which are so apt to grow in Childrens Mouths, and are first discoverable by white Specks: the way is to rub them with it upon a Rag ty'd to a Probe, or a piece of Stick. In Venereal Ulcerations likewise in the throat, i.e., about the *Uvula* and *Tonsils*, it does great Service." (J. Quincy, *A Compleat English Dispensatory*, 1718, p. 453)
DATE OF MANUFACTURE: 1662
PLACE OF MANUFACTURE: London
DIMENSIONS: Height 190 mm, maximum width 140 mm
PROVENANCE: Bought in 1957, Howard Collection.
CONDITION: Fair; chip above angel's head, glaze flaked on neck and rim of base.
COMMENT: Howard notes the "cypher" on the right-hand "lozenge" of the cartouche, and links this to other jars including KBG3 (Cat. 72), KAG11 (Cat. 68), KAE1 (Cat. 62) and KDG10 (Cat. 105). It seems unlikely that these jars were by the same artist, but there are two jars which probably are by the same hand: one in the Grendel Collection, Holland, and one in the Sheffield City Museum. (Lipski and Archer, Dated English Delftware No. 1604 and No. 1607)
REFERENCES: Howard, English Delftware Drug Jars, No. 9.
Lipski and Archer, Dated English Delftware, No. 1606.

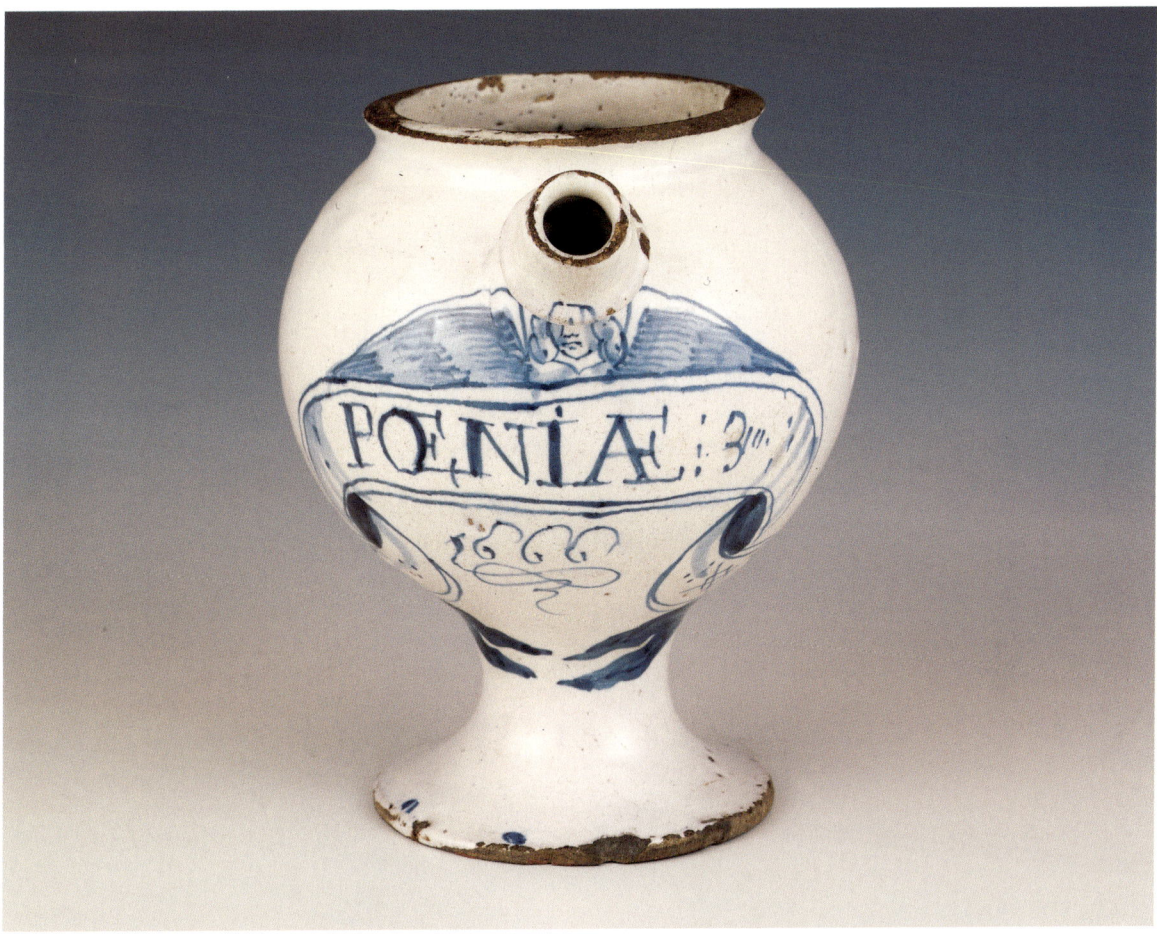

Wet drug jar (Cat.70)

ACCESSION NUMBER: KBG5

DESCRIPTION: Bulbous jar on spreading foot, with spout and fluted strap-like looped handle. White glaze with pinkish tinge and design in blue. Label panel curved slightly upwards with even outline. Neck everted, with unglazed rim, flanged spout, hollowed unglazed base.

DESIGN: Angel with outspread wings.

INSCRIPTION: S POENIAE 1666

MEANING OF INSCRIPTION: *Syrupus paeoniae*, syrup of peony (*Paeonia officinalis*).

CONTEMPORARY ACCOUNT: "'Take Roots of fresh Pioney, Male and Female, ana ℨ iss. infused in White-Wine; of Contrayerva ℨ ss. Bastard-Lovage ℨ vi. Elks-Hoof ℨ i. Rosemary with the Flowers m.i. Betony, Origanum, Hyssop, Ground-Pine, and Rue ana ℨ iii. Wood of Aloes, Cloves and the lesser Cardamoms, ana ℨ ii. Ginger and Spikenard, ana ℨ ii. Staechas and Nutmegs, ana ℨ iiss. Water of Pioney-Root ℔ vi. Digest them together some hours, and boil to ℔ iv. To the straining add ℔ ivss. of Sugar, and make into a Syrup.' This is much prescribed in extemporaneous Forms, either to sweeten Liquors, or to give due Consistence, in all nervous Intentions; but very little good can be expected from it." (J. Quincy, *A Compleat English Dispensatory*, 1718, p. 379)

DATE OF MANUFACTURE: 1666

PLACE OF MANUFACTURE: London

DIMENSIONS: Height 160 mm, maximum width 135 mm

PROVENANCE: Bought in 1957, Howard Collection. Previously in the Hodgkin Collection.

CONDITION: Good; small crack descending from neck, base chipped, glaze flaked on spout and handle.

COMMENT: Howard describes the angel on this jar as a "distinctly Puritan type" and suggests a resemblance to Oliver Cromwell. He also notes the unusual design with the head elongated upwards onto the spout (p. 14).

Five jars are known from this set: this jar, one in the Jephcott Collection in New Zealand, one in the Gardiner Museum, Toronto, one in the Longridge Collection, and one sold from the Price Glover Collection, by Christies, 14/6/1988 (lot 2).

REFERENCES: Hodgkin, Examples of Early English Pottery, p. 89.

Howard, English Delftware Drug Jars, No. 13.

Lipski and Archer, Dated English Delftware, No. 1615C.

Angel with outspread wings

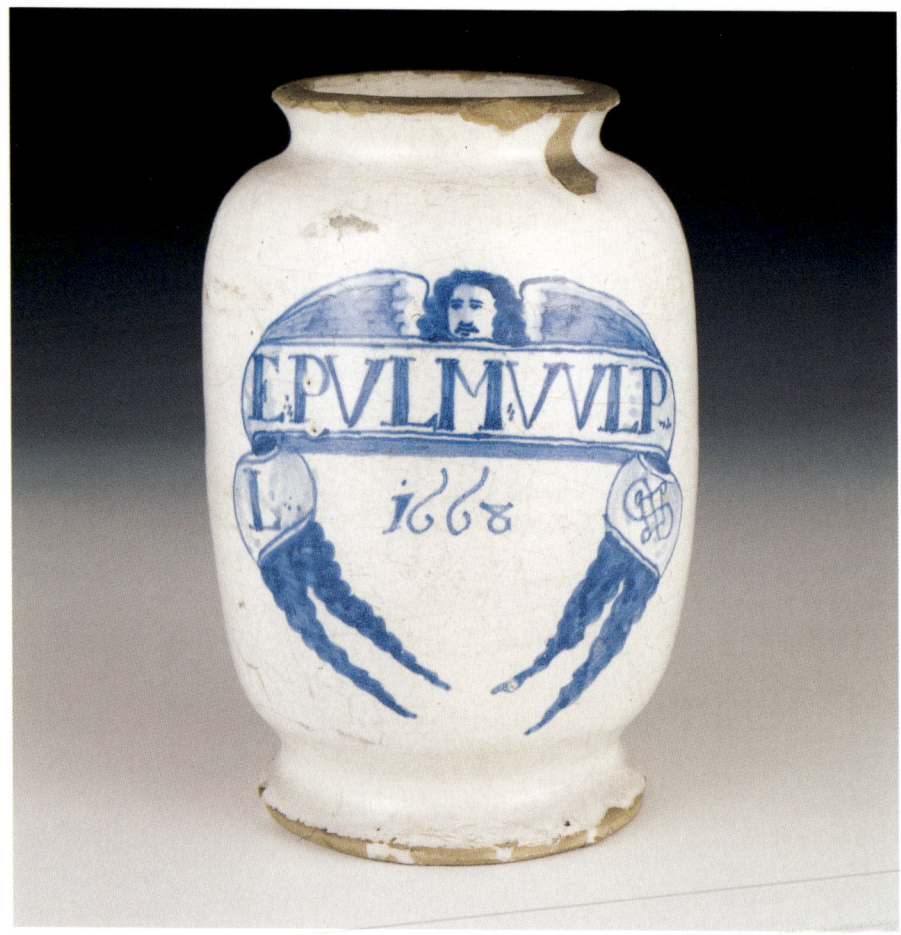

Dry drug jar (Cat.71)

ACCESSION NUMBER: KAG5

DESCRIPTION: Ovoid jar with splayed base. White glaze with pinkish tinge and design in blue. Label panel curved slightly upwards with even outline. Neck everted, with unglazed rim, slightly concave unglazed base.

DESIGN: Angel with outspread wings.

INSCRIPTION: L E.PVLM.VVLP 1668

MEANING OF INSCRIPTION: *Lohoch e pulmone vulpis*, lohoch of fox lungs

CONTEMPORARY ACCOUNT: "Colledg. *Take of Fox Lungs rightly prepared, juyce of Liquoris, Maiden-hair, Anniseeds, Sweet Fennel seeds, of each equal parts, sugar dissolved in Coltsfoot and Scabious water, and boyled in a Syrup, three times of their weight; the rest being in fine powder, let them be put to it and strongly stirred together, that it may be made into a Lohoch according to art...."*

"It cleanseth and uniteth Ulcers in the Lungs and Breast, and is a present remedy in Ptisicks." (Culpeper, *The Physicians Library*, 1667, p. 140)

DATE OF MANUFACTURE: 1668

PLACE OF MANUFACTURE: London

DIMENSIONS: Height 200 mm, maximum width 140 mm

PROVENANCE: Bought in 1951. Previously Sir John Evans' collection, sold at Christies, 14/2/1911, lot 24.

CONDITION: Good; large chip off neck rim, glaze crazed and chipped below neck and at rim of base.

REFERENCES: Hodgkin, Examples of Early English Pottery.
Lipski and Archer, Dated English Delftware, No. 1622.
Lothian. Angels p. 732.
Lothian. English Delftware in the Pharmaceutical Society's Collection. p. 3 and Plate 5a.
Lothian. Vessels for Apothecaries. p. 4 and Plate No. XVII.
Lothian Short. Apothecary Jar Inscriptions, pp. 145–146.

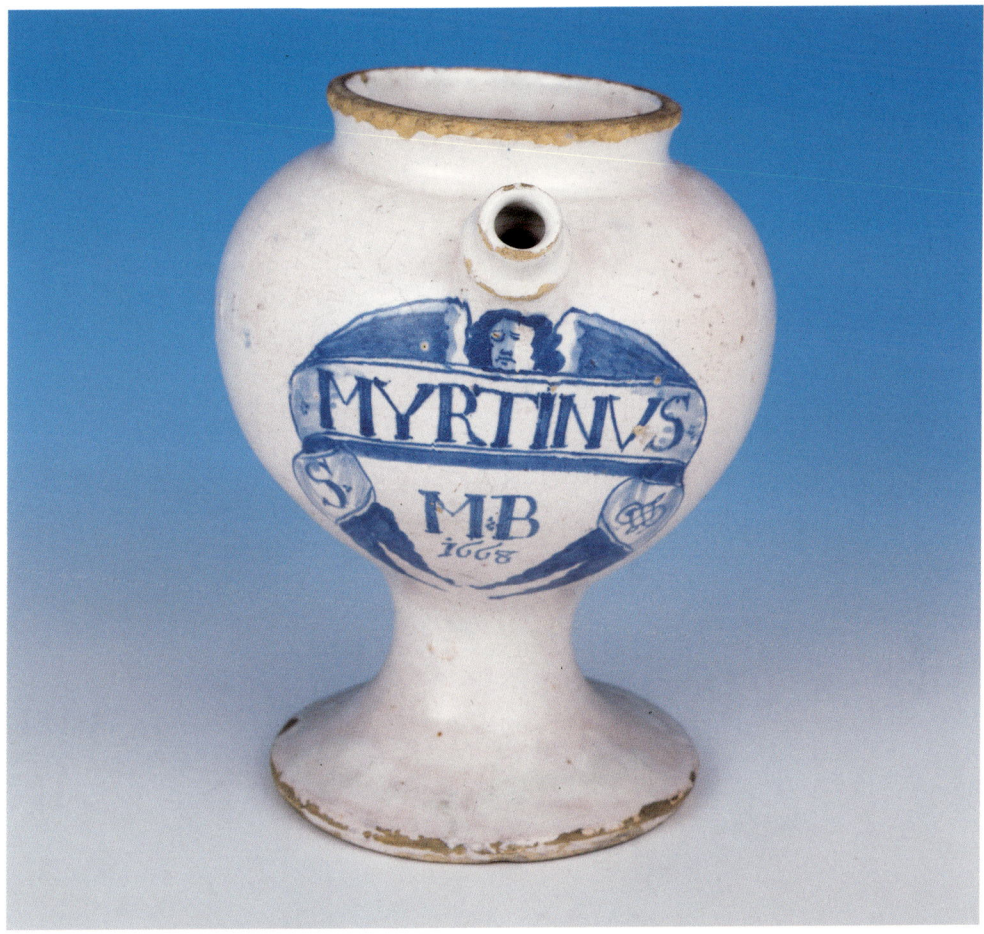

Wet drug jar (Cat.72)

ACCESSION NUMBER: KBG3

DESCRIPTION: Bulbous jar on spreading foot, with spout and fluted strap-like looped handle. White glaze with pinkish tinge and design in blue. Label panel curved slightly upwards with even outline. Neck slightly everted, unglazed, flanged spout, hollowed unglazed base.

DESIGN: Angel with outspread wings.

INSCRIPTION: S MYRTINVS MB 1668

MEANING OF INSCRIPTION: *Syrupus myrtinus*, syrup of myrtle berries (*Myrtus communis*). 'MB' are the initials of the apothecary who commissioned the jar.

CONTEMPORARY ACCOUNT: "These are very rough and astringent. They are not much in Composition for inward use, the Syrup is the chief: but they are in several of the strengthening Plaisters. The Syrup is esteem'd good against Abortion, and used in Fluxes of all kinds." (J. Quincy, *A Compleat English Dispensatory*, 1718, p. 100)

DATE OF MANUFACTURE: 1668

PLACE OF MANUFACTURE: London

DIMENSIONS: Height 210 mm, maximum width 170 mm

PROVENANCE: Bought in 1957, Howard Collection. Previously F. Bennett-Goldney's collection, sold by Puttick and Simpson, 4/3/1920 (lot 94).

CONDITION: Good; two cracks ascending from base, glaze crazed and flaked on neck, spout, handle and base.

COMMENT: Howard claims that this is the first jar on which the angel has a fashionable wig. He also notes the "cypher" on the right-hand "lozenge" of the cartouche, and links this to other jars including KAG11 (Cat. 68), KAG6 (Cat. 69), KAE1 (Cat. 62) and KDG10 (Cat. 105).

REFERENCES: Howard, G. E. English Delftware Drug Jars, No. 12. Lipski and Archer, Dated English Delftware, No. 1621.

Angel with outspread wings

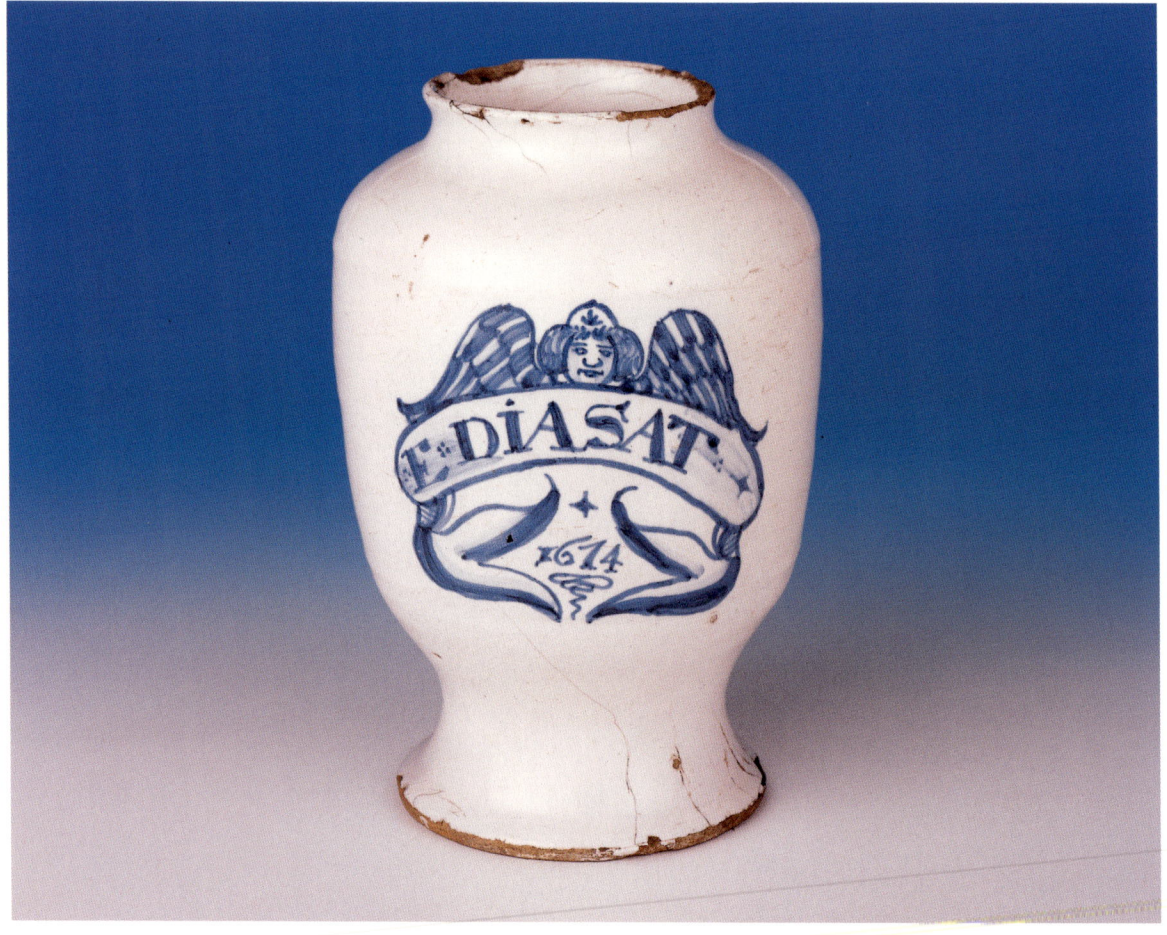

Dry drug jar (Cat.73)

ACCESSION NUMBER: KAG9

DESCRIPTION: Ovoid jar, tapering slightly towards splayed base, with two faint ridges encircling bowl, one below the neck the other below the label. White glaze with pinkish tinge and design in blue. Label panel curved slightly upwards with even outline. Neck everted with glazed rim, slightly concave unglazed base.

DESIGN: Angel with outspread wings.

INSCRIPTION: E DIASAT 1674

MEANING OF INSCRIPTION: *Electuarium diasatyrion*, electuary of satyrion (*Orchis mascula*).

CONTEMPORARY ACCOUNT: "The *Electuarium Diasatyrion*, which is in many Dispensatories, and which takes its name from this Root [satyrion], is certainly with good reason commended for a great Strengthener; and it wonderfully warms and titillates the Nerves, whereby such Desires are excited: and on the like account in many Constitutions may cure Barrenness, and promote Conception. But as there are some warm *Aromaticks* in that Compositions besides, it is to be doubted whether they do not come in for the greatest share in these Effects." (J. Quincy, *A Compleat English Dispensatory*, 1718, p. 86)

DATE OF MANUFACTURE: 1674

PLACE OF MANUFACTURE: London

DIMENSIONS: Height 195 mm, maximum width 143 mm

PROVENANCE: Bought in 1957, Howard Collection.

CONDITION: Good; cracks descending from neck and ascending from base, neck chipped, glaze flaked from neck and base rims.

COMMENT: Howard suggests that this is one of a set by the same artist with KBG6 (Cat. 74) and KAG10 (Cat. 75). There are seven jars from this set dated 1674, and an undated dry jar, in a private collection, painted by two different hands.

REFERENCES: Howard, English Delftware Drug Jars, No. 18.
   Lipski and Archer, Dated English Delftware, No. 1634A.

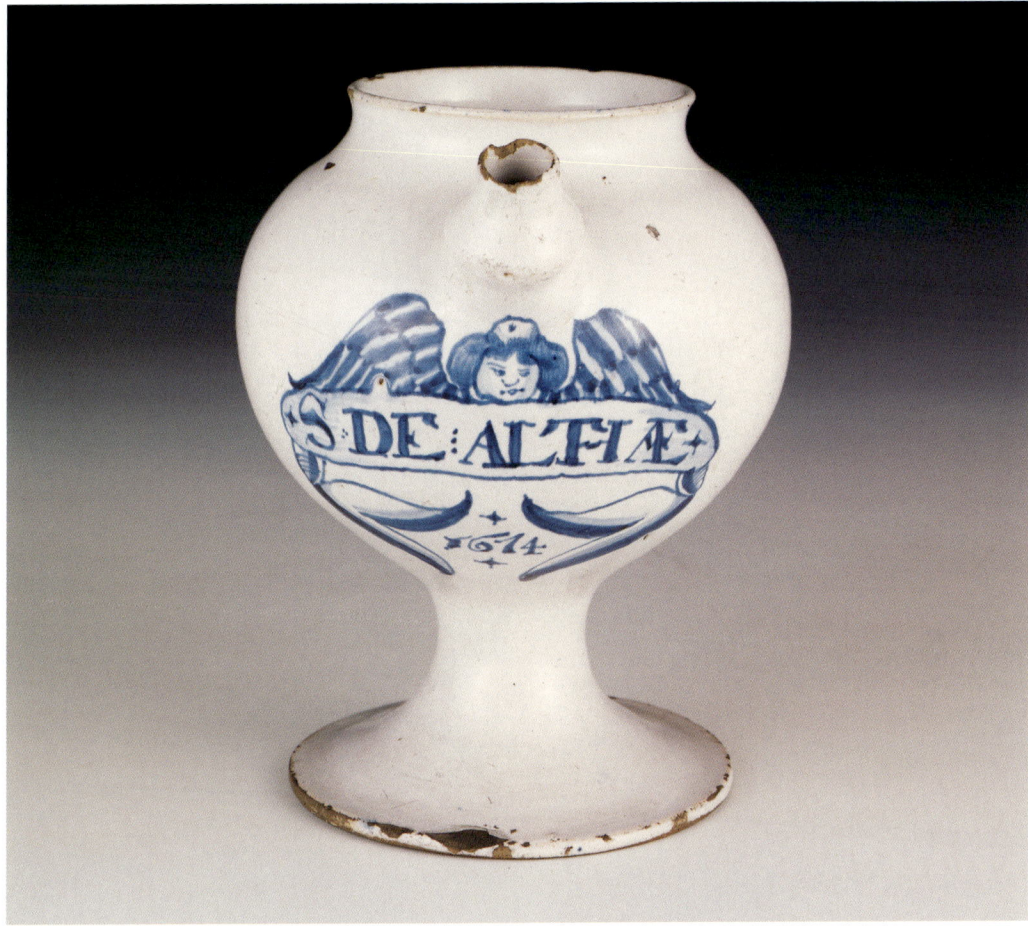

Wet drug jar (Cat.74)

ACCESSION NUMBER: KBG6

DESCRIPTION: Bulbous jar on spreading foot, with spout and slightly fluted strap-like looped handle. White glaze with pinkish tinge and design in dark blue. Label panel curved slightly upwards with even outline. Neck everted with glazed rim, flanged spout, hollowed unglazed base.

DESIGN: Angel with outspread wings.

INSCRIPTION: S:DE:ALTHAE 1674

MEANING OF INSCRIPTION: *Syrupus de althaea*, syrup of marshmallow (*Althaea officinalis*).

CONTEMPORARY ACCOUNT: "This Syrup is originally ascrib'd to *Fernelius*, and hath remain'd un-alter'd in all the *College Dispensatories*; but 'tis by many though a very indifferent Medicine, tho' greatly us'd, and much prescrib'd: for what can be expected from two or three Spoonfuls of a Syrup, when the Decoction, of which ℔ v. or thereabouts of Syrup is made, which is near an hundred times as much, may be taken at one Dose, or drank in the space of an Hour or two, to give but tolerable hopes of any Effect? Instead therefore of trifling with such a Medicine by Spoonfuls, where a *Diuretic* is wanted (for this is given only as such) as Decoction ought to be made with those of the Ingredients that are at all to the purpose, which the *Chiches* and *cool Seeds* are not; and large Draughts of it should be pour'd down, until they have manifestly made their way by the Increase of Urine, and Abatement of the Symptoms." (J. Quincy, *A Compleat English Dispensatory*, 1718, pp. 394–395)

DATE OF MANUFACTURE: 1674

PLACE OF MANUFACTURE: London

DIMENSIONS: Height 160 mm, maximum width 135 mm

PROVENANCE: Bought in 1957, Howard Collection. Previously T. Boynton collection, sold by C. Butters and Sons, Stoke-on-Trent, 23/3/1920 (lot 104).

CONDITION: Good; large chip off base, spout and neck rims chipped, glaze pitted.

COMMENT: Howard suggests that this is one of a set by the same artist with KAG9 (Cat. 73) and KAG10 (Cat. 75). There are seven jars from this set dated 1674, and an undated dry jar, in a private collection, painted by two different hands.

REFERENCES: Howard, English Delftware Drug Jars, No. 16.
Lipski and Archer, Dated English Delftware, No. 1635A.

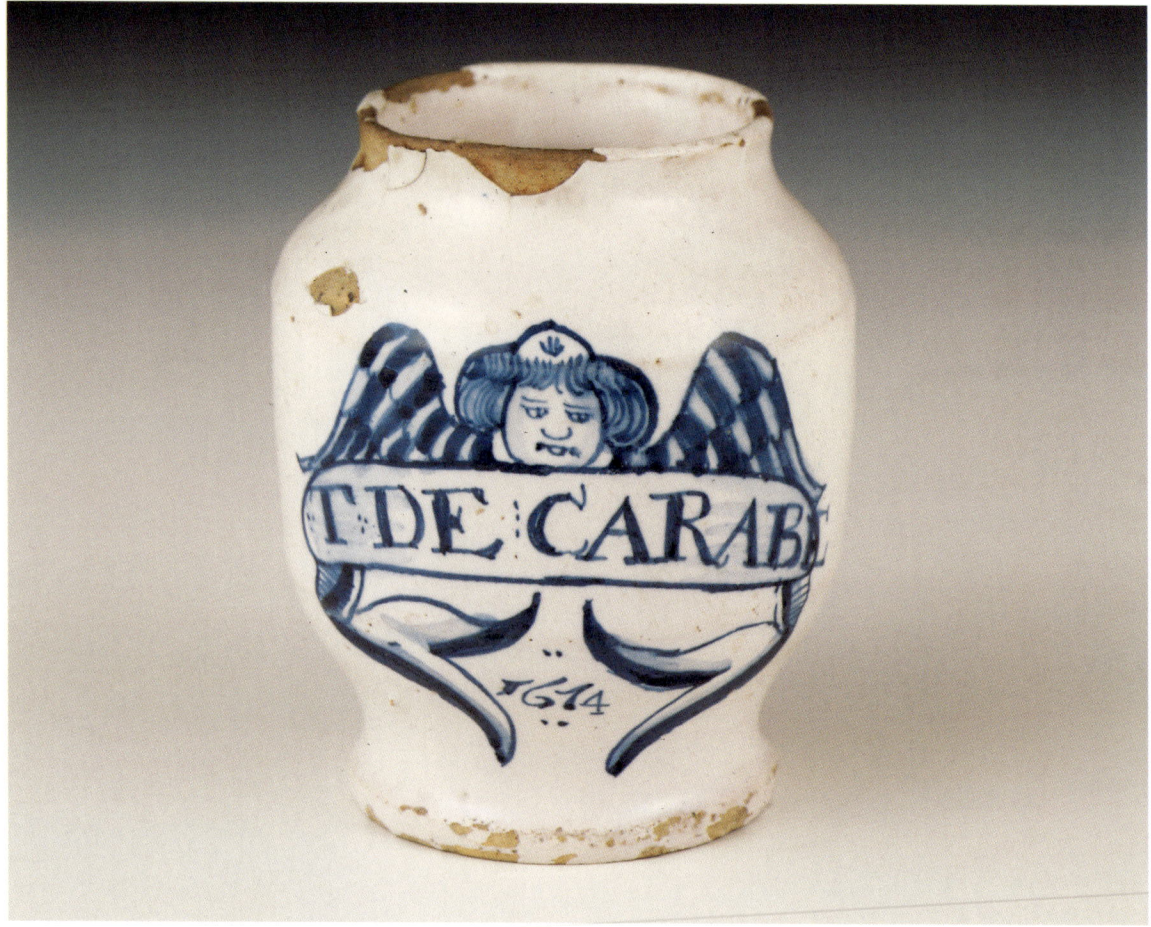

Dry drug jar (Cat.75)

ACCESSION NUMBER: KAG10

DESCRIPTION: Ovoid jar, tapering slightly towards splayed base, with two faint ridges encircling bowl, one below the neck the other below the label. White glaze with pinkish tinge and design in blue. Label panel curved slightly upwards with even outline. Neck slightly ridged with glazed rim, slightly concave unglazed base.

DESIGN: Angel with outspread wings.

INSCRIPTION: T DE:CARABE 1674

MEANING OF INSCRIPTION: *Trochisci de carabi*, lozenges of amber (which also contained red coral).

CONTEMPORARY ACCOUNT: "'Take of Amber ℥ i. of burnt Harts-horn, Gum-Arabic, Red Coral, Gum-Tragacanth, Acaia, Hypocistis, Balustines, Mastich, Gum-Lacca washed, and black Poppy-seeds, ana ℥ ii. ℈ ii. of Frankincense and Saffron, ana ℥ ii. of Opium ℥ i. and make them all into Troches with a sufficient quantity of the Mucilage of Fleawort-seeds made in Plaintain-Water.'

"This Composition is ascrib'd to *Mesue*, and seems design'd against Hemorrhages, and chiefly spitting of Blood." (J. Quincy, *A Compleat English Dispensatory*, 1718, p. 448)

DATE OF MANUFACTURE: 1674

PLACE OF MANUFACTURE: London

DIMENSIONS: Height 85 mm, maximum width 75 mm

PROVENANCE: Bought in 1957, Howard Collection.

CONDITION: Fair; glaze peeling from bowl and neck and flaked from base rim.

COMMENT: Howard suggests that this is one of a set by the same artist with KBG6 (Cat. 74) and KAG9 (Cat. 73). There are seven jars from this set dated 1674, and an undated dry jar, in a private collection, painted by two different hands. Note that the artist ran out of room in the cartouche to paint the final letter.

REFERENCES: Howard, English Delftware Drug Jars, p. 15 and No. 15.

Lipski and Archer, Dated English Delftware, No. 1634C.

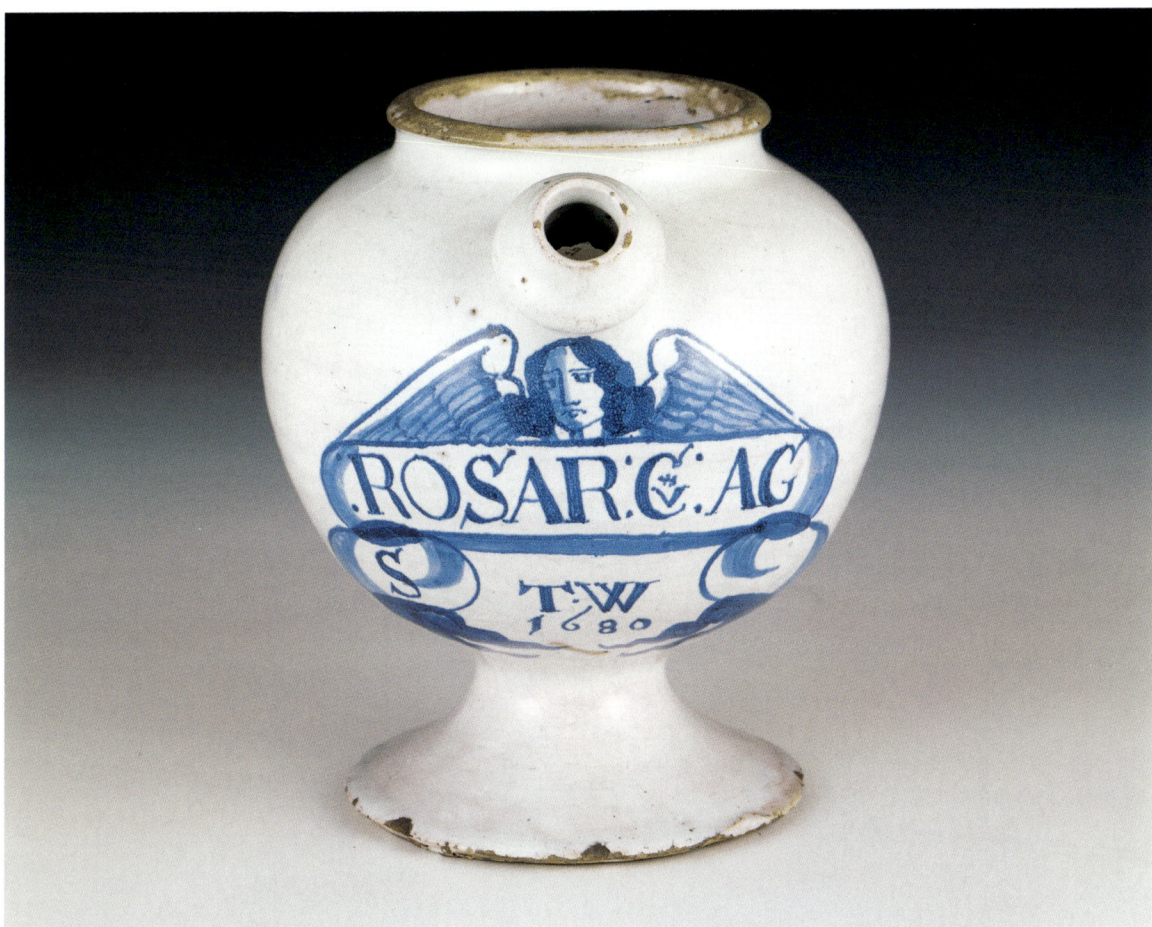

Wet drug jar (Cat.76)

ACCESSION NUMBER: KBG4

DESCRIPTION: Bulbous jar on spreading foot, with spout and fluted strap-like looped handle. White glaze with pinkish tinge and design in blue. Label panel straight, with even outline. Neck everted with unglazed rim, flanged spout, hollowed unglazed base.

DESIGN: Angel with outspread wings.

INSCRIPTION: S:ROSAR:C:AG T.W 1680

MEANING OF INSCRIPTION: *Syrupus rosarum cum agarico*, syrup of red roses with agaric. 'T.W' are the initials of the apothecary who commissioned the jar.

CONTEMPORARY ACCOUNT: "Take of Agarick cut thin an ounce, Ginger two drachms, Sal-Gem one drachm, Polypodium bruised two ounces, sprinkle them with white wine and steep them two daies over warm ashes, in a pound and a half of the infusion of Damask Roses prescribed before, and with one pound of sugar boyl it into a syrup according to Art....'

"It purgeth flegm from the head, relieves the sences oppressed by it, it provokes the terms in women, it purgeth the stomach and Liver, and provoketh urin. Some hold it an universal purge for all parts of the body" (Culpeper, *Pharmacopoeia Londoniensis or London Dispensatory*, 1653, p. 110)

DATE OF MANUFACTURE: 1680

PLACE OF MANUFACTURE: London

DIMENSIONS: Height 160 mm, maximum width 145 mm

PROVENANCE: Bought in 1957, Howard Collection.

CONDITION: Good; base chipped, glaze crazed.

COMMENT: Howard writes: "it is amusing to notice that the celestial coiffure continues to follow the fashions of the day by a progressive spread of the tresses." He states that this jar was decorated by the same artist as KCG9 (Cat. 100), KBG2 (Cat. 85), KBG8 (Cat. 81), KAG8 (Cat. 84), and KAG2 (Cat. 78) (pp. 15–16).

Six jars from this set are known: this jar, one in the Wilkinson Collection, one from the Blumbery Collection sold by Sotheby Parke Bernet in New York, 26/4/1973, one in the British Museum, one in the Manfield Collection, Central Museum and Art Gallery, Northampton, and one other (Lipski and Archer, Dated English Delftware, Nos. 1648, 1648A, 1648B, 1648C and 1648D).

Leslie Matthews attributed this jar to Thomas Warner, Master of the Society of Apothecaries, 1678.

REFERENCES: Howard, English Delftware Drug Jars, p. 15 and No. 24.
Lipski and Archer, Dated English Delftware, No. 1648D.

Angel with outspread wings

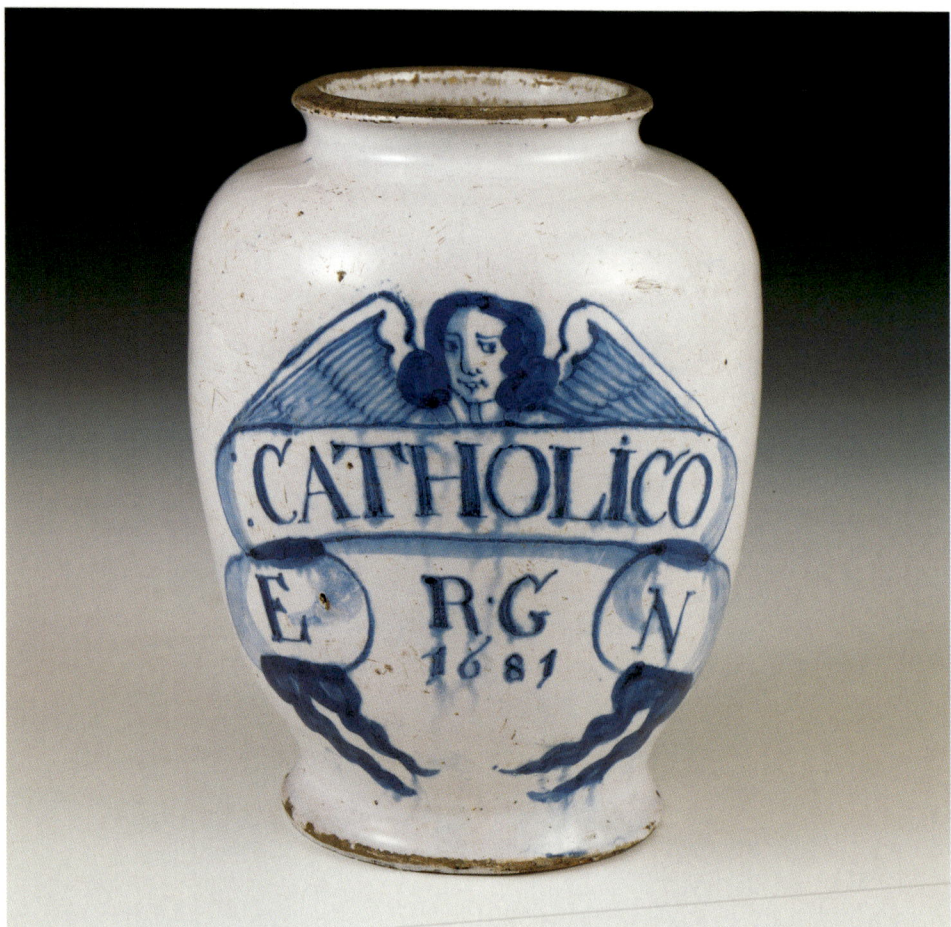

Dry drug jar (Cat.77)

ACCESSION NUMBER: KAG4
DESCRIPTION: Ovoid jar, tapering slightly towards splayed base. White glaze with pinkish tinge and design in blue. Label panel curved slightly upwards with even outline. Neck everted with unglazed rim, slightly concave unglazed base.
DESIGN: Angel with outspread wings.
INSCRIPTION: E : CATHOLICON R.G 1681
MEANING OF INSCRIPTION: *Electuarium diacatholicon*, a universal purging electuary. 'R.G' are the initials of the apothecary who commissioned the jar.
CONTEMPORARY ACCOUNT: "*From the College.* Catholicon. 'Take Polypody of the Oak ℥ iii. Sweet Fennel-Seeds ℥ vi. Boil in a sufficient quantity of Water to ℔ ii. to the strain'd Liquor put Sugar ℔ ii. and boil to the Consistence of a thick Syrup, to which add Sena in Powder ℥ ii. Violets, Polypody, Rhubarb, ana ℥ i. Aniseeds, Penydates, Sugar-Candy, Liquorice, and of the four greater cold Seeds, ana ℥ ii. Pulps of Cassia and Tamarinds, ana ℥ ii. and stir them all together.'

  "This is used as a gentle Lenitive, but wears much out of practice, and is now seldom order'd. Its Dose from ℥ ii. to ℥ i. The two Drams of cold Seeds, Sugar-Candy &c. make a very simple part of the Medicine, and are as well left out." (J. Quincy, *A Compleat English Dispensatory*, 1718, p. 402)
DATE OF MANUFACTURE: 1681
PLACE OF MANUFACTURE: London
DIMENSIONS: Height 170 mm, maximum width 140 mm
PROVENANCE: Bought in 1957, Howard Collection.
CONDITION: Good; glaze crazed and flaked on rim of base.
COMMENT: There is a second jar from this set in the Harris Museum, Preston.
REFERENCE: Lipski and Archer, Dated English Delftware, No. 1649A.

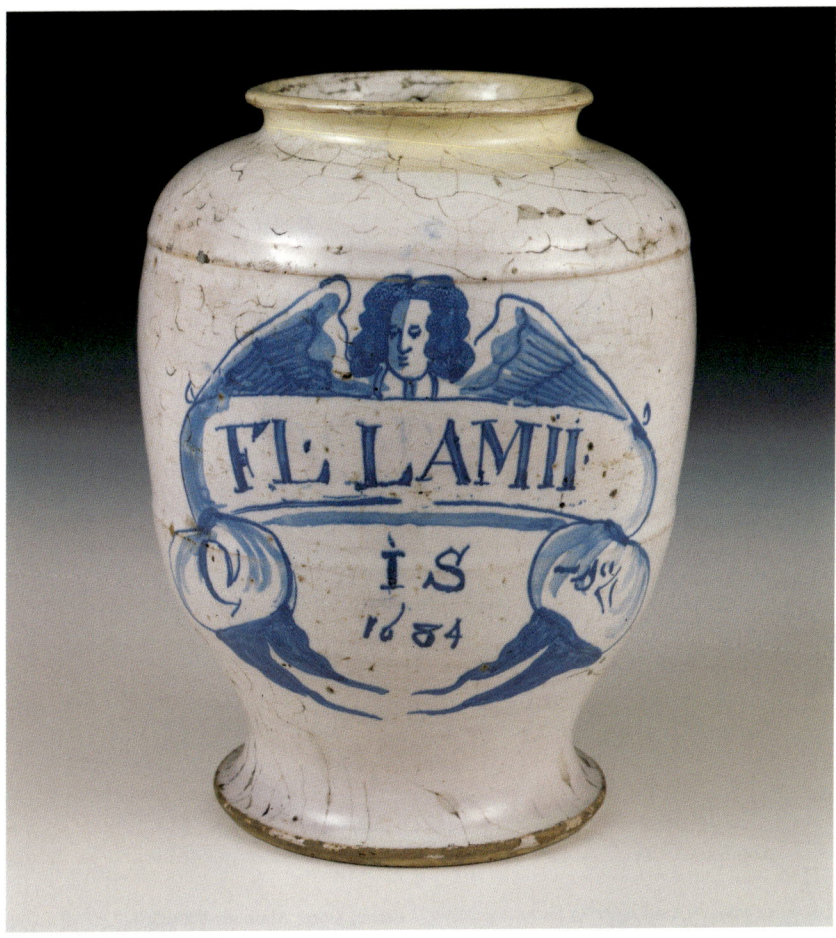

Dry drug jar (Cat.78)

ACCESSION NUMBER: KAG2
DESCRIPTION: Ovoid jar, tapering slightly towards splayed base, with two narrow ridges encircling bowl, one below the neck and the other above the base. White glaze with pinkish tinge. Glazed rim, slightly concave unglazed base.
DESIGN: Angel with outspread wings.
INSCRIPTION: C FL:LAMII IS 1684
MEANING OF INSCRIPTION: *Conserva de floribus lamii*, conserve of the flowers of deadnettle (*Lamium album*). 'IS' are the initials of the apothecary who commissioned the jar.
CONTEMPORARY ACCOUNT: "This Plant has been already mention'd... under the name of *Galeopsis*. But the Flowers, which blow about *June*, are chiefly in use. They are accounted not only soft and lubricating, but also strengthening, and are therefore given in some female Weaknesses, as the *Whites*, and in Heat and Difficulty of Urine. A Conserve is made of them in the Shops, but not often prescribed; and upon that account seldom to be met with fresh and good." (J. Quincy, *A Compleat English Dispensatory*, 1718, p. 113)

DATE OF MANUFACTURE: 1684
PLACE OF MANUFACTURE: London
DIMENSIONS: Height 185 mm, maximum width 150 mm
PROVENANCE: Bought in 1957, Howard Collection. Previously J. H.Taylor collection, sold at Sotheby's 11/11/1930 (lot 376).
CONDITION: Good; glaze crazed and flaked.
COMMENT: Howard states that this jar was decorated by the same artist as KCG9 (Cat. 100), KBG2 (Cat. 85), KBG8 (Cat. 81), KAG8 (Cat. 84), and KBG4 (Cat. 76) (pp. 15–16)
REFERENCES: Howard, English Delftware Drug Jars, p. 16 and No. 23.

Lipski and Archer, Dated English Delftware, No. 1652.

Angel with outspread wings

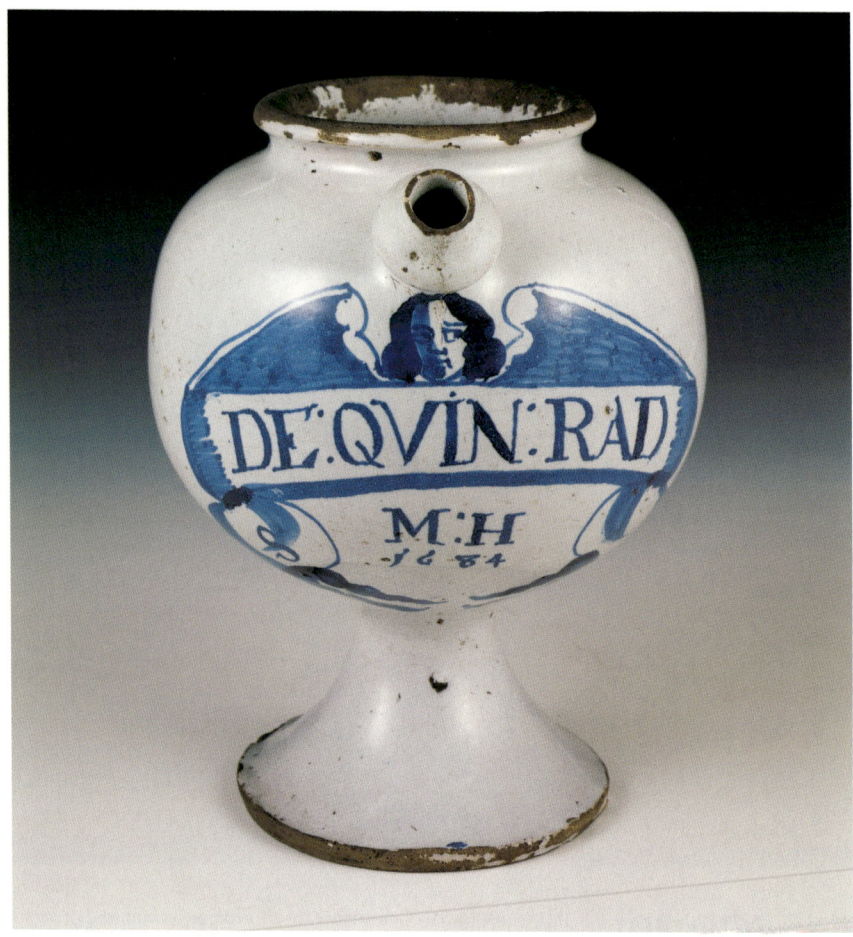

Wet drug jar (Cat.81)

ACCESSION NUMBER: KBG8

DESCRIPTION: Bulbous jar on spreading foot, with spout and fluted strap-like looped handle. White glaze with pinkish tinge and design in blue. Label panel curved slightly upwards with even outline. Neck everted with unglazed rim, flanged spout, hollowed unglazed base.

DESIGN: Angel with outspread wings.

INSCRIPTION: S DE:QVIN:RAD M:H 1684

MEANING OF INSCRIPTION: *Syrupus de quinque radicibus*, syrup of five roots. The ingredients were the roots of smallage, asparagus, parsley, fennel and dyer's or butcher's broom. 'M:H' are the initials of Michael Hastings of Dublin, the apothecary who commissioned the jar.

CONTEMPORARY ACCOUNT: "This is used pretty frequently as a *Diuretick*, and also to promote Expectoration; and had the Ounces of Roots been so many Pounds, there would have been some Chance of Efficacy from it: but as it is, there is very little, unless from the *Vinegar*, which assists it as an Expectorant, and gives it so grateful a Tartness, as makes it a good Ingredient in some extemporaneous Forms; as *Linctus's, Eclegma's* &c." (J. Quincy, *A Compleat English Dispensatory*, 1718, p. 379)

DATE OF MANUFACTURE: 1684

PLACE OF MANUFACTURE: London

DIMENSIONS: Height 200 mm, maximum width 168 mm

PROVENANCE: Bought in 1957, Howard Collection.

CONDITION: Good; glaze crazed and flaked on body and handle and rims of neck, spout and base.

COMMENT: Michael Hastings, the apothecary who is believed to have commissioned this jar as part of a set (at least 15 of which survive), was the founder of the business at 49 Dawson Street, Dublin, in 1684, the year on the jar. Some of the jars remained in the business into the 20th century.

Howard states that this jar was decorated by the same artist as KCG9 (Cat. 100), KBG2 (Cat. 85), KBG4 (Cat. 76), KAG8 (Cat. 84), and KAG2 (Cat. 78) (pp. 15–16).

REFERENCES: Howard, English Delftware Drug Jars, p. 14 and No. 21.

Lipski and Archer, Dated English Delftware, No. 1655C.

'Old Irish Pharmacies', Chemist and Druggist, Vol. 53, July 30 1898, p. 201.

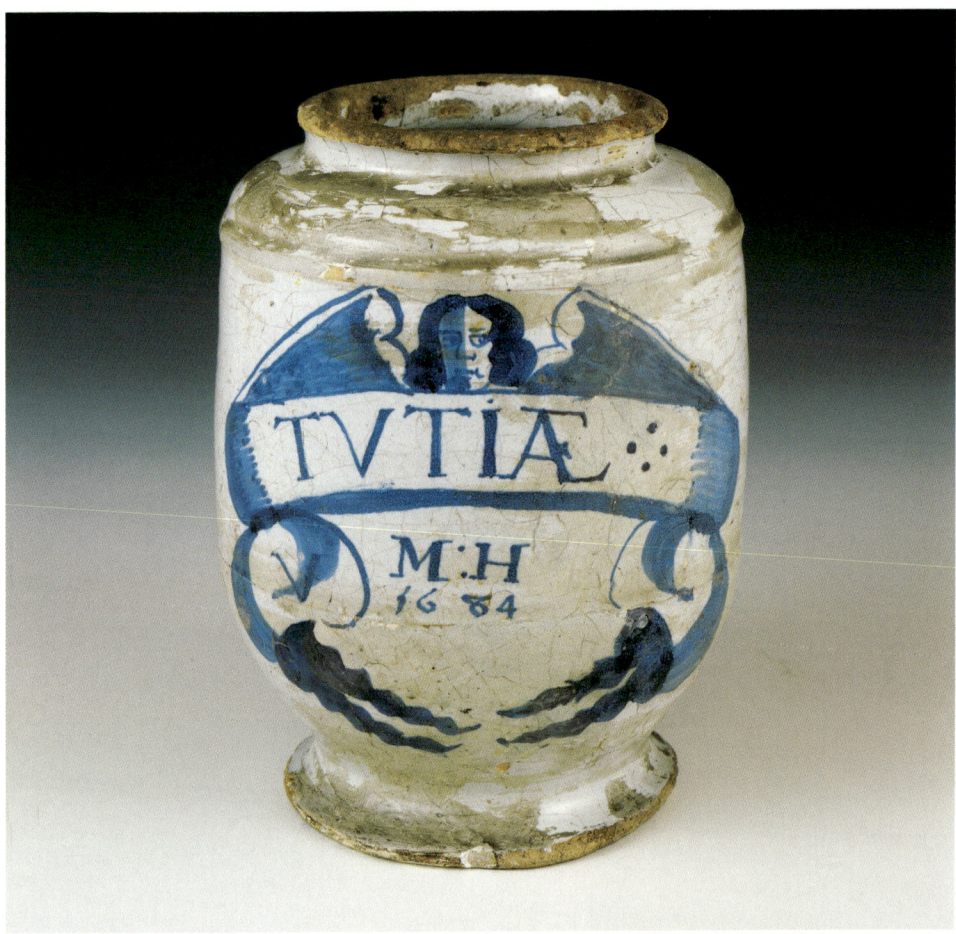

Dry drug jar (Cat.82)

ACCESSION NUMBER: KAG12

DESCRIPTION: Ovoid jar with splayed base and two narrow ridges encircling bowl, one below the neck and the other below the label. White glaze with bluish tinge and design in blue. Label panel curved slightly upwards with even outline. Neck everted with unglazed rim; flat unglazed base.

DESIGN: Angel with outspread wings.

INSCRIPTION: V TVTIAE M:H 1684

MEANING OF INSCRIPTION: *Unguentum tutiae*, ointment of tutty. Tutiae, impure zinc oxide, is a Latinisation of an unknown word of Sanskrit origin. It is an emollient used in unguents or collyria. 'M:H' are the initials of Michael Hastings of Dublin, the apothecary who commissioned the jar.

CONTEMPORARY ACCOUNT: "Take of prepared Tutty, ℥ ii. of Calamine burnt and quenched two or three times in Plaintain Water ℥ i. Let them be reduced to a very fine Powder, and mixed with ℔ iss. of the *Unguentum Rosaceum*, so as to make them into an Ointment....this is not very often referred to in Prescription, but it is in great esteem amongst the common

People." (J. Quincy, *A Compleat English Dispensatory*, 1718, p. 506)

DATE OF MANUFACTURE: 1684

PLACE OF MANUFACTURE: London

DIMENSIONS: Height 190 mm, maximum width 155 mm

PROVENANCE: Bought in 1957, Howard Collection.

CONDITION: Poor; has been restored, glaze badly crazed and flaked from bowl and neck and base rims.

COMMENT: Michael Hastings, the apothecary who is believed to have commissioned this jar as part of a set (of which at least 15 survive), was the founder of the business at 49 Dawson Street, Dublin, in 1684, the year on the jar. Some of the jars remained in the business into the 20th century.

REFERENCES: Howard, English Delftware Drug Jars, referred to in Plate VII, but not illustrated.

Lipski and Archer, Dated English Delftware, No. 1655I.

'Old Irish Pharmacies', Chemist and Druggist, Vol. 53, July 30 1898, p. 201.

Angel with outspread wings

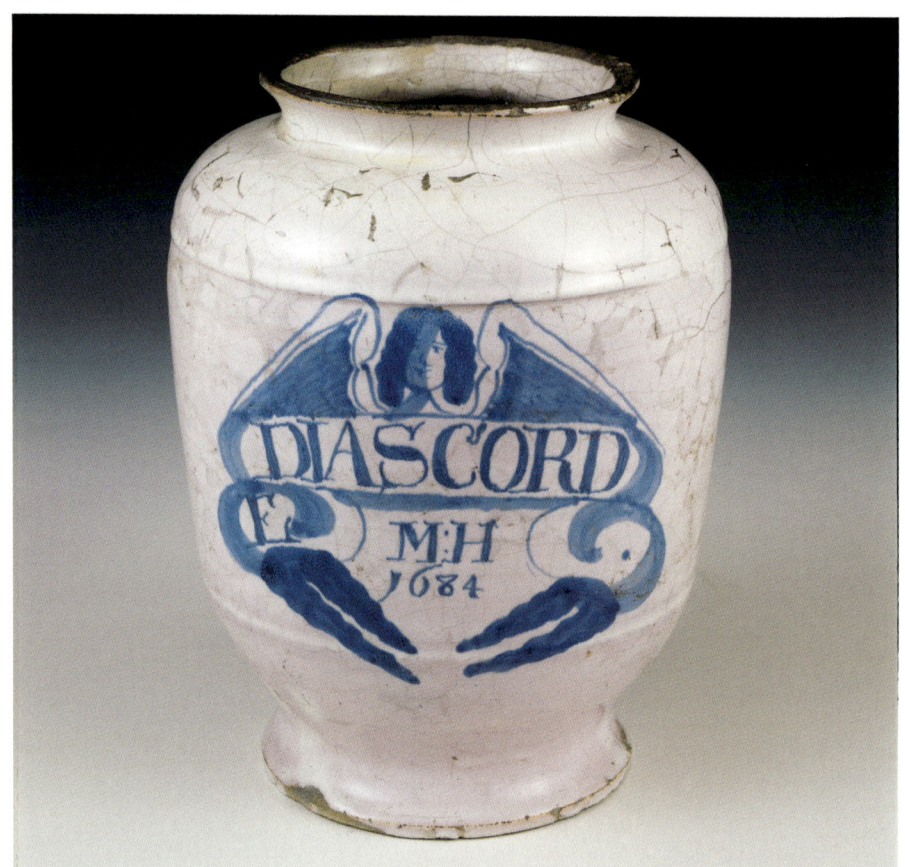

Dry drug jar (Cat.83)

ACCESSION NUMBER: KAG1
DESCRIPTION: Ovoid jar, tapering slightly towards splayed base, with two narrow ridges encircling bowl, one below the neck and the other above the base. White glaze with pinkish tinge and design in blue. Label panel curved slightly upwards with even outline. Neck everted with unglazed rim, slightly concave base.
DESIGN: Angel with outspread wings.
INSCRIPTION: E DIASCORD M:H 1684
MEANING OF INSCRIPTION: *Electuarium diascordium*, diascordium electuary. 'M:H' are the initials of Michael Hastings of Dublin, the apothecary who commissioned the jar. The medicine is traced back to Frascatorius in the 1500s, as a remedy of great importance, chiefly used for the plague.
CONTEMPORARY ACCOUNT: "Take of Cinnamon, and Cassia Wood, ana ℥ ss. of true Scordium ℥ i. of *Cretan* Dittany, Tormentil, Bistort, Galbanum, and Gum Arabic, ana ℥ iss. of Storax ℥ ivss. of Opium and Seeds of Sorrel, ana ℥ iss. of Gentian ℥ ss. of *Armenian* Bole ℥ iss. of *Lemnian* Sealed Earth ℥ ss. of long Pepper and Ginger, ana ℥ ii. of clarif'd Honey ℔ iiss. of Sugar of Roses ℔ i. of generous Canary ℥ viii. Take it into an Electuary, S.A...."
"Everyone knows how much this is of use, and for what purposes, and indeed if the several Ingredients be nicely selected, and the Medicine fresh made, it is excellent in all Fluxes whatsoever, and a great Strengthener both of the Stomach and Bowels. In its influence on the Fluxes, the Opium has no small share, as may be well conceiv'd from the Virtues of that Drug... A very mischievous way some Nurses have got, of giving their Children this Medicine to make them sleep, more for their own Ease than any thing else..." (J. Quincy, *A Compleat English Dispensatory*, 1718, p. 429)
DATE OF MANUFACTURE: 1684
PLACE OF MANUFACTURE: London
DIMENSIONS: Height 190 mm, maximum width 165 mm
PROVENANCE: Bought in 1957, Howard Collection.
CONDITION: Fair; has been restored, glaze crazed.
COMMENT: Michael Hastings, the apothecary who is believed to have commissioned this jar as part of a set (of which at least 15 have survived), was the founder of the business at 49 Dawson Street, Dublin, in 1684, the year on the jar. Some of the jars remained in the business into the 20th century.
REFERENCES: Howard, English Delftware Drug Jars, p. 16, referred to in Plate VII, but not illustrated.
Lipski and Archer, Dated English Delftware, No. 1655G.
'Old Irish Pharmacies', Chemist and Druggist, Vol. 53, July 30 1898, p. 201.

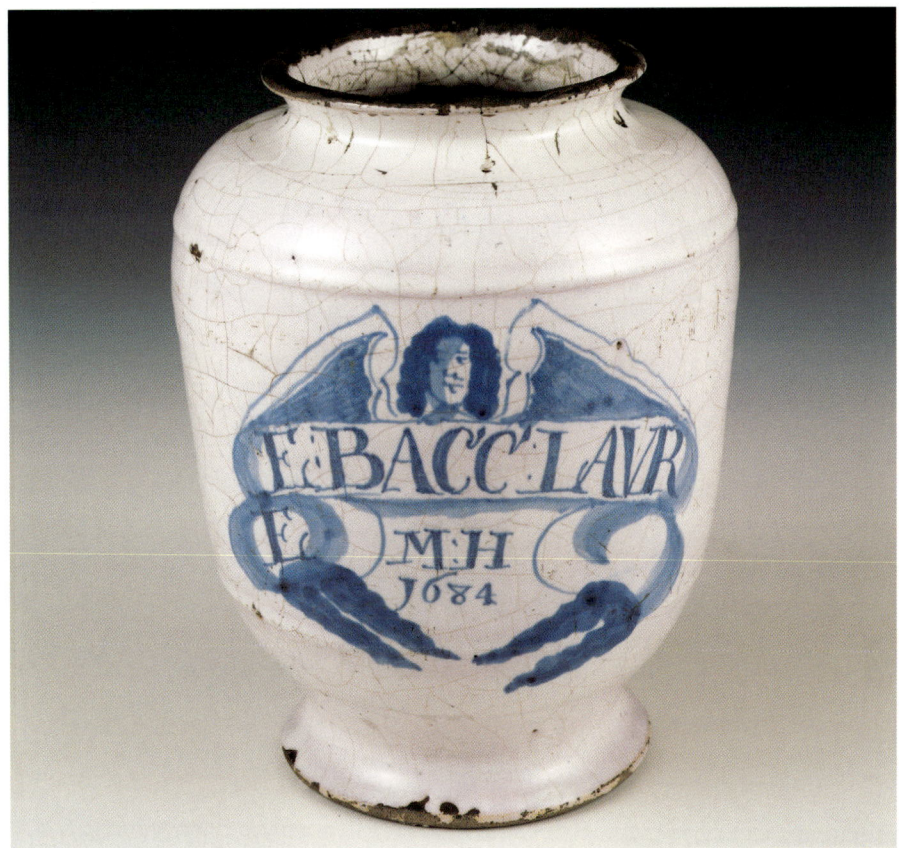

Dry drug jar (Cat.84)

ACCESSION NUMBER: KAG8

DESCRIPTION: Ovoid jar, tapering slightly towards splayed base, with two narrow ridges encircling bowl, one below the neck and the other below the label. White glaze with pinkish tinge and design in blue. Label panel curved slightly upwards with even outline. Neck everted with unglazed rim, slightly concave unglazed base.

DESIGN: Angel with outspread wings.

INSCRIPTION: E E:BACC:LAVR M:H 1684

MEANING OF INSCRIPTION: *Emplastrum e baccis lauri*, plaster of bay berries (*Laurus nobilis*). 'M:H' are the initials of Michael Hastings of Dublin, the apothecary who commissioned the jar.

CONTEMPORARY ACCOUNT: "*Colledg.* Take of Bay-berries husked, Turpentine of each two ounces; Frankincense, Mastich, Mirrh, of each an ounce; Cyperus, Costus, of each half an ounce; Honey warmed and * not scummed [*and why not scummed? I had forgot, the Colledg is not bound to give a reason for what they do] four ounces; make it into a plaister according to Art."

"It is an excellent plaister to ease any pains coming of cold of wind, in any part of the body, whether Stomach, Liver, Belly, Reins or Bladder." (Culpeper, *The Physicians Library*, 1667, p. 237)

DATE OF MANUFACTURE: 1684

PLACE OF MANUFACTURE: London

DIMENSIONS: Height 190 mm, maximum width 160 mm

PROVENANCE: Bought in 1957, Howard Collection

CONDITION: Good; glaze crazed and flaked from body and neck and base rims.

COMMENT: Michael Hastings, the apothecary who is believed to have commissioned this jar as part of a set (of which at least 15 survive), was the founder of the business at 49 Dawson Street, Dublin, in 1684, the year on the jar. Some of the jars remained in the business into the 20th century.

Howard states that this jar was decorated by the same artist as KCG9 (Cat. 100), KBG2 (Cat. 85), KBG8 (Cat. 81), KBG4 (Cat. 76), and KAG2 (Cat. 78) (pp. 15–16).

REFERENCES: Howard, English Delftware Drug Jars, p. 16 and No. 22.

Lipski and Archer, Dated English Delftware, No. 1655J.

'Old Irish Pharmacies', Chemist and Druggist, Vol. 53, July 30 1898, p. 201.

Angel with outspread wings

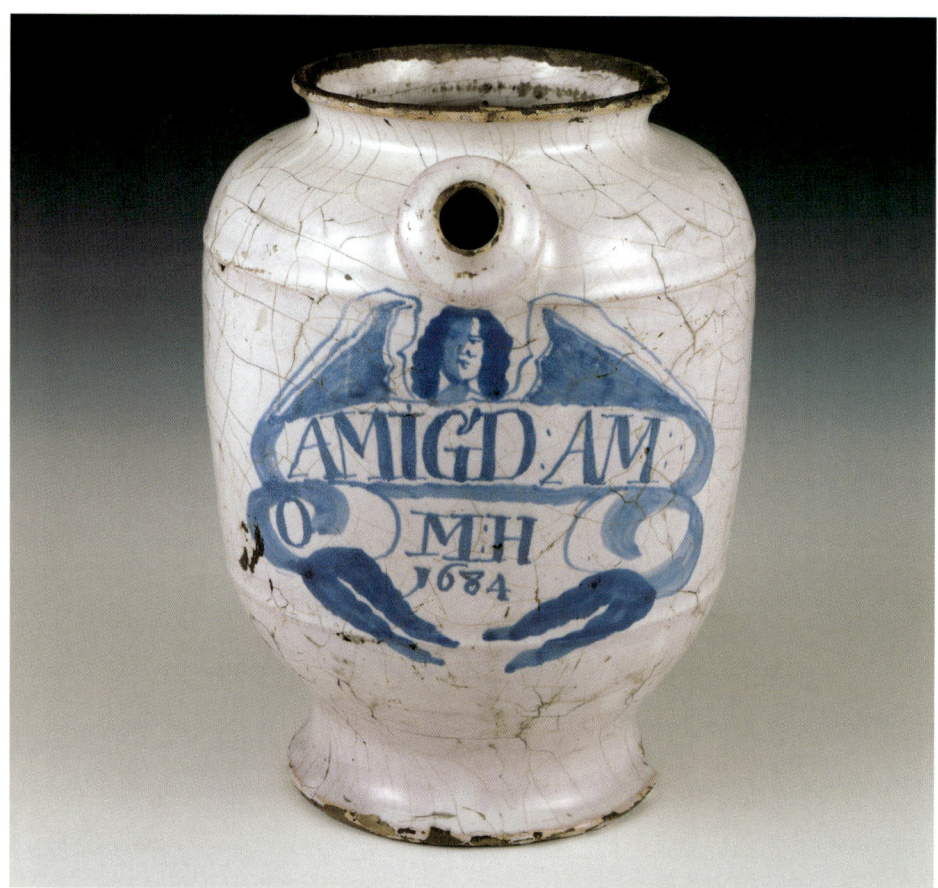

Wet drug jar (Cat.85)

ACCESSION NUMBER: KBG2

DESCRIPTION: Ovoid jar, tapering slightly towards base, with two narrow ridges encircling bowl, one below the neck and the other above the foot, and with spout and (broken) strap-like handle. White glaze with pinkish tinge and design in blue. Label panel curved slightly upwards with even outline. Neck everted with unglazed rim, spout with wide flange, slightly concave unglazed base.

DESIGN: Angel with outspread wings.

INSCRIPTION: O AMIGD:AM: M:H 1684

MEANING OF INSCRIPTION: *Oleum amigdala amara*, oil of bitter almonds (*Prunus amygdalus amara*). 'M:H' are the initials of Michael Hastings of Dublin, the apothecary who commissioned the jar.

CONTEMPORARY ACCOUNT: "These are *aperient*, *detersive*, and *diuretick*; and therefore commended in Obstructions of the *Liver, Spleen, Mesentery,* and *Womb*. They are by some said to take off the Effects of Drunkenness, and also to expel Wind... Their expressed *Oil* is now much in use to soften and deterge the *Wax* out of the *Ears*; and they are of very little account in the present Practice for any thing else..." (J. Quincy, *A Compleat English Dispensatory*, 1718, p. 133)

DATE OF MANUFACTURE: 1684

PLACE OF MANUFACTURE: London

DIMENSIONS: Height 198 mm, maximum width 158 mm

PROVENANCE: Bought in 1957, Howard Collection.

CONDITION: Fair; glaze crazed, base chipped, fragments of broken handle remaining.

COMMENT: Michael Hastings, the apothecary who is believed to have commissioned this jar as part of a set (of which at least 15 survive), was the founder of the business at 49 Dawson Street, Dublin, in 1684, the year on the jar. Some of the jars remained in the business into the 20th century.

Howard states that this jar was decorated by the same artist as KCG9 (Cat. 100), KBG4 (Cat. 76), KBG8 (Cat. 81), KAG8 (Cat. 84), and KAG2 (Cat. 78) (pp. 15–16).

REFERENCES: Howard, English Delftware Drug Jars, p. 16 and No. 20.

Lipski and Archer, Dated English Delftware, No. 1655L.

'Old Irish Pharmacies', Chemist and Druggist, Vol. 53, July 30 1898, p. 201.

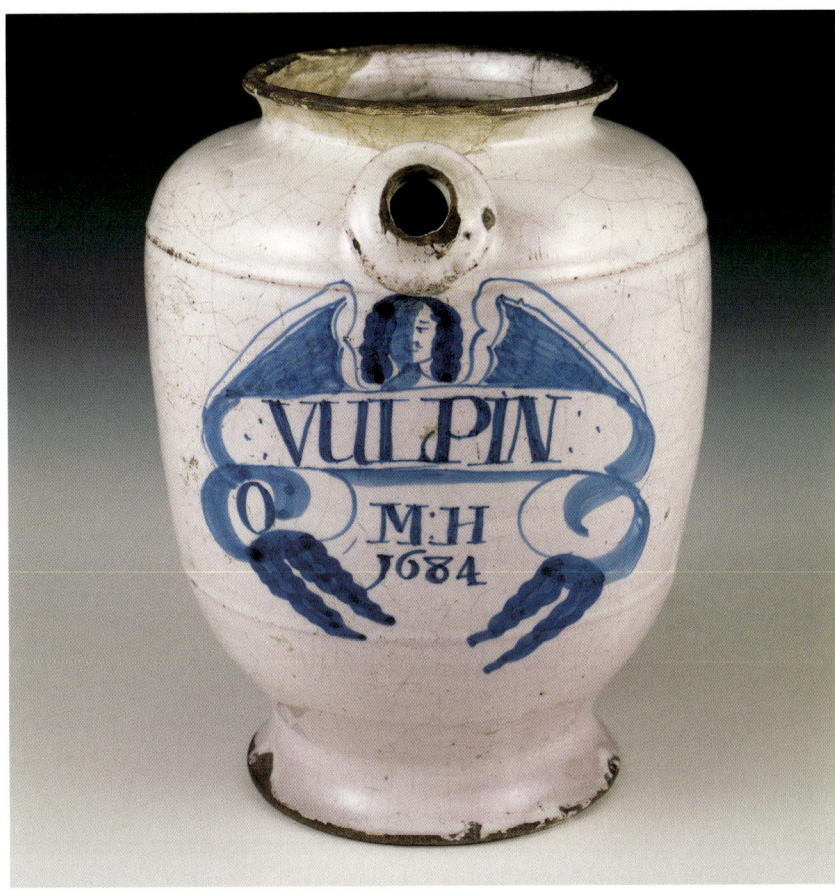

Angel with outspread wings

Wet drug jar (Cat.86)

ACCESSION NUMBER: KBG1

DESCRIPTION: Ovoid jar, tapering slightly towards base, with two narrow ridges encircling bowl, one below the neck and the other above the foot, and with spout and (broken) strap-like handle. White glaze with pinkish tinge and design in blue. Label panel curved slightly upwards with even outline. Neck everted with unglazed rim, spout with wide flange, slightly concave unglazed base.

DESIGN: Angel with outspread wings.

INSCRIPTION: O VULPIN: M:H 1684

MEANING OF INSCRIPTION: *Oleum vulpinum*, oil of fox. 'M:H' are the initials of Michael Hastings of Dublin, the apothecary who commissioned the jar.

CONTEMPORARY ACCOUNT: "*Colledg. Take a fat Fox, of a middle age, *(if you can get such an one)* [*that was wel put in, therefore when you have caught a Fox, bring him alive to the Colledg, and let them look in his mouth first, and tell you how old he is, so shall your Oil be* cum privilegio] *caught by hunting about Autumn, cut in pieces, the skin and bowels taken away, the bones broken, boyl him (scumming it diligently) in white wine and spring water, of each six pound, till half be consumed: with three ounces of Sea salt, the tops of Dill, Time and Chamepitys, of each one handful;*

after straining boil it again with four pound of the best old Oil, the flowers of Sage and Rosemary, of each one handful; the water being consumed, strain it again, and keep the pure Oil for use."

"It is exceeding good in pains of the joynts, Gouts, pains in the Back and Reins; it heats the body being afflicted by cold, and hard lodging in the Aire, whereby the joynts are stiff, a disease incident to many in these times." (Culpeper, *The Physicians Library*, 1667, p. 220)

DATE OF MANUFACTURE: 1684

PLACE OF MANUFACTURE: London

DIMENSIONS: Height 198 mm, maximum width 165 mm

PROVENANCE: Bought in 1957, Howard Collection.

CONDITION: Fair; glaze crazed with glaze missing below handle, base and spout rim chipped, fragments of broken handle remaining.

COMMENT: Michael Hastings, the apothecary who is believed to have commissioned this jar as part of a set (of which at least 15 survive), was the founder of the business at 49 Dawson Street, Dublin, in 1684, the year on the jar. Some of the jars remained in the business into the 20th century.

REFERENCES: Howard, English Delftware Drug Jars, referred to in Plate VII, but not illustrated.

Lipski and Archer, Dated English Delftware, No. 1655K.

'Old Irish Pharmacies', Chemist and Druggist, Vol. 53, July 30 1898, p. 201.

Angel with outspread wings

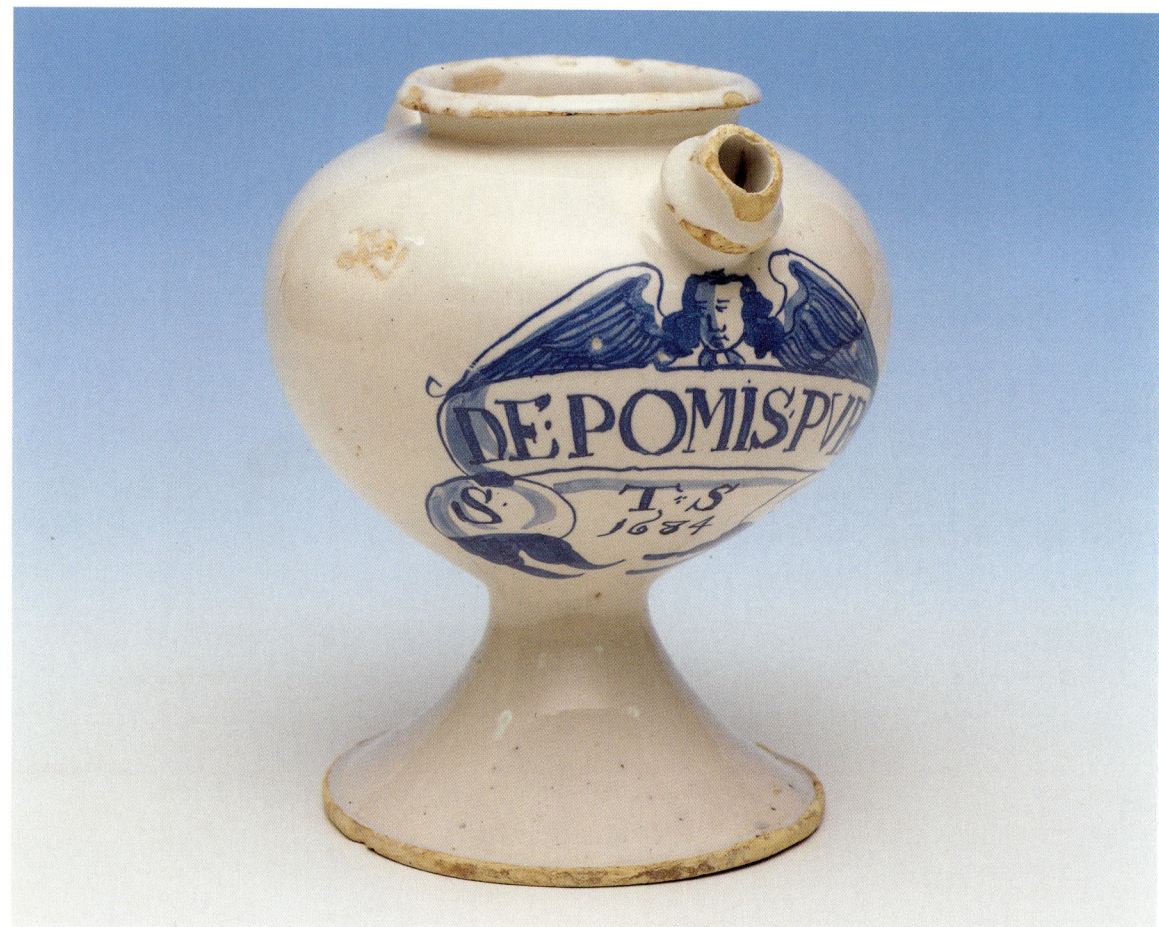

Wet drug jar (Cat.87)

ACCESSION NUMBER: KBG11

DESCRIPTION: Bulbous jar on spreading foot, with spout and fluted strap-like looped handle. White glaze with pinkish tinge and design in blue. Label panel curved slightly upwards with even outline. Neck everted with glazed rim, flanged spout, hollowed unglazed base.

DESIGN: Angel with outspread wings.

INSCRIPTION: S DE POMIS PVRG T S 1684

MEANING OF INSCRIPTION: *Syrupus de pomis purgans*, purging syrup of apples. 'T S' are the initials of the apothecary who commissioned the jar.

CONTEMPORARY ACCOUNT: "*Colledg* Take of the juyce of sweet smelling Apples two pound, the juyce of Borrage and Bugloss, of each one pound and a half; Senna 2 ounces, Aniseeds half an ounce, Saffron one dram. Let the Senna be steeped in the Juyces twenty four hours, and after a warm or two strain it, and with two pound of white Sugar boil it to a Syrup according to art, the Saffron being tied up in a rag, and often crushed in the boiling."

Culpeper: "The syrup is a pretty cooling Purge, and tends to rectifie the distempers of the blood, it purgeth Choler and Melancholy, and therefore must needs be effectual both in yellow and black Jaundice, Madness, Scurf, Leprosie and Scabs. It is very gentle, and for that I commend both the Receipt, and *Mesue* the Author of it. The dose is from one ounce to three, according as the body is in age and strength. An ounce of it in the morning is excellent for such Children as break out in scabs." (Culpeper, *The Physicians Library*, 1667, p. 128)

DATE OF MANUFACTURE: 1684

PLACE OF MANUFACTURE: London

DIMENSIONS: Height 175 mm, maximum width 160 mm

PROVENANCE: Bought in 1957, Howard Collection.

CONDITION: Good; neck chipped, glaze flaked on bowl (three patches to right of label) on handle and neck.

COMMENT: There is an oil jar from this set in the Wilkinson Collection, Thackray Museum, Leeds.

REFERENCES: Howard, English Delftware Drug Jars, No. 25.
   Lipski and Archer, Dated English Delftware, No. 1654A.

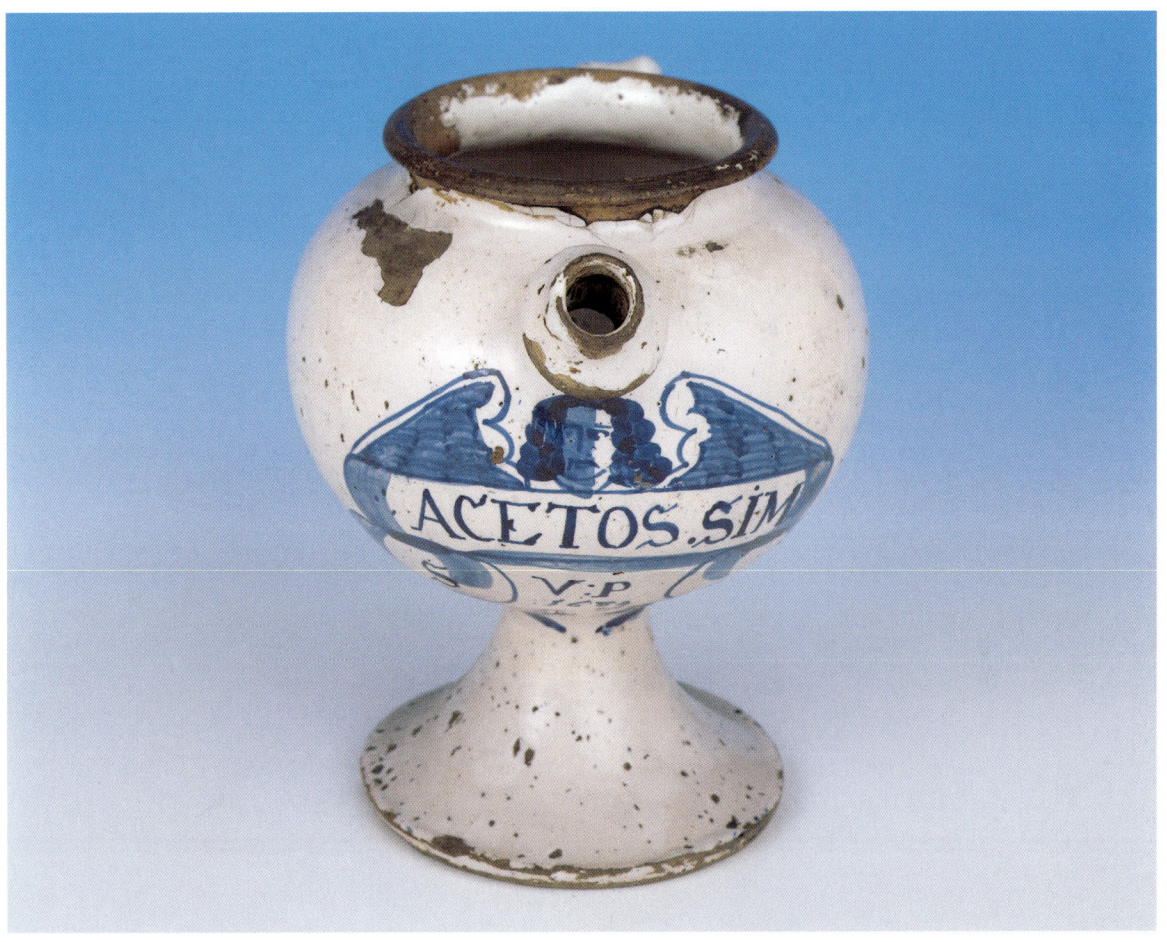

Wet drug jar (Cat.88)

ACCESSION NUMBER: KBG13

DESCRIPTION: Bulbous jar on spreading foot with spout and fluted strap-like looped handle. White glaze with pinkish tinge and design in blue. Label panel straight with even outline. Neck everted with unglazed rim, flanged spout, hollowed and glazed base with unglazed edge.

DESIGN: Angel with outspread wings.

INSCRIPTION: S ACETOS.SIM V:P 1684

MEANING OF INSCRIPTION: *Syrupus acetosus simplex* or *simplicior*, syrup of vinegar simple or mere simple. 'V:P' are the initials of the apothecary who commissioned the jar.

CONTEMPORARY ACCOUNT: "Of these two Syrups let every one use which he finds by Experience to be best, the difference is but little. I hold the last [*Syrupus acetos simplicior*] to be the best of the two, and would give my reasons for it, but I fear the book wil swel too big. They both of them cut flegm, as also tough, hard, viscous humors in the Stomach: they cool the body, quench thirst, provoke urin, and prepare the stomach before the taking of a Vomit. If you take it as a Preparative for a Vomit, take half an ounce of it when you go to bed, the night before you intend to vomit, it wil make you to vomit the earlier: but if for any of the foregoing occasions, take it with a Liquoris stick." (Culpeper, *The Physicians Library*, 1667, pp. 112–113)

DATE OF MANUFACTURE: 1684

PLACE OF MANUFACTURE: Lambeth, London

DIMENSIONS: Height 165 mm, maximum width 150 mm

PROVENANCE: Bought in 1957, Howard Collection.

CONDITION: Poor; glaze badly pitted and flaked from body, handle, spout and neck and base rims.

COMMENT: There are six surviving jars from this set, almost certainly painted by the same hand as the syrup jars in the Michael Hastings 1684 set. The six jars are this jar, KBG14 (Cat. 89), three jars in the Wilkinson Collection, Thackray Museum, Leeds, and one jar recorded by Garner as "in a private collection in Norwich before the Second World War".

REFERENCE: Lipski and Archer, Dated English Delftware, No. 1653A.

Angel with outspread wings

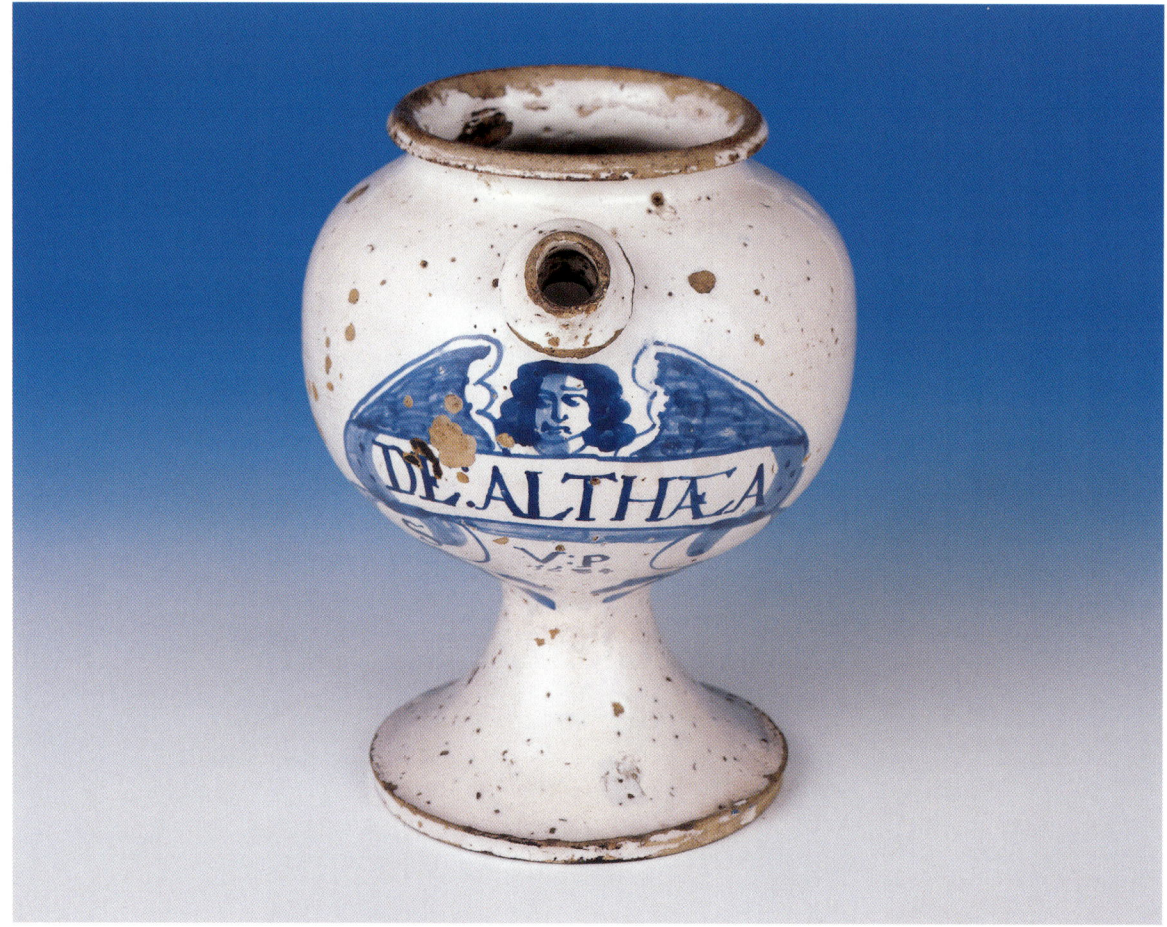

Wet drug jar (Cat.89)

ACCESSION NUMBER: KBG14

DESCRIPTION: Bulbous jar on spreading foot, with spout and fluted strap-like looped handle. White glaze with pinkish tinge and design in blue. Label panel straight with even outline. Neck everted with unglazed rim, flanged spout, hollowed glazed base.

DESIGN: Angel with outspread wings.

INSCRIPTION: S DE:ALTHAEA V:P 1684

MEANING OF INSCRIPTION: *Syrupus de althaea*, syrup of marshmallow (*Althaea officinalis*). 'V.P' are the initials of the apothecary who commissioned the jar.

CONTEMPORARY ACCOUNT: "'Take Marsh-Mallow Roots ℥ ii. of Grass, Asparagus, Liquorise, Roots and Raisins ston'd, ana ℥ ss. Leaves of Marsh-Mallows, common Mallows, Pellitory of the Wall, Pimpernel, Saxifrage, Plantain, white and black Maidenhair, ana m.i. red Chiches ℥ i. The four greater and lesser cold Seeds, ana ℥ iii. Boil them in a Sufficient quantity of Water, strain the Liquor out hard and boil it up when clarify'd into a Syrup, with ℔ iiiss. of white Sugar.'

"This Syrup is originally ascrib'd to *Fernelius*, and hath remain'd un-alter'd in all the *College Dispensatories*; but 'tis by many though a very indifferent Medicine, tho' greatly us'd, and much prescrib'd." (J. Quincy, *A Compleat English Dispensatory*, 1718, pp. 394–395)

DATE OF MANUFACTURE: 1684

PLACE OF MANUFACTURE: Lambeth, London

DIMENSIONS: Height 170 mm, maximum width 150 mm

PROVENANCE: Bought in 1957, Howard Collection.

CONDITION: Fair; badly pitted, glaze flaked on body, handle and spout and on neck and base rims.

COMMENT: There are six surviving jars from this set, almost certainly painted by the same hand as the syrup jars in the Michael Hastings 1684 set. The six jars are this jar, KBG13 (Cat. 88), three jars in the Wilkinson Collection, Thackray Museum, Leeds, and one jar recorded by Garner as "in a private collection in Norwich before the Second World War".

REFERENCE: Lipski and Archer, Dated English Delftware, No. 1653B.

Angel with outspread wings

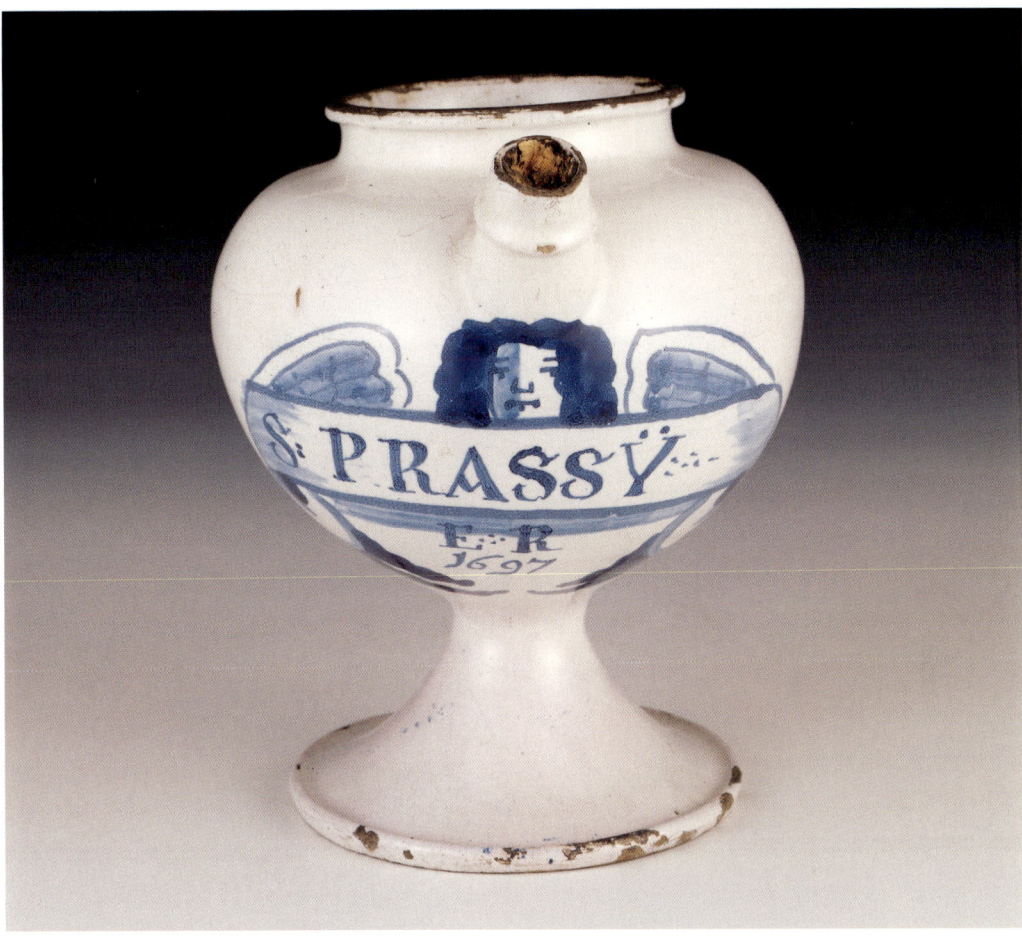

Wet drug jar (Cat.90)

ACCESSION NUMBER: KBG7

DESCRIPTION: Bulbous jar on spreading foot, with spout and fluted strap-like looped handle. White glaze with pinkish tinge and design in blue. Label panel straight with even outline. Neck everted with unglazed rim, flanged spout, hollowed and ridged base, glazed. Cork remnant remains in jar's spout.

DESIGN: Angel with outspread wings.

INSCRIPTION: S:PRASSY E:R 1697

MEANING OF INSCRIPTION: *Syrupus de prassio*, syrup of horehound (*Marrubium vulgare*). 'E:R' are the initials of the apothecary who commissioned the jar.

CONTEMPORARY ACCOUNT: "It flowers in *July*. This is reckcon'd a very great *Pectoral* and *Vulnerary*. It is also call'd *Prassium*, under which Name there is a *Syrup* made of it in the Shops. *Diascorides* advis'd its Juice to be boil'd up into a *Syrup* with *Honey*, and given in Asthma's and Consumptive *Coughs*. It is by some esteem'd good against Spitting of Blood. The most convenient Form to give it in, is in *Decoction*, which ought to be made very strong." (J. Quincy, *A Compleat English Dispensatory*,

1718, p. 124)

DATE OF MANUFACTURE: 1697

PLACE OF MANUFACTURE: London

COMMENT: Howard suggests that this jar is part of a set, with KAG3 (Cat. 91). There seem to be five jars in a set dated 1697, with the initials 'E.R', two wet and three dry, and all in the same style.

DIMENSIONS: Height 180 mm, maximum width 150 mm

PROVENANCE: Bought in 1957, Howard Collection.

CONDITION: Good; glaze crazed and flaked from handle and neck and base rims.

REFERENCES: Howard, English Delftware Drug Jars, pp. 16–17 and No. 29.

Lipski and Archer, Dated English Delftware, No. 1661C.

Angel with outspread wings

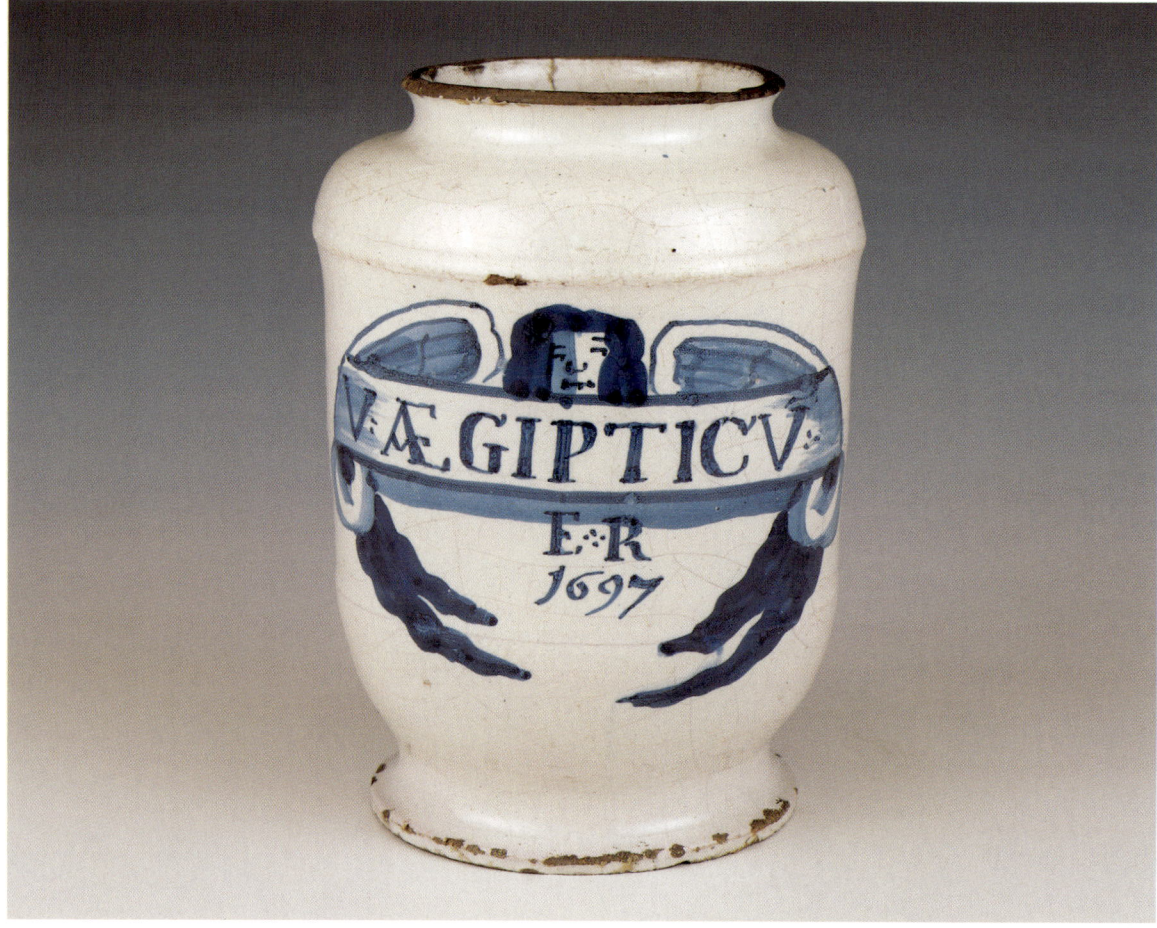

Dry drug jar (Cat.91)

ACCESSION NUMBER: KAG3
DESCRIPTION: Ovoid jar, tapering slightly towards splayed base, with two narrow ridges encircling bowl, one below the neck and the other above the base. White glaze with pinkish tinge. Unglazed rim and unglazed flat base.
DESIGN: Angel with outspread wings.
INSCRIPTION: V:AEGIPTICV E:R 1697
MEANING OF INSCRIPTION: *Unguentum Egiptiacum*, Egyptian ointment. This remedy had a universal reputation, from the 1500s to the 1700s, as an application for wounds. It was included in the London Pharmacopoeia until 1721. Verdigris ointment is mentioned in the ancient Egyptian papyrus, Ebers, which dates from 2500 BC. 'E:R' are the initials of the apothecary who commissioned the jar.
CONTEMPORARY ACCOUNT: "'Take Verdigrease in fine Powder ℥ v. Honey ℥ xiv. Vinegar ℥ vii. Boil all together till it is of a deep red, and as thick as Honey.'

"This is a Prescription of *Mesue*, but many Authors have given it more compounded, but have thereby made it rather worse than better.

Fabricus Hildanus, in a Discourse concerning a Gangrene and Mortification, gives this Medicine an extraordinary Recommendation, for deterging or eating off rotten Flesh, and cleansing to admiration foul Ulcers. This is of great Use to destroy those cankerous Erosions which are so apt to grow in Childrens Mouths, and are first discoverable by white Specks: the way is to rub them with it upon a Rag ty'd to a Probe, or a piece of Stick. In Venereal Ulcerations likewise in the throat, i.e., about the *Uvula* and *Tonsils*, it does great Service." (J. Quincy, *A Compleat English Dispensatory*, 1718, p. 453)
DATE OF MANUFACTURE: 1697
PLACE OF MANUFACTURE: London
DIMENSIONS: Height 180 mm, maximum width 143 mm
PROVENANCE: Bought in 1957, Howard Collection.
CONDITION: Good; glaze crazed and chipped at base.
COMMENT: Howard describes this angel as "a winged portrait of the King [William III]" (p. 17). Howard also suggests that this jar is part of a set with KBG7 (Cat. 90). There seem to be five jars in a set dated 1697, with the initials 'E.R', two wet and three dry and all the same style.
REFERENCES: Howard, English Delftware Drug Jars, pp. 16–17 and No. 28.

Lipski and Archer, Dated English Delftware, No. 1661B.

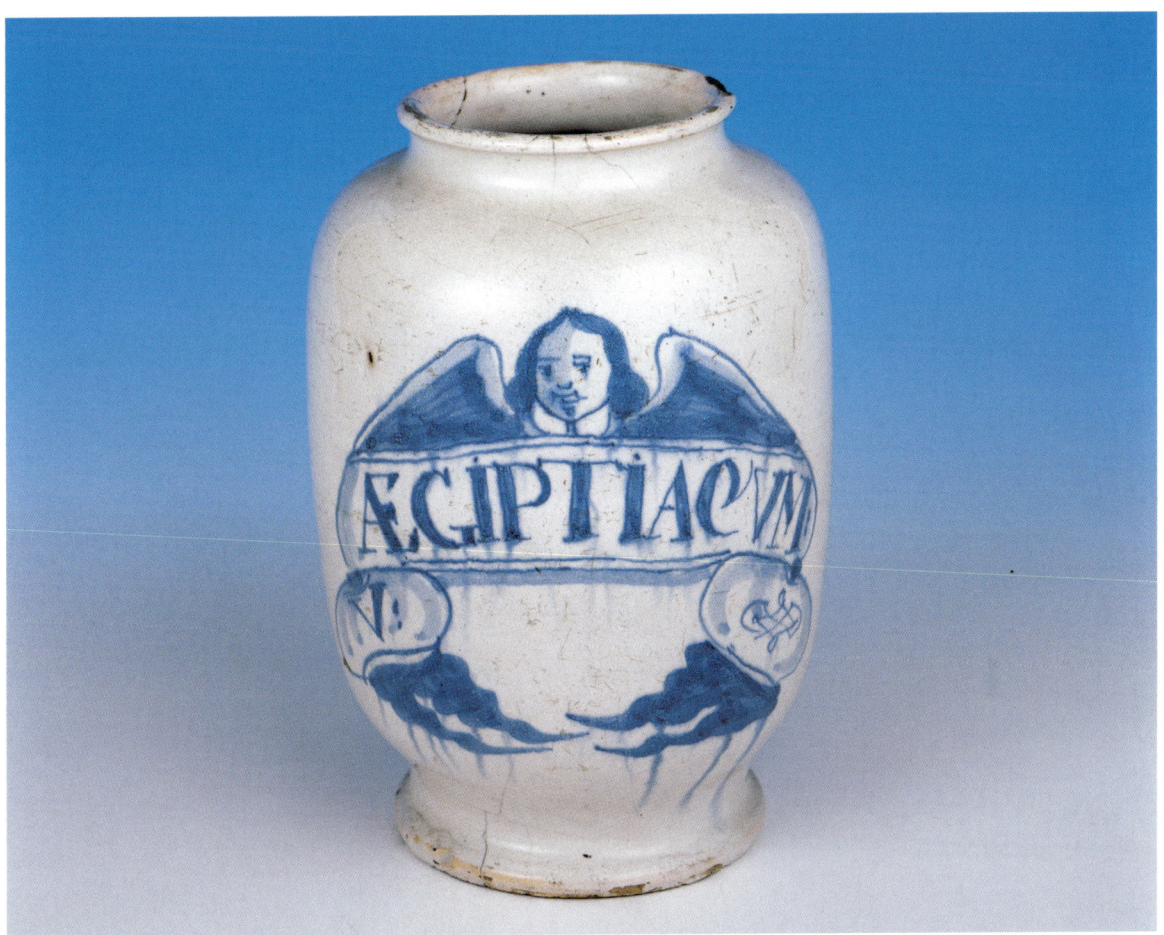

Angel with outspread wings

Dry drug jar (Cat.92)

ACCESSION NUMBER: KCG4

DESCRIPTION: Ovoid jar, tapering slightly towards splayed base. White glaze with pinkish tinge and design in blue. Label panel curved slightly upwards with thin even outline. Neck everted with glazed rim, flat unglazed base.

DESIGN: Angel with outspread wings.

INSCRIPTION: V AEGIPTIACVM

MEANING OF INSCRIPTION: *Unguentum Egiptiacum*, Egyptian ointment. This remedy had a universal reputation, from the 1500s to the 1700s, as an application for wounds. It was included in the London Pharmacopoeia until 1721. Verdigris ointment is mentioned in the ancient Egyptian papyrus, Ebers, which dates from 2500 BC.

CONTEMPORARY ACCOUNT: "'Take Verdigrease in fine Powder ℥ v. Honey ℥ xiv. Vinegar ℥ vii. Boil all together till it is of a deep red, and as thick as Honey.'

"This is a Prescription of *Mesue*, but many Authors have given it more compounded, but have thereby made it rather worse than better. *Fabricus Hildanus*, in a Discourse concerning a Gangrene and Mortification, gives this Medicine an extraordinary Recommendation, for deterging or eating off rotten Flesh, and cleansing to admiration foul Ulcers. This is of great Use to destroy those cankerous Erosions which are so apt to grow in Childrens Mouths, and are first discoverable by white Specks: the way is to rub them with it upon a Rag ty'd to a Probe, or a piece of Stick. In Venereal Ulcerations likewise in the throat, i.e., about the *Uvula* and *Tonsils*, it does great Service." (J. Quincy, *A Compleat English Dispensatory*, 1718, p. 453)

DATE OF MANUFACTURE: c. 1660

PLACE OF MANUFACTURE: London

DIMENSIONS: Height 180 mm, maximum width 133 mm

PROVENANCE: Bought in 1947.

CONDITION: Good; neck chipped, glaze crazed and flaked from base rim.

REFERENCE: Lothian, Seventeenth Century English History Reflected in Pharmaceutical Antiques, no date, p. 9, Plate 7.

Angel with outspread wings

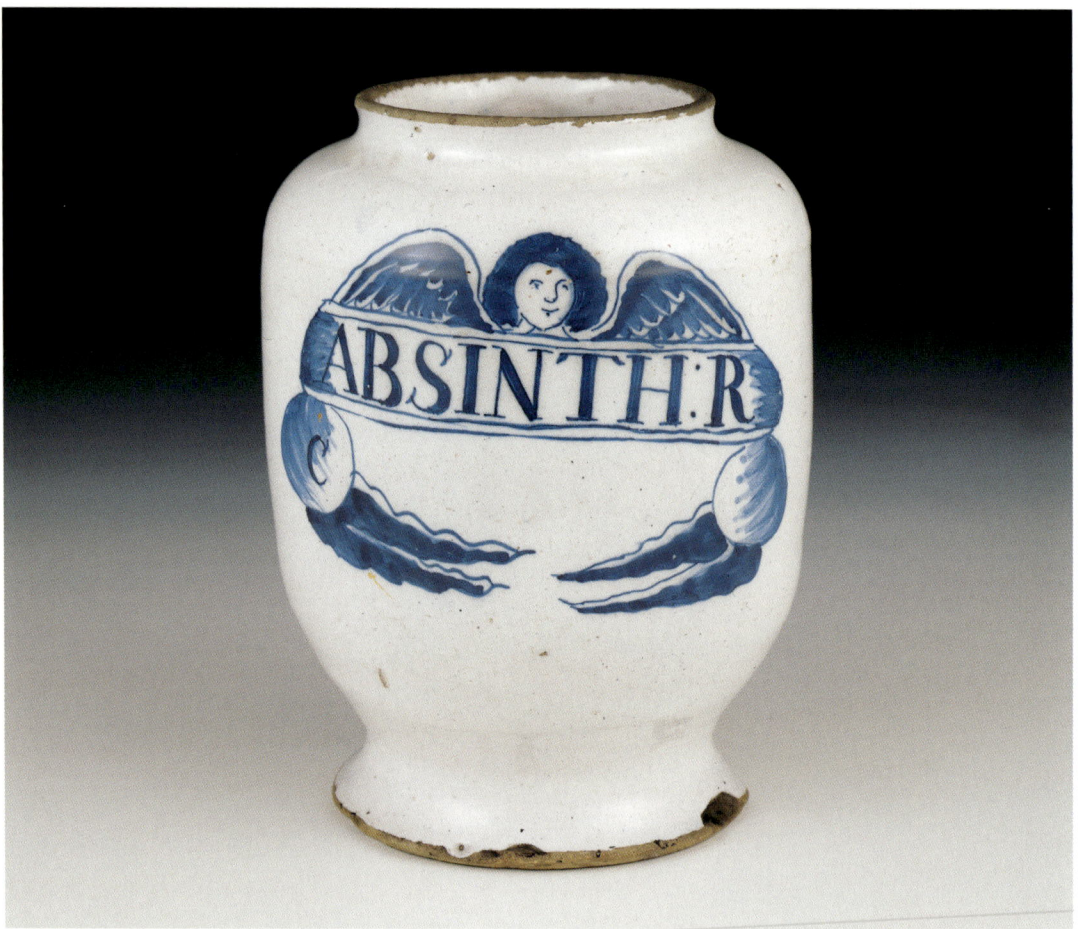

Dry drug jar (Cat.93)

ACCESSION NUMBER: KCG12
DESCRIPTION: Ovoid jar, with splayed base and two faint ridges encircling bowl, one below the neck and the other below the label. White glaze with pinkish tinge and design in blue. Label panel straight but sloping upwards to left, framed in two thin lines. Neck straight with unglazed rim, slightly concave unglazed base.
DESIGN: Angel with outspread wings.
INSCRIPTION: C ABSINTH:R
MEANING OF INSCRIPTION: *Conserva absinth romanum*, conserve of Roman wormwood (*Artemisia pontica*).
CONTEMPORARY ACCOUNT: "It is not by much so bitter as the *common Wormwood*, but is a much more grateful *Stomatick*. It astringes, incides, discusses, prevents Putrefaction, and carries off *Choler* by *Urine*; whereupon it is good in all Disorders of the *Liver*, and abates Pains and Wind in the Stomach and Bowels… A Conserve made of it, is now much in use in the Shops."
(J. Quincy, *A Compleat English Dispensatory*, 1718, p. 109)
DATE OF MANUFACTURE: 1660–1680

PLACE OF MANUFACTURE: London
DIMENSIONS: Height 190 mm, maximum width 150 mm
PROVENANCE: Bought in 1957, Howard Collection.
CONDITION: Good; base chipped, glaze crazed and flaked from rim of base.
REFERENCE: Howard, English Delftware Drug Jars, No. 26.

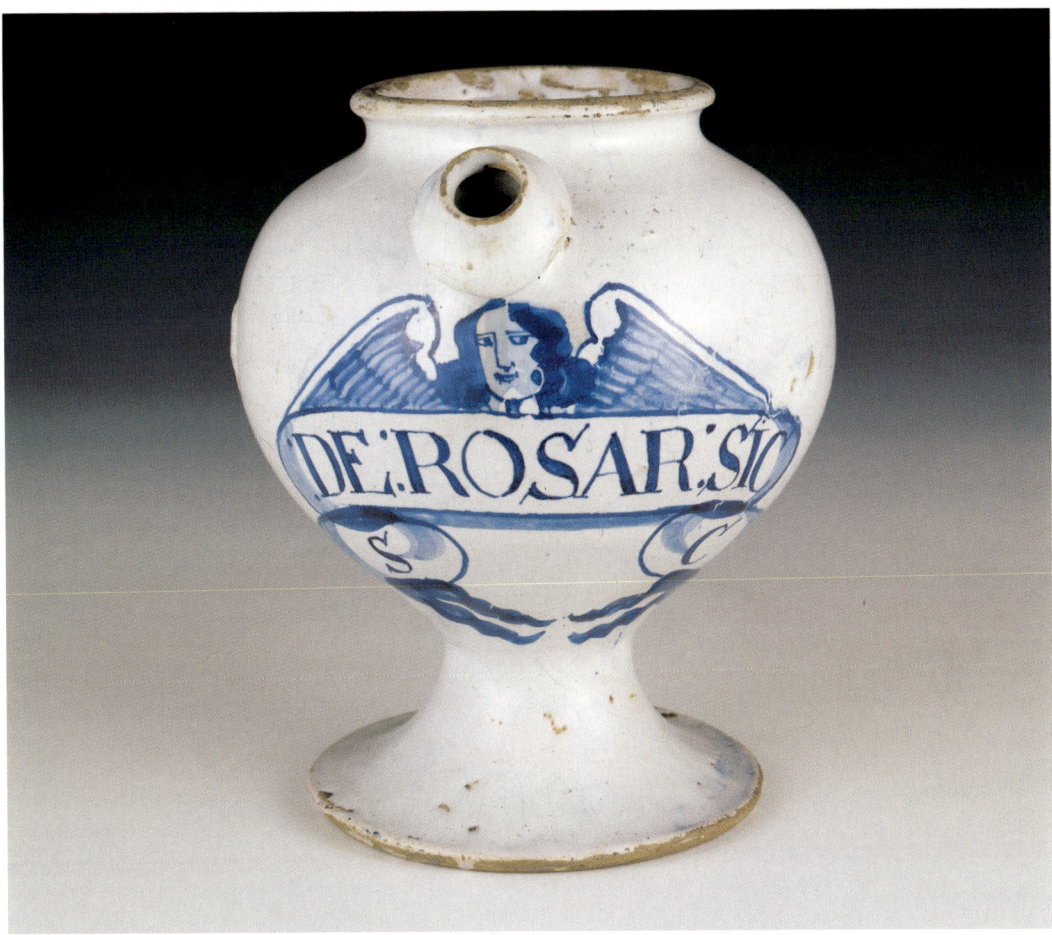

Wet drug jar (Cat.94)

ACCESSION NUMBER: KDG14

DESCRIPTION: Bulbous jar on spreading foot with spout and fluted strap-like handle. White glaze with pinkish tinge and design in blue. Label panel straight with even outline. Neck ridged with unglazed rim, spout with wide flange, hollowed and partly glazed base.

DESIGN: Angel with outspread wings.

INSCRIPTION: S :DE:ROSAR:SIC C

MEANING OF INSCRIPTION: *Syrupus de rosis siccis*, syrup of dried roses.

CONTEMPORARY ACCOUNT: "'Take red Roses ℔ ss. Infuse them in ℔ iv. of Water, which press out hard, and boil up to a Syrup with ℔ ii. of Sugar.'

"This is but little used, tho as much as it deserves; for the Roses are in too mean a quantity to give any Expectations from them. This also may be made from the Residuum after Distillation, if any distil this sort, which has been shewn to be needless." (J. Quincy, *A Compleat English Dispensatory*, 1718, p. 380)

DATE OF MANUFACTURE: 1660–1680

PLACE OF MANUFACTURE: London

DIMENSIONS: Height 180 mm, maximum width 150 mm

PROVENANCE: Bequest, Saville Peck, 1955. Museum records suggest that this came from Prior's collection.

CONDITION: Good; crack ascending from base, glaze crazed and flaked from spout, handle, neck and base rims.

Angel with outspread wings

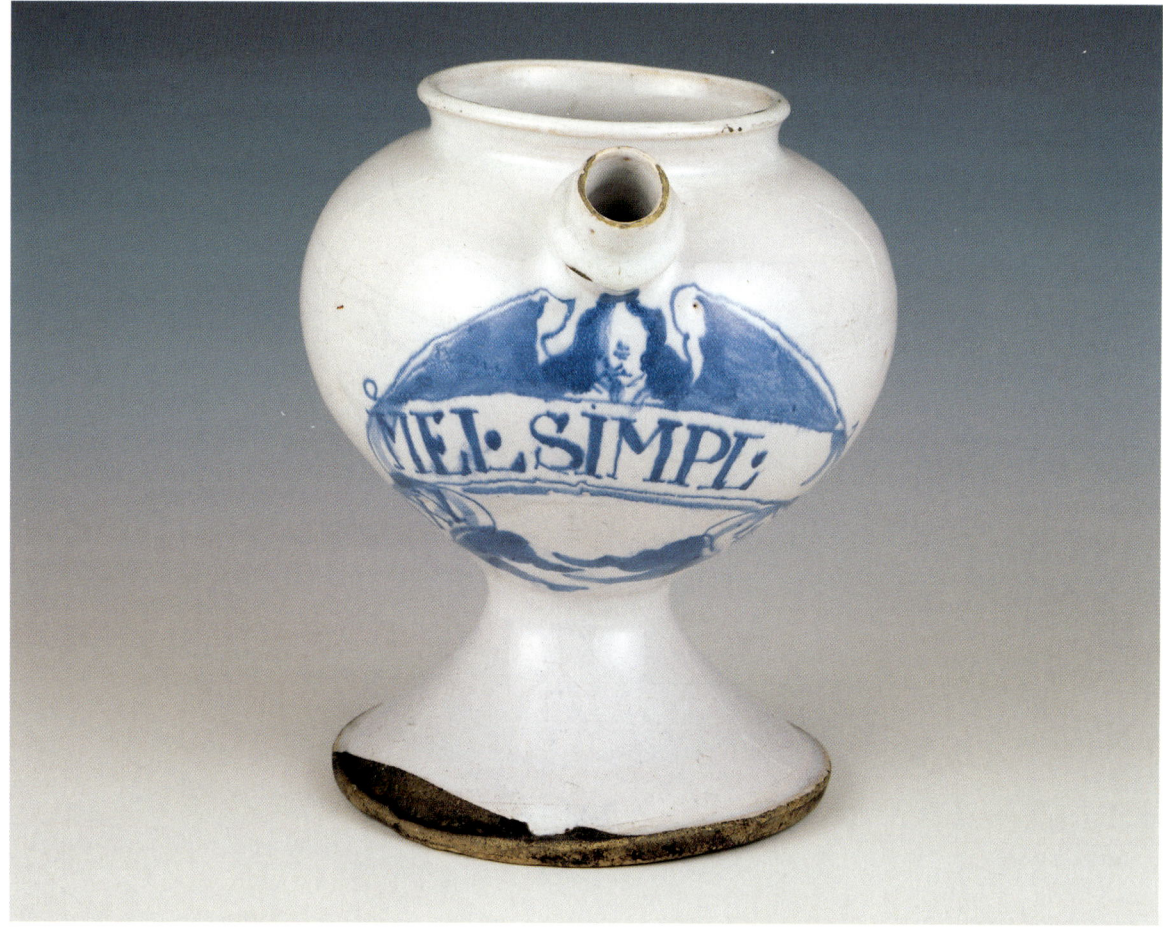

Wet drug jar (Cat.95)

ACCESSION NUMBER: KDG1

DESCRIPTION: Bulbous jar on spreading foot, with spout and strap-like looped handle. White glaze with pinkish tinge and design in blue. Label panel curved slightly upwards with even outline. Neck everted with glazed rim, flanged spout, hollowed, unglazed base.

DESIGN: Angel with outspread wings.

INSCRIPTION: MEL SIMPL

MEANING OF INSCRIPTION: *Mel simplex*, simple oxymel

CONTEMPORARY ACCOUNT: "Take of clarified honey two pounds; of vinegar a pint. Boil them in a glazed earthen vessel with a gentle fire, to the consistence of a syrup.

"Remark. In all the Oxymels a metalline vessel must be avoided, lest it should be corroded by the vinegar." (H. Pemberton, *The Dispensatory*, 1746, p. 307)

DATE OF MANUFACTURE: 1665–1685

PLACE OF MANUFACTURE: London

DIMENSIONS: Height 170 mm, maximum width 150 mm

PROVENANCE: Bought in 1949, as a pair with KDG2

(Cat. 116).

CONDITION: Good; part of foot lost glaze, glaze crazed.

COMMENT: There is a third jar from this group in the Wilkinson Collection, Thackray Museum, Leeds.

Angel with outspread wings

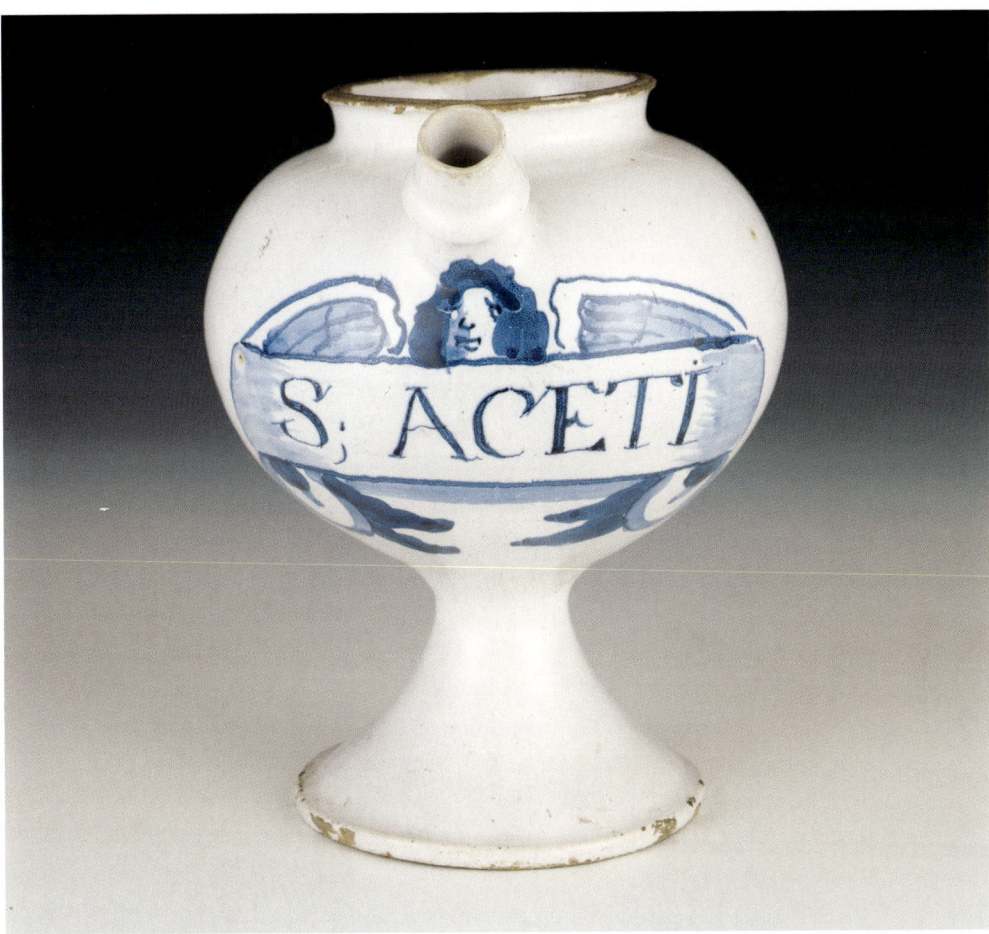

Wet drug jar (Cat.96)

ACCESSION NUMBER: KDG7

DESCRIPTION: Bulbous jar on spreading foot, with spout and strap-like looped handle. White glaze with pinkish tinge and design in blue. Label panel straight with even outline. Neck everted with unglazed rim, flanged spout, hollowed, glazed base with unglazed edge.

DESIGN: Angel with outspread wings.

INSCRIPTION: S; ACETI

MEANING OF INSCRIPTION: *Syrupus acetosus*, syrup of vinegar

CONTEMPORARY ACCOUNT: "This is made by dissolving with a gentle Heat Sugar ℔ v. in the best White-Wine Vinegar ℔ ii.

"This, as all other acid Syrups, must not be made in Brass or Copper Vessels, because it will erode enough of the Metal to nauseate the Stomach. They are best done in Earthen or *Silver*. This is reckon'd good to expectorate and cut Phlegm; and in such Intentions any other Syrup may be helpful, because the Sugar it self has a Tendency that way." (J. Quincy, *A Compleat English Dispensatory*, 1718, p. 372)

DATE OF MANUFACTURE: 1670–1690

PLACE OF MANUFACTURE: London

DIMENSIONS: Height 185 mm, maximum width 155 mm

PROVENANCE: Bought in 1954 from the collection of Mrs Robert Sargeant (previously Howard Collection).

CONDITION: Good; glaze crazed and flaked from handle, neck and base rims.

REFERENCE: Howard, English Delftware Drug Jars, No. 31.

Angel with outspread wings

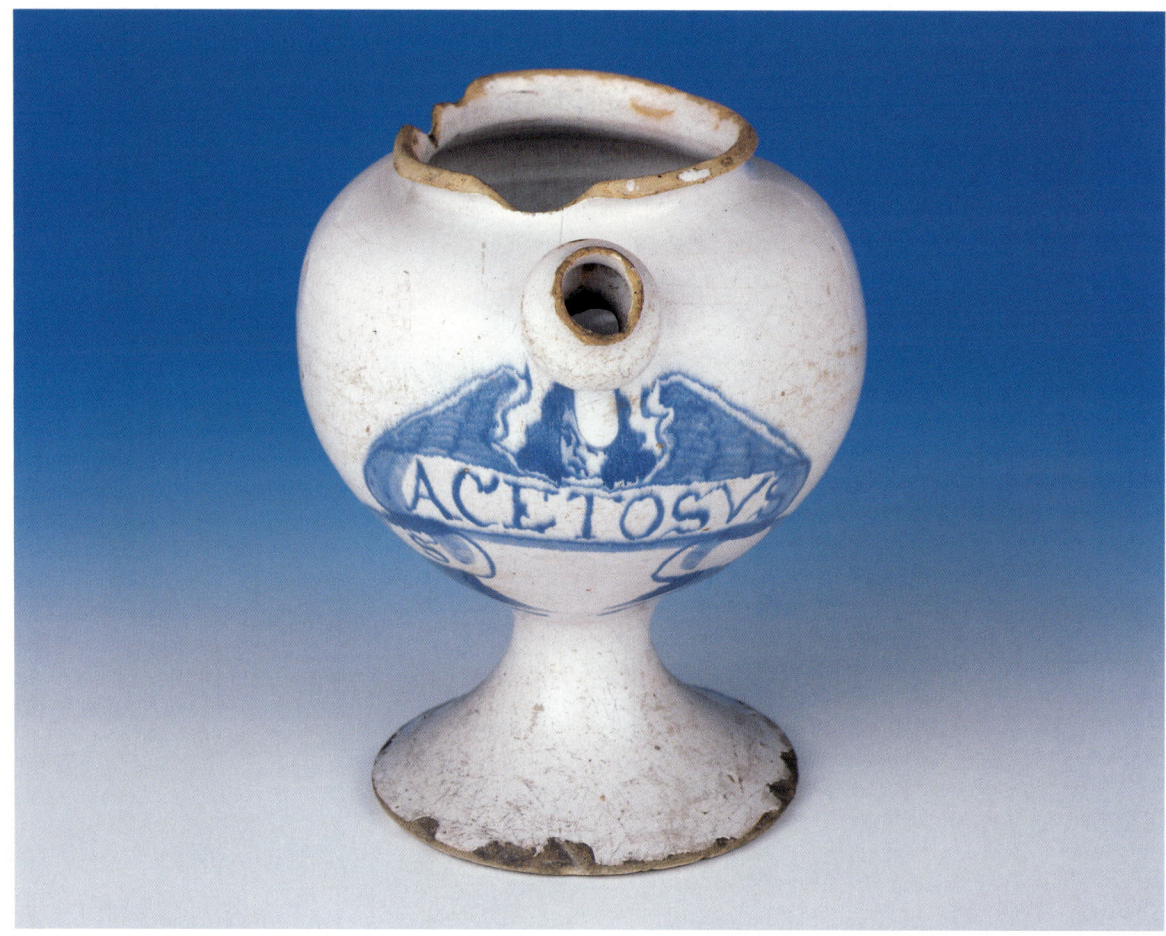

Wet drug jar (Cat.97)

ACCESSION NUMBER: KDG8

DESCRIPTION: Bulbous jar on spreading foot, with spout and fluted strap-like looped handle. White glaze with pinkish tinge and design in blue. Label panel straight with even outline. Neck everted with unglazed rim, spout with large flange, hollowed, unglazed base.

DESIGN: Angel with outspread wings.

INSCRIPTION: S ACETOSVS

MEANING OF INSCRIPTION: *Syrupus acetosus*, syrup of vinegar

CONTEMPORARY ACCOUNT: "This is made by dissolving with a gentle Heat Sugar ℔ v. in the best White-Wine Vinegar ℔ ii.

"This, as all other acid Syrups, must not be made in Brass or Copper Vessels, because it will erode enough of the Metal to nauseate the Stomach. They are best done in Earthen or *Silver*. This is reckon'd good to expectorate and cut Phlegm; and in such Intentions any other Syrup may be helpful, because the Sugar it self has a Tendency that way." (J. Quincy, *A Compleat English Dispensatory*, 1718, p. 372)

DATE OF MANUFACTURE: 1670–1690

PLACE OF MANUFACTURE: London

DIMENSIONS: Height 170 mm, maximum width 150 mm

PROVENANCE: Bequest, Saville Peck, 1955.

CONDITION: Fair; large crack descending from neck and another ascending from base, neck chipped in three places, glazed and flaked from spout and handle and rim of base.

REFERENCE: Walker, Ancient pharmacy jars pp. 253–254, No. VI, 6.

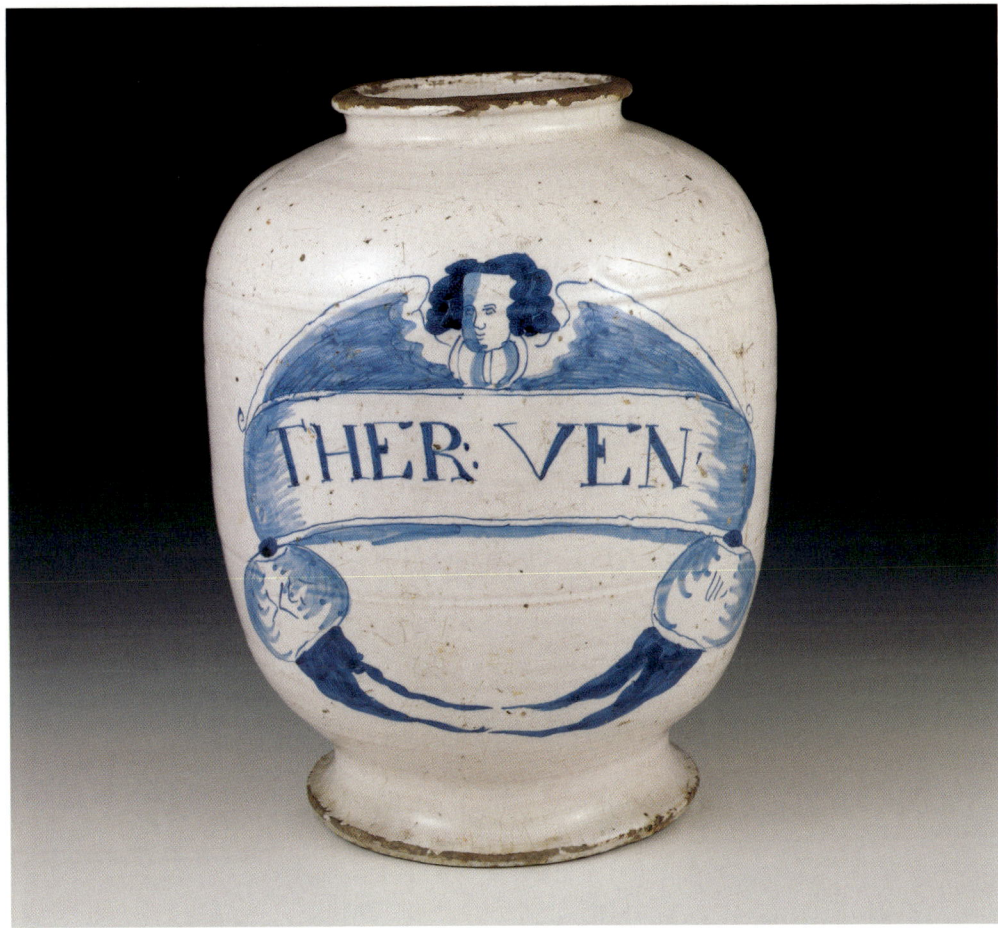

Dry drug jar (Cat.98)

ACCESSION NUMBER: KCG2

DESCRIPTION: Ovoid jar, tapering towards splayed base, with two narrow ridges encircling bowl, one below the neck and the other above the base. White glaze with pinkish tinge and design in blue. Label panel curved slightly upwards, with even outline. Neck everted and unglazed, flat unglazed base.

DESIGN: Angel with outspread wings.

INSCRIPTION: THER:VEN

MEANING OF INSCRIPTION: *Theriaca Veneta*, Venice treacle, also known as *Theriaca Andromachi*

CONTEMPORARY ACCOUNT: "'Take *Troches of Squills* ʒ vi. Troches of Vipers, long Pepper, *Opium*, and Troches of Hedycroi, ana ʒ iii. *Red Rose Buds dry'd, Orrice, Juice of Liquorice, Seeds of Sweet Navew*, Tops of Scordium, Opobalsam, *Troches of Agarick*, Cinnamon, ana ʒ iss. Myrrh, Zedoary, Saffron, *Cassia-Bark*, Spikenard, Schoenanth, white and black Pepper, *Frankincense, Dittany of Crete, Rhapontick*, Staecha's, *Hore-Hound, Parsley-Seeds*, Calaminth, *Cyprus* Turpentine, *Roots of Cinque-foil*, and Ginger, ana ʒ vi. *Tops of Polymountain*, Ground-Pine, *Celtick*

Spikenard, *Amomus*, Styrax, Meum-Root, Tops of Germander, *Phu-Root, Earth of* Lemnos, Indian Leaf, *Calcanthum, Gentian Root, Gum-Arabick, Juice of Hypocistis*, Cubebs, Seeds of Anise, Cardomoms, Fennel, of *Hartwort, German Acacia*, Seeds of Treacle-Mustard, Tops of St John's-wort, *Seeds of Bishop's-weed*, Sagapenum, ana ʒ iv. Castor, *long Birthwort, Amber*, or *Bitumen Judaicum, Seeds of Daucus*, Opoponax, *Centaury the lesser*, and Galbanum, ana ʒ ii. Canary ʒ xl. Honey, three times the weight of the whole Species when powder'd; and mix all into an Electuary.'

"This is not only the Capital Alexipharmick of our Shops, but of all *Europe*; and has a great deal more wrote about it, than could be contain'd in the largest Volume" (J. Quincy, *A Compleat English Dispensatory*, 1718, p. 409)

DATE OF MANUFACTURE: c. 1680

PLACE OF MANUFACTURE: London

DIMENSIONS: Height 310 mm, maximum width 250 mm

PROVENANCE: Bought in 1950.

CONDITION: Good; base chipped and with four small holes, glaze crazed and flaked on body, neck and base.

COMMENT: From the same set as KCG8 (Cat. 104).

REFERENCE: Lothian, Vessels for Apothecaries. p. 4 and Plate No. XX.

Angel with outspread wings

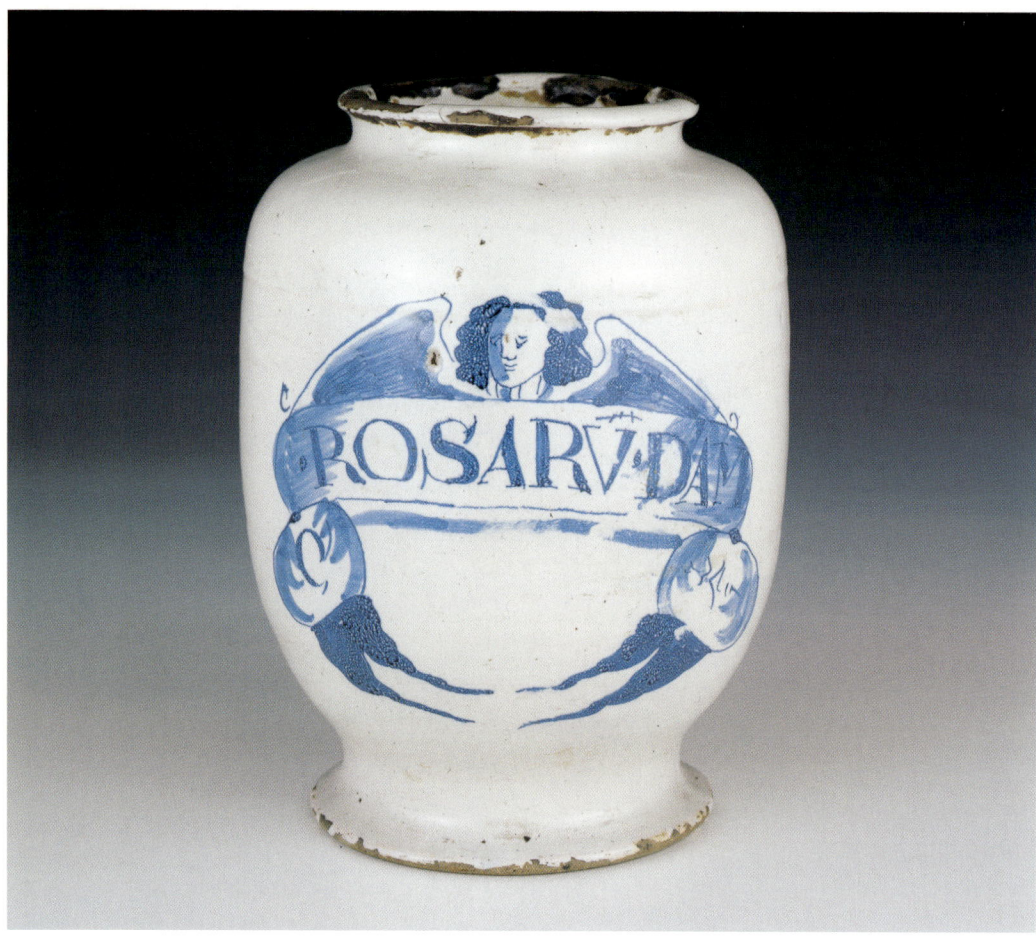

Dry drug jar (Cat.99)

ACCESSION NUMBER: KCG3

DESCRIPTION: Ovoid jar, tapering slightly towards splayed base, with two narrow ridges encircling bowl, one below the neck and the other above the base. White glaze with pinkish tinge and design in blue. Label panel curved slightly upwards with even outline. Neck everted, with partly glazed rim, slightly concave unglazed base.

DESIGN: Angel with outspread wings.

INSCRIPTION: C ROSARV DAM

MEANING OF INSCRIPTION: *Conserva rosarum Damascena*, conserve of *Rosa damascena* or damask rose.

CONTEMPORARY ACCOUNT: "They blow in *May* and *June*, and are much in use both in the Shops and amongst the common People, who are well enough acquainted with them as a *Purge*. They work gently enough, as to be safe to Infants in a proper Dose, but it may be increas'd so as to make it very ruffling and strong." (J. Quincy, *A Compleat English Dispensatory*, 1718, p. 181)

DATE OF MANUFACTURE: c. 1680

PLACE OF MANUFACTURE: London

DIMENSIONS: Height 190 mm, maximum width 150 mm

PROVENANCE: Bequest, Saville Peck, 1955.

CONDITION: Good; glaze flaked on rim of neck and base.

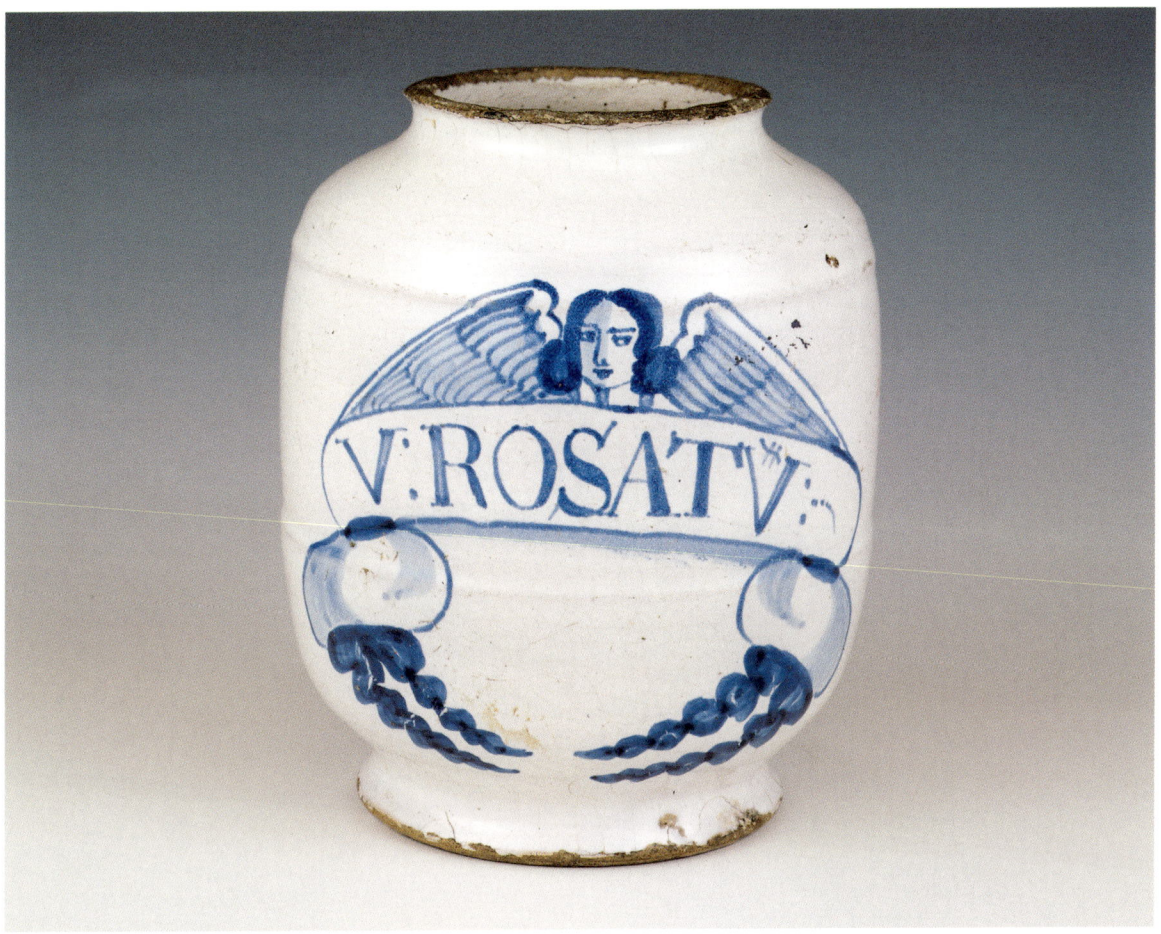

Angel with outspread wings

Dry drug jar (Cat.100)

ACCESSION NUMBER: KCG9
DESCRIPTION: Ovoid jar with splayed base, with two narrow ridges encircling bowl, one below the neck and the other below the label. White glaze with pinkish tinge and design in blue. Label panel curved slightly upwards with even outline. Neck everted with unglazed rim, slightly concave unglazed base.
DESIGN: Angel with outspread wings.
INSCRIPTION: V:ROSATV
MEANING OF INSCRIPTION: *Unguentum rosatum*, rose ointment.
CONTEMPORARY ACCOUNT: "'Take fresh red Rose-Leaves and Hog's-Lard, ana ℔ i. Bruise the Roses, and let them stand in Maceration with the Lard for some days; then put to it ℥ vi. of Juice of Roses, and ℥ ii. of Oil of sweet Almonds, and boil together till the Juice is exhaled, then Strain for use.'

...In this last the addition of the *Oil of Almonds* and the *Rose-Juice*, is mere trifling; and the whole is but an indifferent Medicine, intended for a Cooler: but it is so little acknowledg'd, as to be very seldom heard of." (J. Quincy, *A Compleat English Dispensatory*, 1718, p. 459)
DATE OF MANUFACTURE: c. 1680
PLACE OF MANUFACTURE: London
DIMENSIONS: Height 170 mm, maximum width 148 mm
PROVENANCE: Bought in 1957, Howard Collection.
CONDITION: Good; glaze crazed and flaked from rim of base.
COMMENT: Howard suggests this jar was decorated by the same artist as KBG4 (Cat. 76), KBG2 (Cat. 85), KBG8 (Cat. 81), KAG8 (Cat. 84), and KAG2 (Cat. 78) (pp. 15–16). Although of a similar date, the painting on this jar a different style.
REFERENCE: Howard, English Delftware Drug Jars, p. 15 and No. 19.

Angel with outspread wings

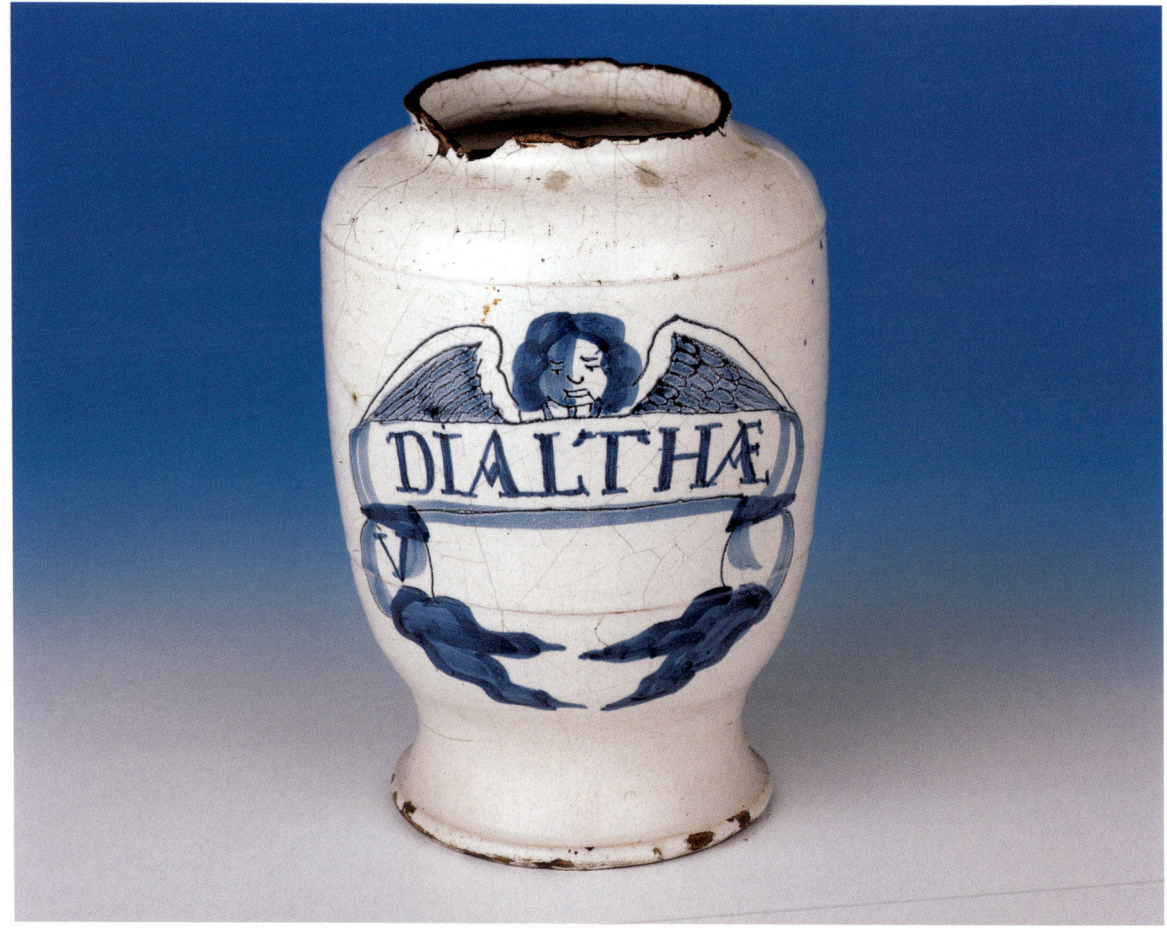

Dry drug jar (Cat.101)

ACCESSION NUMBER: KCG10

DESCRIPTION: Ovoid jar, tapering slightly towards splayed base, with two narrow ridges encircling bowl, one below the neck and the other below the label. White glaze with pinkish tinge and design in blue. Label panel curved slightly upwards with even outline. Neck everted and unglazed, slightly concave glazed base with unglazed edge.

DESIGN: Angel with outspread wings.

INSCRIPTION: V DIALTHAE

MEANING OF INSCRIPTION: *Unguentum dialthae*, ointment made with marshmallow (*Althaea officinalis*)

CONTEMPORARY ACCOUNT: "Take the thick Mucilage made with Marshmallow-Roots, and Foenugreek and Linseed, ana ℔ ii. Oil of Olives ℔ iv. Wax ℔ i. Resin ℔ ss. Turpentine ℥ ii. Mix S.A.

...This is reckon'd Emollient and Suppurative, and for such purposes is much used in extemporaneous Liniments and Cataplasms. By its Warmth, join'd with a relaxing Property, in such Forms, it greatly helps to rarefy the inclos'd Humours, and dispose them either for Transpiration or Revulsion, but most commonly for Maturation i.e. ripening into Matter: So as to render them fit for Discharge, either by Incision or Caustick." (J. Quincy, *A Compleat English Dispensatory*, 1718, p. 454)

DATE OF MANUFACTURE: c. 1680

PLACE OF MANUFACTURE: London

DIMENSIONS: Height 190 mm, maximum width 143 mm

PROVENANCE: Bought in 1957, Howard Collection.

CONDITION: Fair; part of neck missing, many hair cracks, glaze crazed and flaked from rim of base.

COMMENT: This preparation had an official formula in the first London Pharmacopoeia, 1618.

Angel with outspread wings

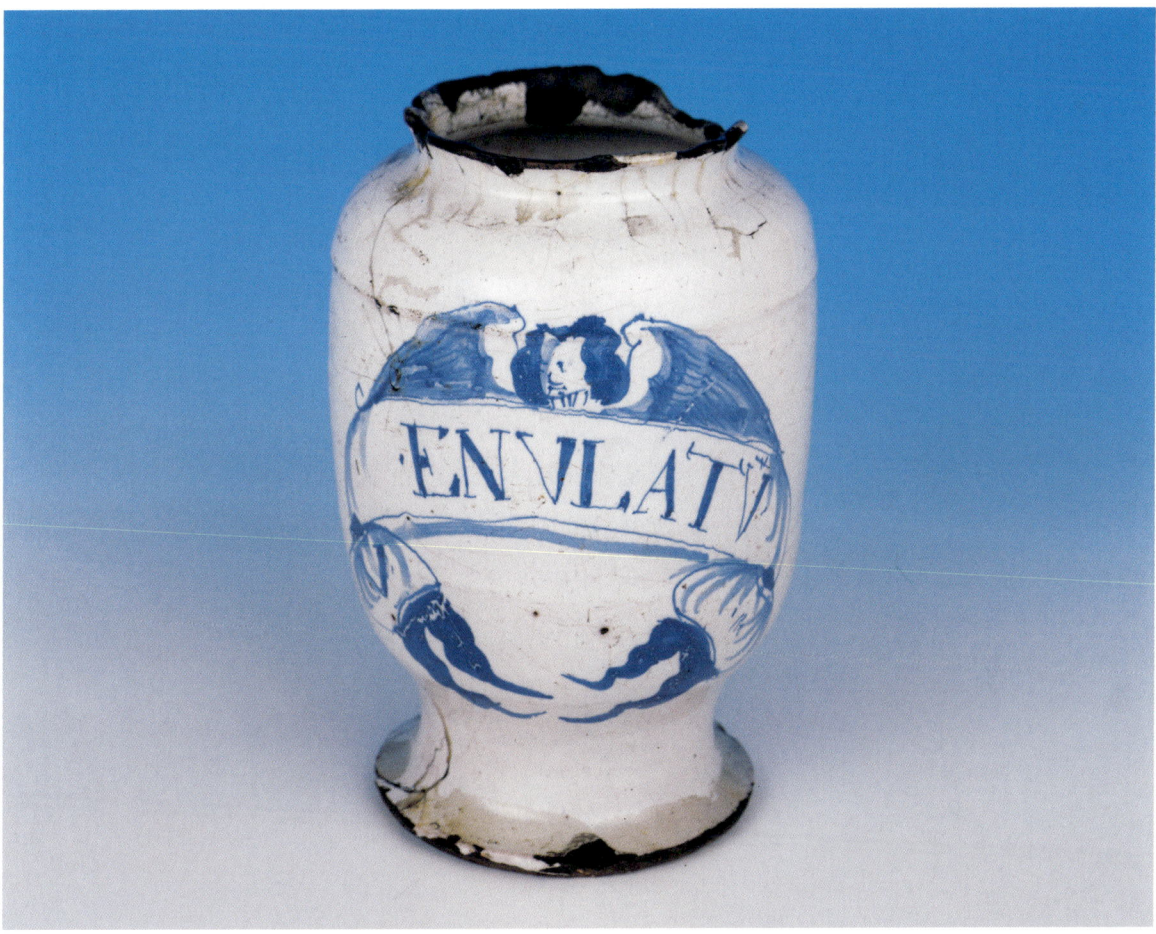

Dry drug jar (Cat.102)

ACCESSION NUMBER: KCG6

DESCRIPTION: Ovoid jar, tapering slightly towards splayed base, with two narrow ridges encircling bowl, one below the neck and the other below the label. White glaze with pinkish tinge and design in blue. Label panel curved slightly upwards with thin even outline. Neck everted with unglazed rim, flat unglazed base.

DESIGN: Angel with outspread wings.

INSCRIPTION: V ENVLATV

MEANING OF INSCRIPTION: *Unguentum enulatum*, enula ointment. Made with *Enula campana*, the root of elecampane (*Inula helenium*). An ointment to treat itching, an expectorant, diuretic, diaphoretic, cathartic, stomachic and emmenagogue.

CONTEMPORARY ACCOUNT: "'Take Elecampane Root, boiled in Vinegar, beat and pulped thro' a Sieve, ℔ i. of Turpentine washed in the same Decoction, ℥ ii. of yellow Wax, ℥ i. of Old Hogs Lard salted, and of old Oil, ana ℥ iv, of common Salt, ℥ ss. Let the Lard, Wax, and Oil melt together, and afterwards add the Turpentine, the Pulp of Elecampane, and Salt, finely powdered, so as to make all together into an Ointment, S.A.'

"This is continued in the last, as the former Dispensatories of the *College*, with a very little Alteration in some of the Quantities of the Ingredients; but it is little used." (J. Quincy, *A Compleat English Dispensatory*, 1718, pp. 502–503)

DATE OF MANUFACTURE: 1660–1700

PLACE OF MANUFACTURE: London

DIMENSIONS: Height 180 mm, maximum width 130 mm

PROVENANCE: Donation, 1953, Austen Collection.

CONDITION: Poor; 5 cm of neck rim missing, remainder chipped, base chipped, cracks descending from neck and ascending from base, glaze crazed and flaked from neck and base rims.

COMMENT: A label on the base of the jar reads 'U.S. Customs, serial 567'.

REFERENCE: Lothian, 'The John Austen Collection' p. 96 and Figure 9.

Angel with outspread wings

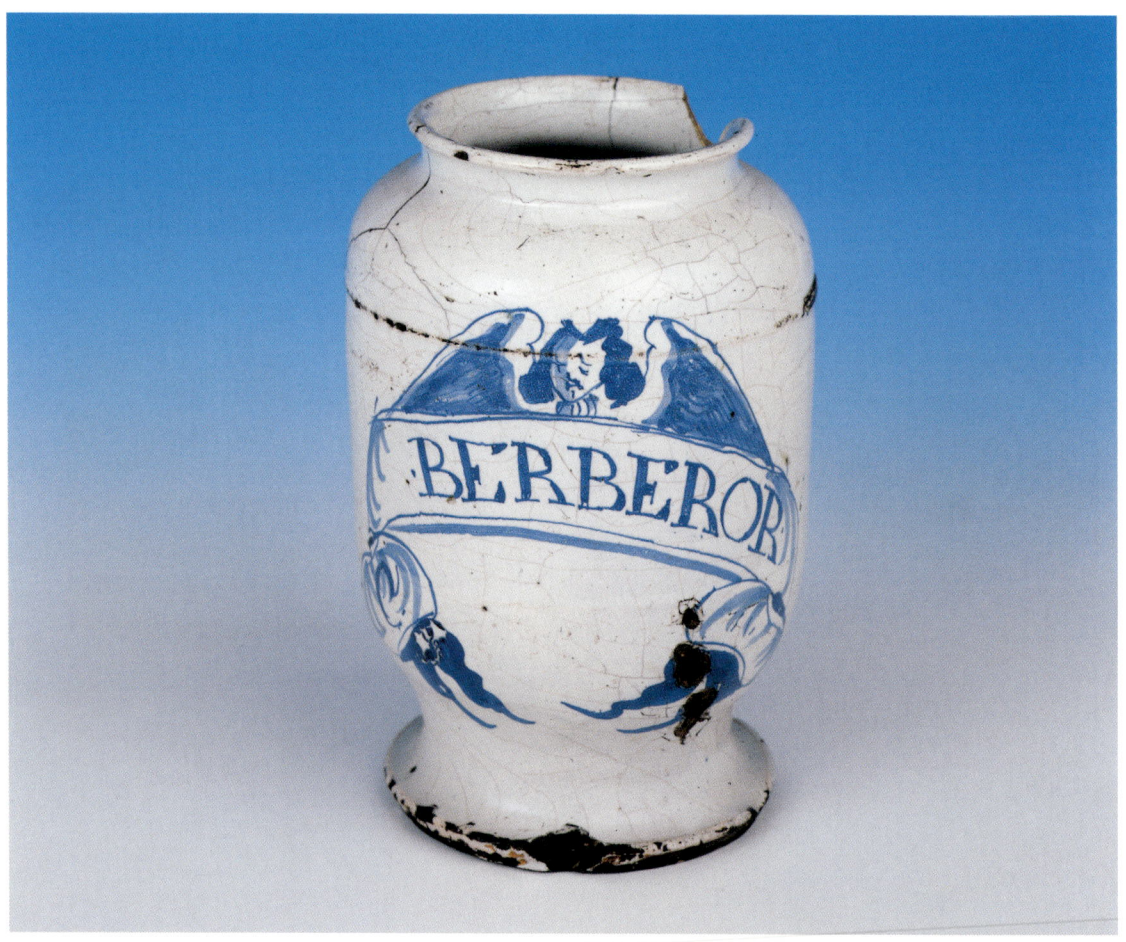

Dry drug jar (Cat.103)

ACCESSION NUMBER: KCG7

DESCRIPTION: Ovoid jar, tapering slightly towards splayed and ridged base, with two narrow ridges encircling bowl, one below the neck and the other below the label. White glaze with pinkish tinge and design in blue. Label panel curved slightly upwards framed with thin even outline. Neck everted with glazed rim, flat unglazed base.

DESIGN: Angel with outspread wings.

INSCRIPTION: C BERBEROR

MEANING OF INSCRIPTION: *Conserva berberis*, conserve of the bark and berry juice of the barberry (*Berberis vulgaris*).

CONTEMPORARY ACCOUNT: "Altho the Fruit of this Tree, which is well known to all, is acid, cooling, and astringent; yet constant Experience as found the Bark to be opening and detersive. That part which grows nearest the Tree, is most valu'd. It is hardly in any of the *Dispensatory*-compositions, but very frequent in common Prescription for the *Jaundice*, or any Distempers from Foulness and Obstruction of the *Viscera*." (J. Quincy, *A Compleat English Dispensatory*, 1718, p. 139)

DATE OF MANUFACTURE: 1660–1700.

PLACE OF MANUFACTURE: London

DIMENSIONS: Height 180 mm, maximum width 128 mm

PROVENANCE: Donation, 1953, Austen Collection.

CONDITION: Poor; 4 cm of neck rim missing, cracks descending from neck and encircling bowl, base chipped, glaze crazed and pitted and flaked from bowl and base rim.

REFERENCE: Lothian, 'The John Austen Collection' p. 96 and Figure 9.

Angel with outspread wings

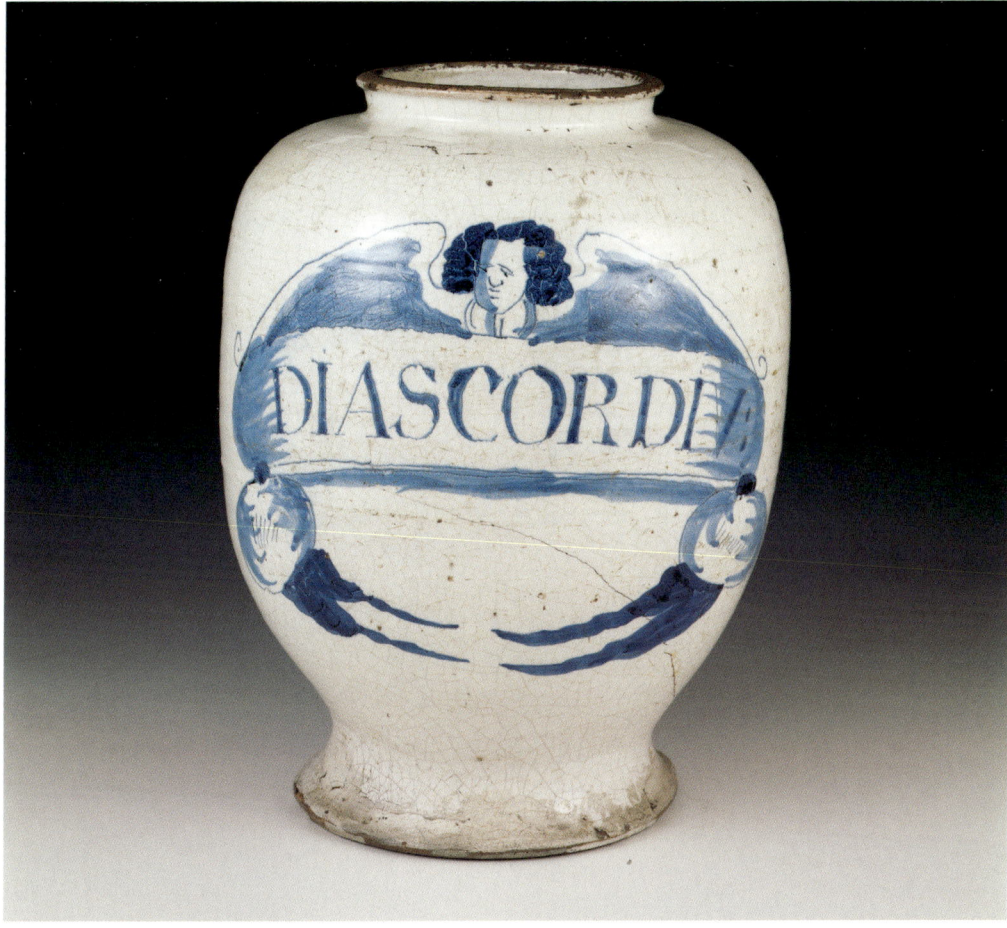

Dry drug jar (Cat.104)

ACCESSION NUMBER: KCG8
DESCRIPTION: Ovoid jar, tapering slightly towards splayed base, with two narrow ridges encircling bowl, one below the neck and the other below the label. White glaze with pinkish tinge and design in blue. Label panel curved slightly upwards with even outline. Neck everted with unglazed rim, flat unglazed base.
DESIGN: Angel with outspread wings.
INSCRIPTION: DIASCORDIV
MEANING OF INSCRIPTION: *Electuarium Diascordium*, electuary of scordium, water germander (*Teucrium scordium*).
CONTEMPORARY ACCOUNT: Quincy includes a substantial entry on this preparation, with the official recipe given and then a long commentary with suggestions of alterations in ingredients and method.

"Diascordium. *A Composition of Scordium*. Take of Cinnamon, and Cassia Wood, ana ℥ ss. of true Scordium ℥ i. of *Cretan* Dittany, Tormentil, Bistort, Galbanum, and Gum Arabic, ana ℥ iss. of Storax ℥ ivss. of Opium and Seeds of Sorrel, ana ℥ iss. of Gentian ℥ ss. of *Armenian* Bole ℥ iss. of *Lemnian* Sealed

Earth ℥ ss. of long Pepper and Ginger, ana ℥ ii. of clarif'd Honey lb iiss. of Sugar of Roses lb i. of generous Canary ℥ viii. Take it into an Electuary, S.A…"

"Everyone knows how much this is of use, and for what purposes, and indeed if the several Ingredients be nicely selected, and the Medicine fresh made, it is excellent in all Fluxes whatsoever, and a great Strengthener both of the Stomach and Bowels. In its influence on the Fluxes, the Opium has no small share, as may be well conceiv'd from the Virtues of that Drug… A very mischievous way some Nurses have got, of giving their Children this Medicine to make them sleep, more for their own Ease than any thing else…" (J. Quincy, *A Compleat English Dispensatory*, 1718, p. 429)
DATE OF MANUFACTURE: 1660–1700
PLACE OF MANUFACTURE: London
DIMENSIONS: Height 310 mm, maximum width 250 mm
PROVENANCE: Bought in 1950.
CONDITION: Fair; crack ascending from base and encircling bowl, glaze crazed and flaked on bowl and neck and base rims.
COMMENT: From the same set as KCG2 (Cat. 98).

Angel with outspread wings

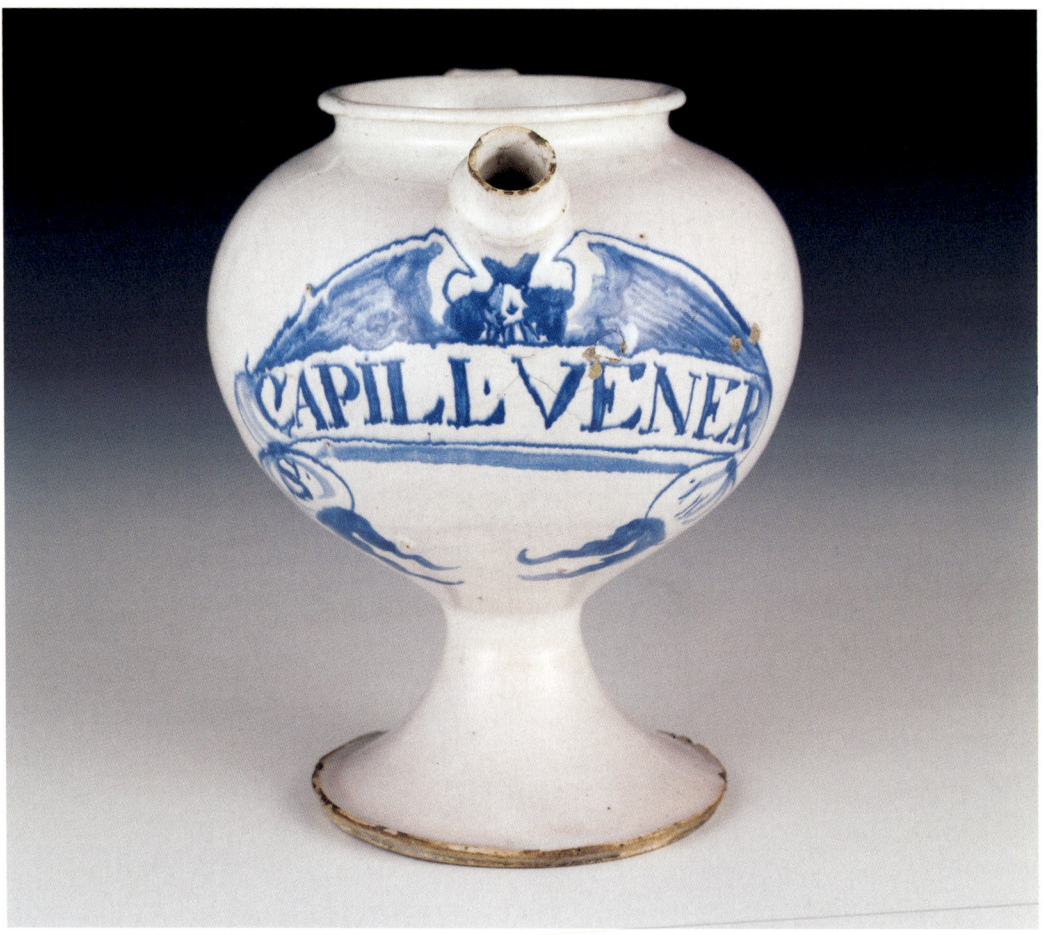

Wet drug jar (Cat.105)

ACCESSION NUMBER: KDG10

DESCRIPTION: Bulbous jar on spreading foot, with spout and strap-like looped handle. White glaze with pinkish tinge and design in blue. Label panel curved slightly upwards with even outline. Neck everted with glazed rim, flanged spout, hollowed, unglazed base.

DESIGN: Angel with outspread wings.

INSCRIPTION: S CAPILL VENER

MEANING OF INSCRIPTION: *Syrupus capillorum veneris*, syrup of maidenhair (*Adiantum capillus-Veneris*)

CONTEMPORARY ACCOUNT: (White) "This is very plentiful about *Narbon* in *France*. It grows likewise in many places in *England*, chiefly on rocky Ground. It is used in Decays of the lungs; and therefore enters much into the Composition of *Pectorals*, both in the Shops and common Prescription. It is also esteem'd as an *Epatick*, and a Remover of Obstructions in the Kidneys, and likewise a Promoter of the *Menses*; but it is not much used in those Intentions."

(Black) "This is also used in the same Intentions as the former, and is reckon'd good in Coughs, Asthma's, Pleurisies, Jaundice, and Obstructions of the Spleen and Kidneys; tho not greatly used for those purposes..." (J. Quincy, *A Compleat English Dispensatory*, 1718, p. 115)

DATE OF MANUFACTURE: 1660–1700

PLACE OF MANUFACTURE: London

COMMENT: Howard notes the "cypher" on the right-hand "lozenge" of the cartouche, and links this to other jars including KBG3 (Cat. 72), KAG11 (Cat. 68), KAG6 (Cat. 69), and KAE1 (Cat. 62).

DIMENSIONS: Height 170 mm, maximum width 145 mm

PROVENANCE: Bought in 1957, Howard Collection.

CONDITION: Good; glaze crazed and flaked from handle, spout and neck and base rims.

REFERENCES: Howard, English Delftware Drug Jars, p. 14 and No. 14.

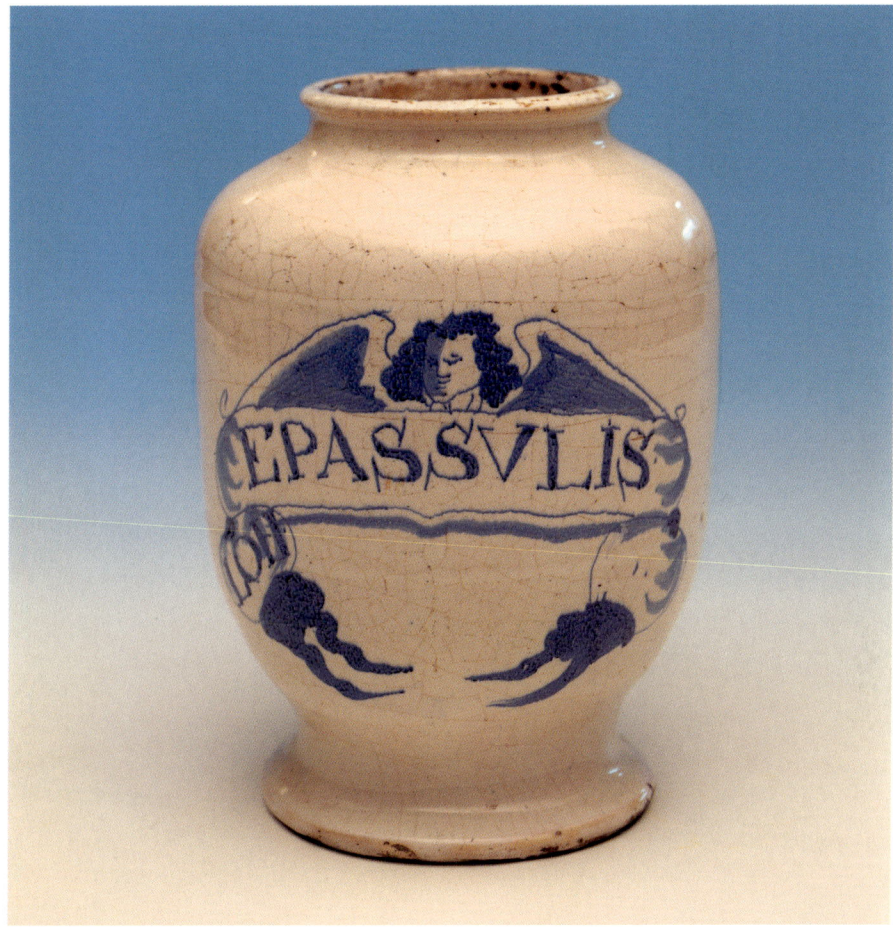

Dry drug jar (Cat.106)

ACCESSION NUMBER: 2002.60.2

DESCRIPTION: Ovoid jar, tapering slightly towards splayed base, with two narrow ridges encircling bowl, one below the neck and the other below the label. White glaze with design in blue. Label panel curved slightly downwards, framed in thin line and thicker outer line. Neck everted with glazed rim, unglazed flat base.

DESIGN: Angel with outspread wings.

INSCRIPTION: LOH EPASSVLIS

MEANING OF INSCRIPTION: *Lohoch e passulae solis*, lohoch of raisins of the sun

CONTEMPORARY ACCOUNT: "These are a Grape dry'd. They are a grateful Fruit, and very *detersive*; for which they are in most Compositions, to promote Expectoration, and dislodge obstructed Viscidities in the *Bronchia*, as also to cleanse the *Viscera*, and particularly the *Kidneys* and *Urinary Passages*." (J. Quincy, *A Compleat English Dispensatory*, 1718, p. 134)

DATE OF MANUFACTURE: 1680–1700

PLACE OF MANUFACTURE: London

DIMENSIONS: Height 195 mm, maximum width 50 mm

PROVENANCE: Bequest, 2002. Originally Saville Peck collection.

CONDITION: Good; some chips to rim.

REFERENCE: Walker, Ancient pharmacy jars p. 251, No. VII 3.

Angel with outspread wings

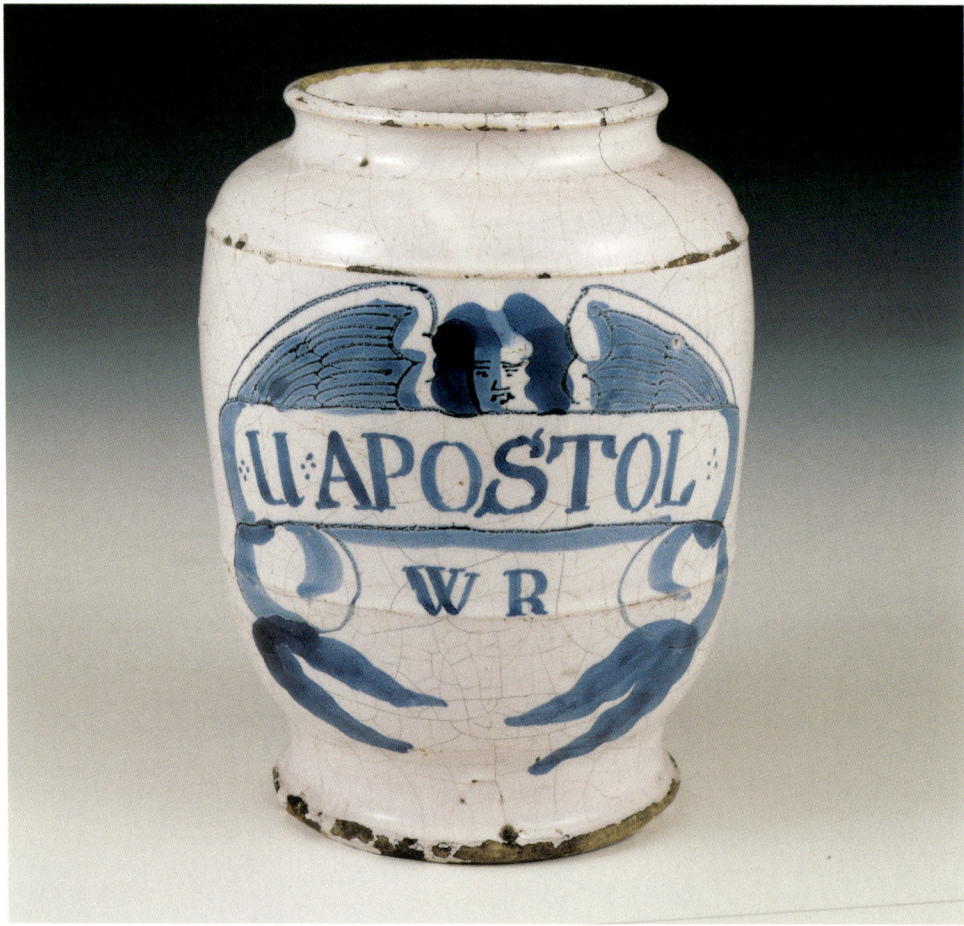

Dry drug jar (Cat.107)

ACCESSION NUMBER: KCG11

DESCRIPTION: Ovoid jar, tapering slightly towards splayed base and two narrow ridges encircling bowl, one below the neck and the other below the label. White glaze with pinkish tinge and design in blue and black. Label panel curved slightly upwards with even outline. Neck everted with glazed rim, slightly concave and partly glazed base.

DESIGN: Angel with outspread wings.

INSCRIPTION: U APOSTOL WR

MEANING OF INSCRIPTION: *Unguentum apostolorum*, ointment of the apostles, as it has 12 ingredients. 'WR' are the initials of the apothecary who commissioned the jar.

CONTEMPORARY ACCOUNT: "Take Turpentine, Resin, Wax, Gum Armoniack, ana ℥ xiv. Roots of long Birth-wort, Olibarium, Bdellium, ana ℥ vi. Myrrh and Galbanum, ana ℥ ss. Opoponax ℥ iii. Verdigrease ℥ ii. Vinegar a sufficient quantity to dissolve the Gums; and make all together into an Ointment S.A.'

In the making this, which is a Prescription of *Avicen*, it must be observ'd to dissolve the Gums in Vinegar; which must after straining be in the greatest part evaporated, and to the *Turpentine*, *Resin*, and *Wax*: and after the *Letharge* has boil'd long enough with the *Oil* to incorporate it, with Water enough to prevent burning, they are to be put together, and then the Ingredients to be powder'd, sifted in, and all mix'd with a Spatule. The *Verdigrease*, if it be rightly order'd, will give it a deep green Colour. This is chiefly intended for a *Detergent*, and it is now pretty much used to cleanse foul Sores and Ulcers, and wear off fungous Excrescences in Wounds, which incarn too fast." (J. Quincy, *A Compleat English Dispensatory*, 1718, pp. 453–454)

DATE OF MANUFACTURE: 1680–1700

PLACE OF MANUFACTURE: London

DIMENSIONS: Height 165 mm, maximum width 125 mm

PROVENANCE: Bought in 1957, Howard Collection.

CONDITION: Good; crack descending from neck, glaze crazed and flaked from body and neck and base rims.

COMMENT: Howard suggests that the initials 'WR' belonged to the apothecary William Richardson (p. 9).

REFERENCE: Howard, English Delftware Drug Jars, No. 27.

Angel with outspread wings

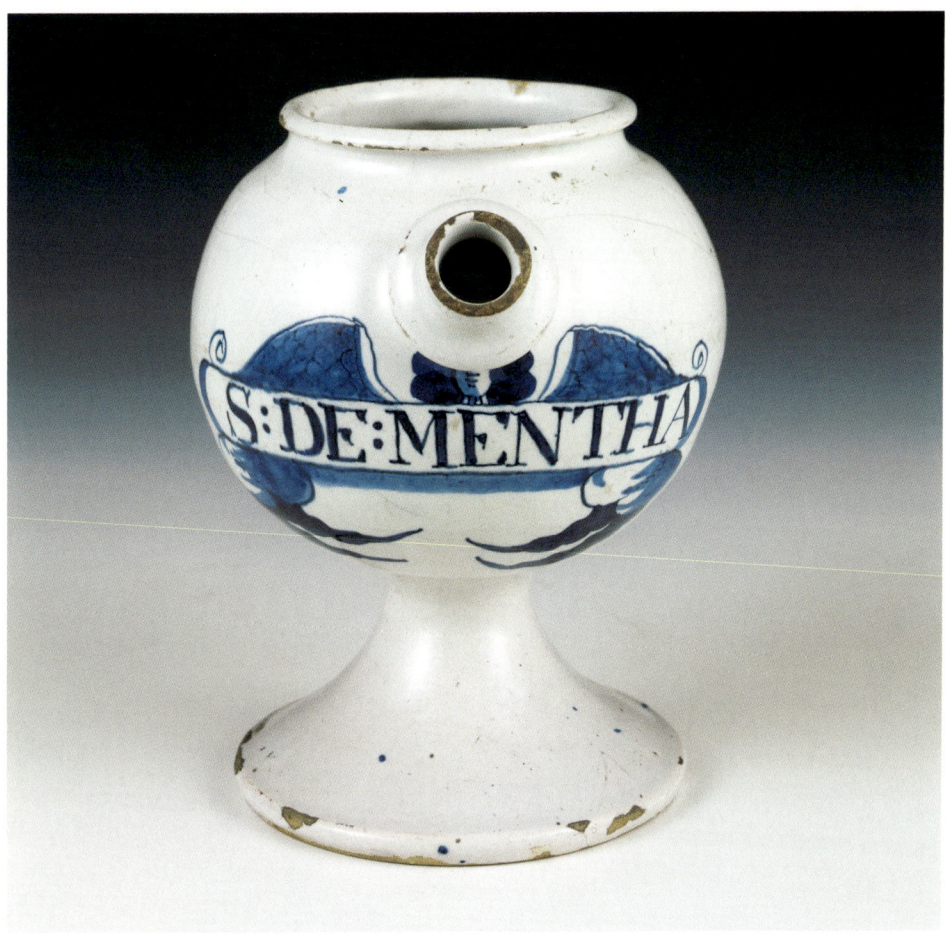

Wet drug jar (Cat.108)

ACCESSION NUMBER: KDG5

DESCRIPTION: Bulbous jar on spreading foot with spout only. White glaze with pinkish tinge and design in blue. Label panel straight with even outline. Neck everted with glazed rim, flanged spout, hollowed, glazed base with unglazed edge.

DESIGN: Angel with outspread wings.

INSCRIPTION: S:DE:MENTHA

MEANING OF INSCRIPTION: *Syrupus de mentha*, syrup of spearmint (*Mentha sperata*)

CONTEMPORARY ACCOUNT: "'Take Juice of Quinces, both of the sweet and sour sort, and of Pomegranates, ana ℔ iss. dry'd Mint ℔ ss. Red Roses ℨ ii. Digest together, press out the Liquor, and boil to a Syrup with ℔ iv. of fine Sugar.'

This is as good a Medicine as this Form could admit of: the Mint must be choicely pick'd from the gross Stalks. It is a good Astringent, and strengthens the Stomach and Bowels against Vomitings and *Diarrhea's*. In which Cases it is very proper to sweeten all Liquids with it, and use it in all convenient extemporary Forms." (J. Quincy, *A Compleat English*

Dispensatory, 1718, p. 378)

DATE OF MANUFACTURE: 1680–1700

PLACE OF MANUFACTURE: London

DIMENSIONS: Height 175 mm, maximum width 140 mm

PROVENANCE: Bought in 1947.

CONDITION: Good; hair cracks encircling bowl, spout and neck chipped, glaze crazed and flaked from neck and base rims.

COMMENT: Part of the same set as KDG6 (Cat. 109)

REFERENCE: Lothian, Vessels for Apothecaries. p. 5 and Plate No. XXIV.

Angel with outspread wings

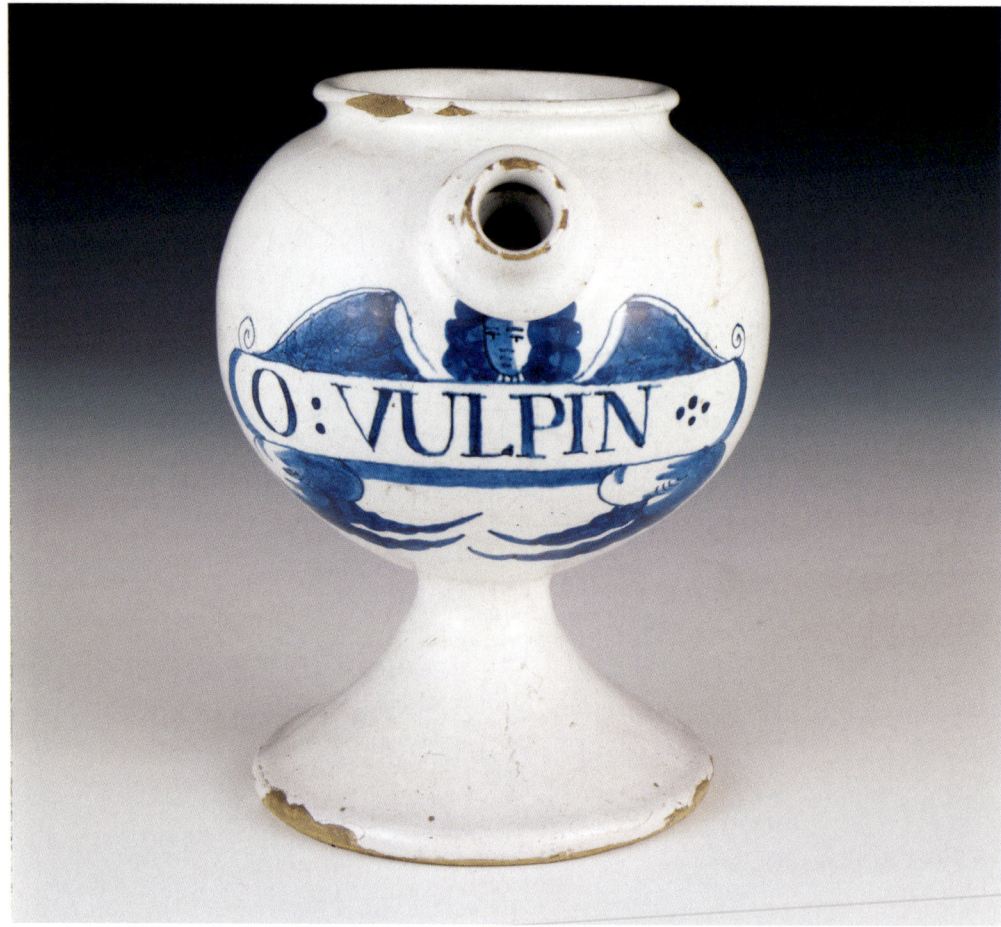

Wet drug jar (Cat. 109)

ACCESSION NUMBER: KDG6
DESCRIPTION: Bulbous jar on spreading foot with spout only. White glaze with pinkish tinge and design in blue. Label panel straight with even outline. Neck everted with glazed rim, flanged spout, hollowed, glazed base with unglazed edge.
DESIGN: Angel with outspread wings.
INSCRIPTION: O:VULPIN
MEANING OF INSCRIPTION: *Oleum vulpinum*, oil of fox
CONTEMPORARY ACCOUNT: "Colledg. *Take a fat Fox, of a middle age, *(if you can get such an one)* [*that was wel put in, therefore when you have caught a Fox, bring him alive to the Colledg, and let them look in his mouth first, and tell you how old he is, so shall your Oil be cum privilegio] caught by hunting about Autumn, cut in pieces, the skin and bowels taken away, the bones broken, boyl him (scumming it diligently) in white wine and spring water, of each six pound, till half be consumed: with three ounces of Sea salt, the tops of Dill, Time and Chamepitys, of each one handful; after straining boil it again with four pound of the best old Oil, the flowers of Sage and Rosemary, of each*

one handful; the water being consumed, strain it again, and keep the pure Oil for use."

Culpeper: "It is exceeding good in pains of the joynts, Gouts, pains in the Back and Reins; it heats the body being afflicted by cold, and hard lodging in the Aire, whereby the joynts are stiff, a disease incident to many in these times." (N. Culpeper, *The Physicians Library*, 1667, p. 220)
DATE OF MANUFACTURE: 1680–1700
PLACE OF MANUFACTURE: London
DIMENSIONS: Height 180 mm, maximum width 143 mm
PROVENANCE: Bought in 1947.
CONDITION: Good; glaze flaked from spout and base rims.
COMMENT: Part of the same set as KDG5 (Cat. 108)
REFERENCE: Lothian, Vessels for Apothecaries. p. 5 and Plate No. XXIV.

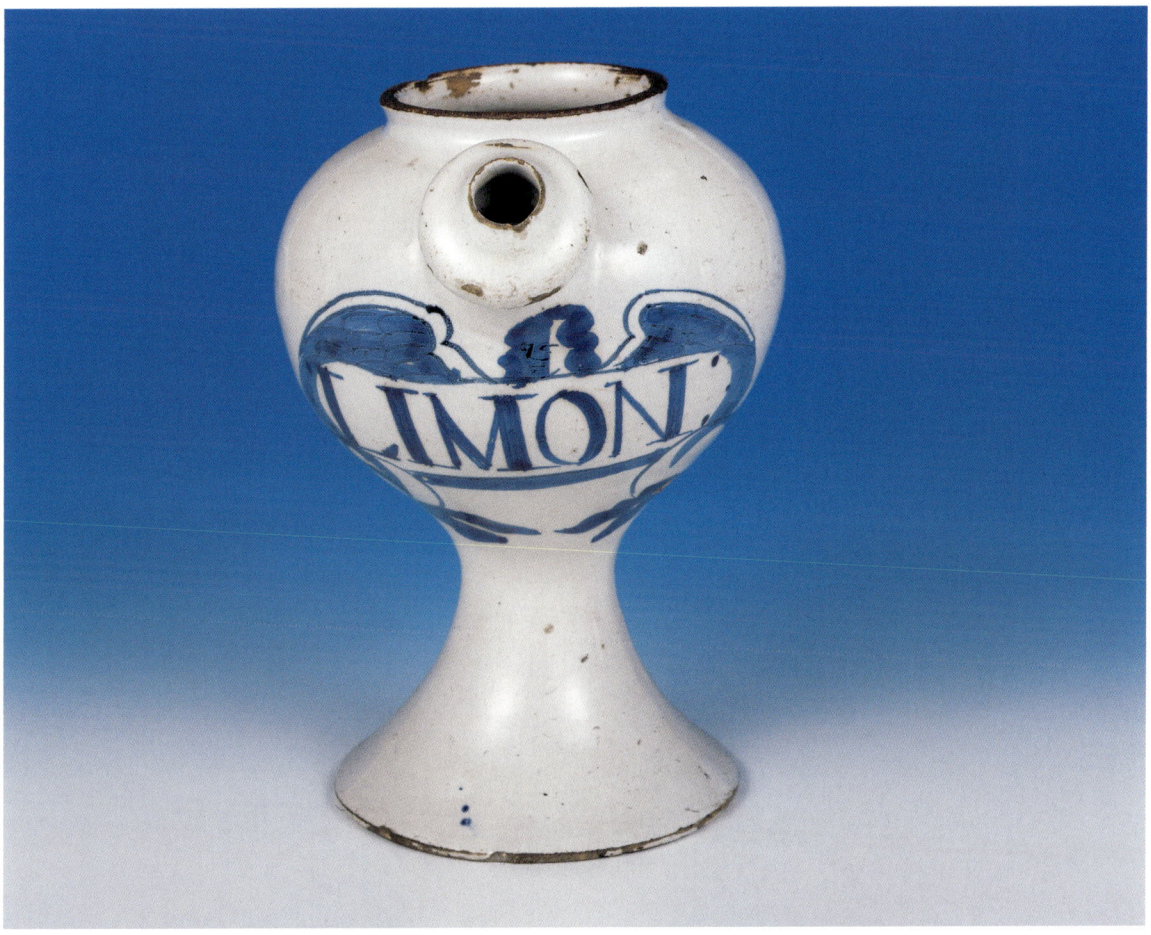

Wet drug jar (Cat.110)

ACCESSION NUMBER: KDG12

DESCRIPTION: Bulbous jar on elongated spreading foot, with spout and fluted strap-like handle. White glaze with pinkish tinge and design in blue. Label panel straight with even outline. Neck slightly everted with unglazed rim, spout with large flange, hollowed, glazed base with unglazed edge.

DESIGN: Angel with outspread wings.

INSCRIPTION: S LIMON:

MEANING OF INSCRIPTION: *Syrupus e succo limonum*, syrup of lemon juice

CONTEMPORARY ACCOUNT: "Take of lemon-juice, after it has stood, till its faeces are subsided, and it has been strained off, a quart; of double refined sugar fifty ounces. Dissolve the sugar in the juice, so as to make the syrup." (H. Pemberton, *The Dispensatory*, 1746, pp. 295–296)

DATE OF MANUFACTURE: 1680–1700

PLACE OF MANUFACTURE: London

DIMENSIONS: Height 190 mm, maximum width 135 mm

PROVENANCE: Bought in 1947.

CONDITION: Good; neck chipped, transverse crack at base of handle, glaze flaked on body (two patches each 1.75 cm diameter), spout, handle, and on rim of neck and base.

Angel with outspread wings

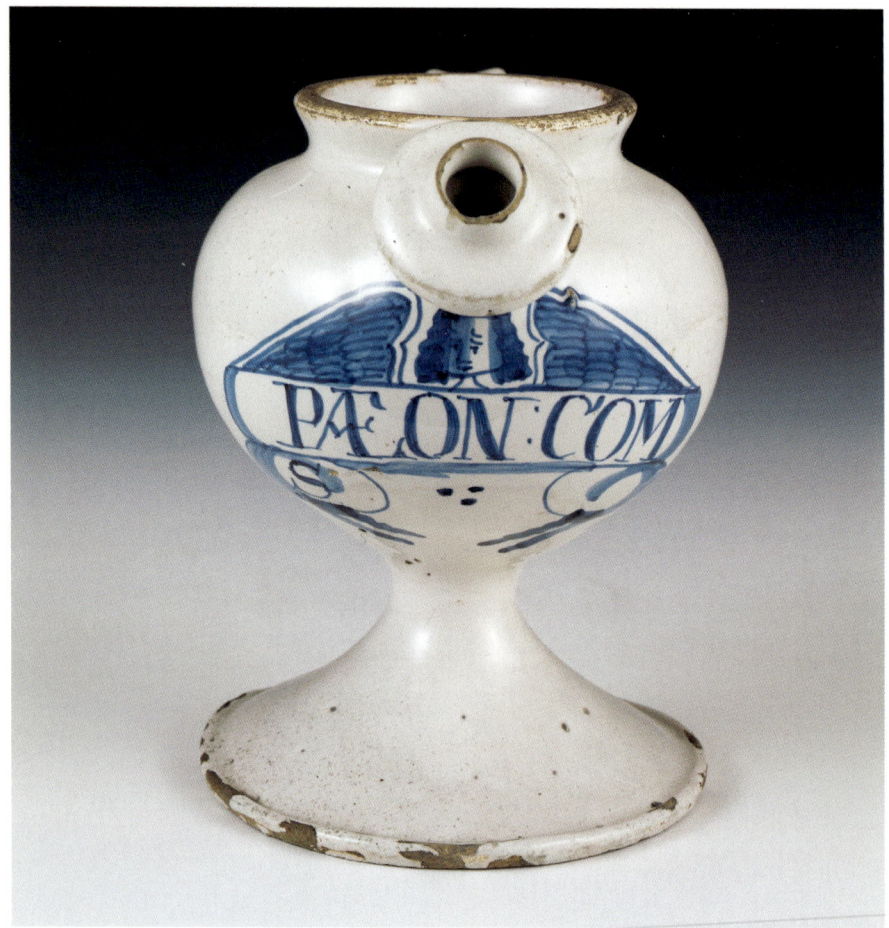

Wet drug jar (Cat.111)

ACCESSION NUMBER: KDG13

DESCRIPTION: Bulbous jar on spreading foot with spout and fluted strap-like looped handle. White glaze with pinkish tinge and design in blue. Label panel straight with even outline. Neck everted with unglazed rim, spout with wide flange, wide and ridged unglazed base.

DESIGN: Angel with outspread wings.

INSCRIPTION: S PAEON:COM

MEANING OF INSCRIPTION: *Syrupus paeonia composita*, compound syrup of peony (*Paeonia officinalis*)

CONTEMPORARY ACCOUNT: "'Take Roots of fresh Pioney, Male and Female, ana ʒ iss. infused in White-Wine; of Contrayerva ʒ ss. Bastard-Lovage ʒ vi. Elks-Hoof ʒ i. Rosemary with the Flowers m.i. Betony, Origanum, Hyssop, Ground-Pine, and Rue ana ʒ iii. Wood of Aloes, Cloves and the lesser Cardamoms, ana ʒ ii. Ginger and Spikenard, ana ʒ ii. Staechas and Nutmegs, ana ʒ iiss. Water of Pioney-Root ℔ vi. Digest them together some hours, and boil to ℔ iv. To the straining add ℔ ivss. of Sugar, and make into a Syrup.' This is much prescribed in extemporaneous Forms, either to sweeten Liquors, or to give due Consistence, in all nervous Intentions; but very little good can be expected from it." (J. Quincy, *A Compleat English Dispensatory*, 1718, p. 379)

DATE OF MANUFACTURE: 1680–1700

PLACE OF MANUFACTURE: London

DIMENSIONS: Height 170 mm, maximum width 133 mm

PROVENANCE: Bought in 1950.

CONDITION: Good; glaze pitted and flaked on spout, handle and rim of base.

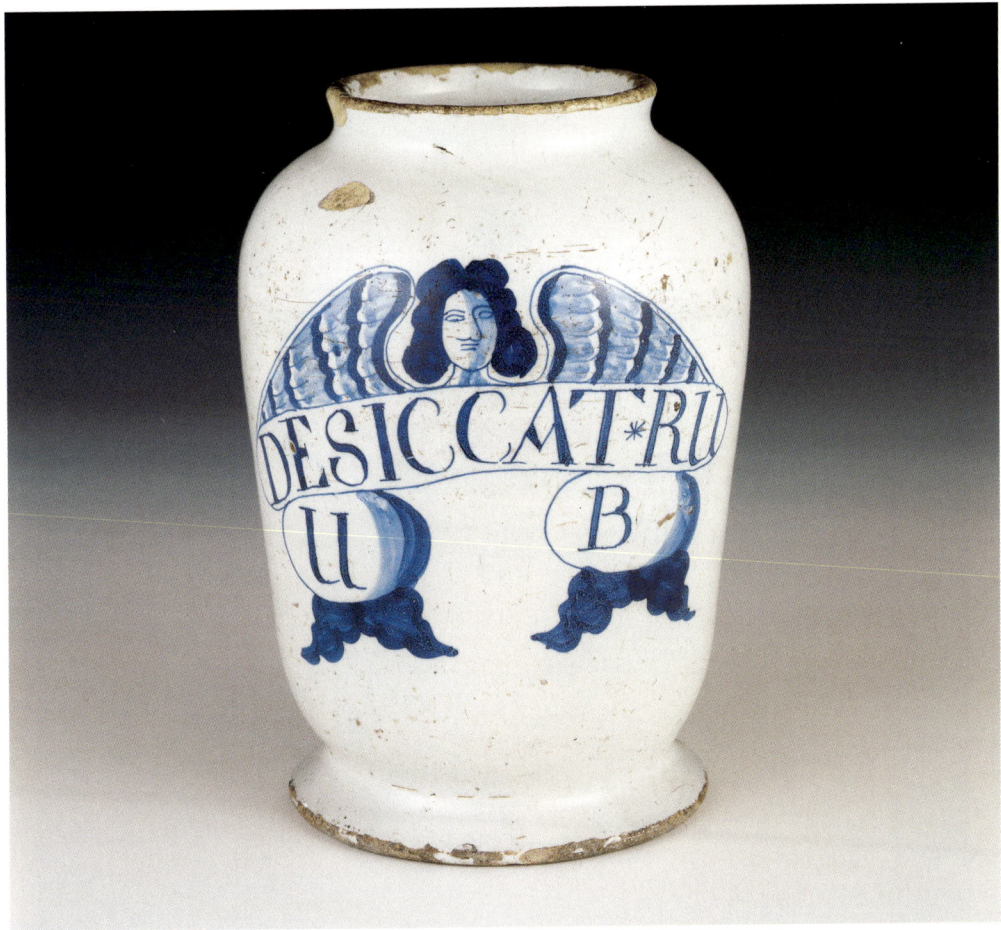

Dry drug jar (Cat.112)

ACCESSION NUMBER: KCG13

DESCRIPTION: Ovoid jar, tapering slightly towards splayed base. White glaze with pinkish tinge and design in blue. Label panel curved slightly upwards with even outline. Neck slightly everted with unglazed rim, very slightly concave glazed base with unglazed edge.

DESIGN: Angel with outspread wings.

INSCRIPTION: U DESICCAT RU B

MEANING OF INSCRIPTION: *Unguent desiccativium rubrum,* red desiccating/drying ointment

CONTEMPORARY ACCOUNT: "'Take Oil of Roses ℔ i. White Wax ʒ v. Melt them together, and mix with them in a Leaden Mortar, finely powder'd, *Lemnian* Earth (or Bole) and Calamine, ana ʒ iv. Letharge and Ceruss, ana ʒ iii. Camphor ʒ i. S.A.'

The Powders in this Medicine are in an Over-proportion, which make it too dry and hard for an Unguent, being almost of the Consistence of a *Cerate*. It drys, cools, and repels, and is pretty much in use for those Intentions; but so much for Kibes, which Children are very subject to in frosty Weather, that it is often ask'd for by the common People by the name of Kibe-Ointment; for it colls and cicatrizes them very soon." (J. Quincy, *A Compleat English Dispensatory*, 1718, p. 459)

DATE OF MANUFACTURE: 1680–1700

PLACE OF MANUFACTURE: London

DIMENSIONS: Height 185 mm, maximum width 138 mm

PROVENANCE: Bought in 1957, Howard Collection.

CONDITION: Good; neck chipped, glaze repaired on back of jar and above label and flaked from rim of base.

COMMENT: Howard suggests that this is "a much finer piece of draughtsmanship than usual". He claims that the angel's wig dates this jar to the reigns of William and Mary, or James II (p. 17). There are two other jars from this very distinctive set in private collections in London (S. AVRANT) and Scotland (O. HYPERICI), and four others (with moustaches that point downwards and straight barred 'A's) in the Wilkinson Collection in the Thackray Museum, Leeds (C. SAMBUC, C. LAMIJ, E. MITHRIDAT and O. HYPERIRI).

REFERENCE: Howard, English Delftware Drug Jars, p. 17 and No. 33.

Angel with outspread wings

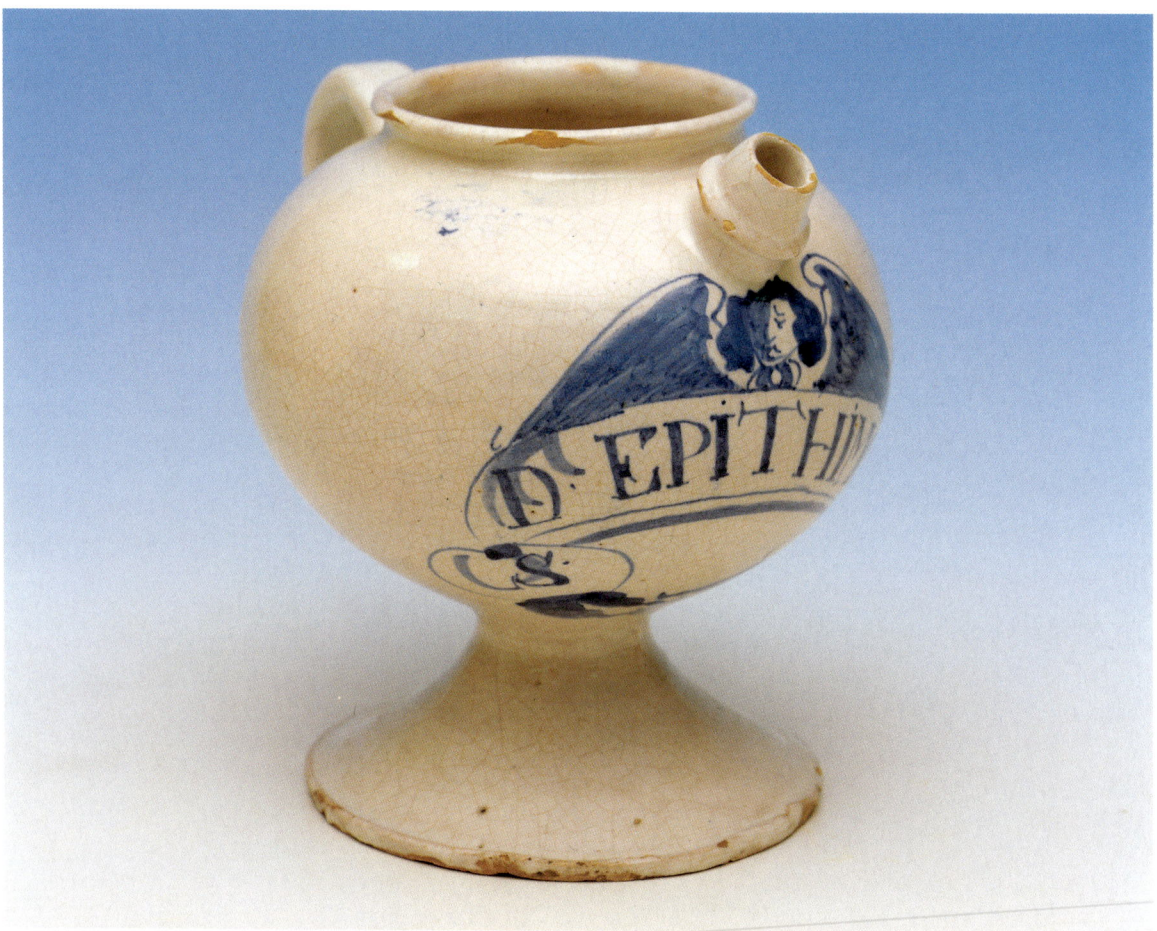

Wet drug jar (Cat.117)

ACCESSION NUMBER: KDG9

DESCRIPTION: Bulbous jar on spreading foot, with spout and strap-like looped handle. White glaze with pinkish tinge and design in blue. Label panel curved slightly upwards with even outline. Neck everted with glazed rim, flanged spout, hollowed, unglazed base.

DESIGN: Angel with outspread wings.

INSCRIPTION: S D EPITHIMO

MEANING OF INSCRIPTION: *Syrupus de epithimo*, syrup of dodder of thyme (*Cuscuta epithymum*)

CONTEMPORARY ACCOUNT: "Take of Epithimum twenty drams, Mirobalans, Citron and Indian of each fifteen drams, Emblicks, Bellericks, Polypodium, Liquoris, Agrick, Time, Calaminth, Bugloss, Stoechas of each six drachms, Dodder, Fumitory, of each ten drachms, red Roses, Annis seeds, and sweet Fennel seeds of each two drachms and a half, sweet Prunes ten, Raisons of the sun stoned four ounces, Tamarinds two ounces and a half; after twenty four hours infusion in ten pints of spring water, boyl it away to six, then take it from the fire and strain it, and with five pound of fine Sugar boyl it into a syrup according to art ... It purgeth Melancholly, and other humours, it strengtheneth the stomach and Liver, clenseth the body of addust choler and addust blood, as also of salt humours, and helps diseases proceeding from these, as scabs, itch, tetters, ringworms, leprosie &c. ..." (N. Culpeper, *Pharmacopoeia Londoniensis*, 1653, p. 109)

DATE OF MANUFACTURE: 1660–1725

PLACE OF MANUFACTURE: London

DIMENSIONS: Height 170 mm, maximum width 165 mm

PROVENANCE: Bequest, Saville Peck, 1955.

CONDITION: Good; 1 cm diameter hole in base, neck chipped, glaze crazed and flaked from spout and neck and base rims.

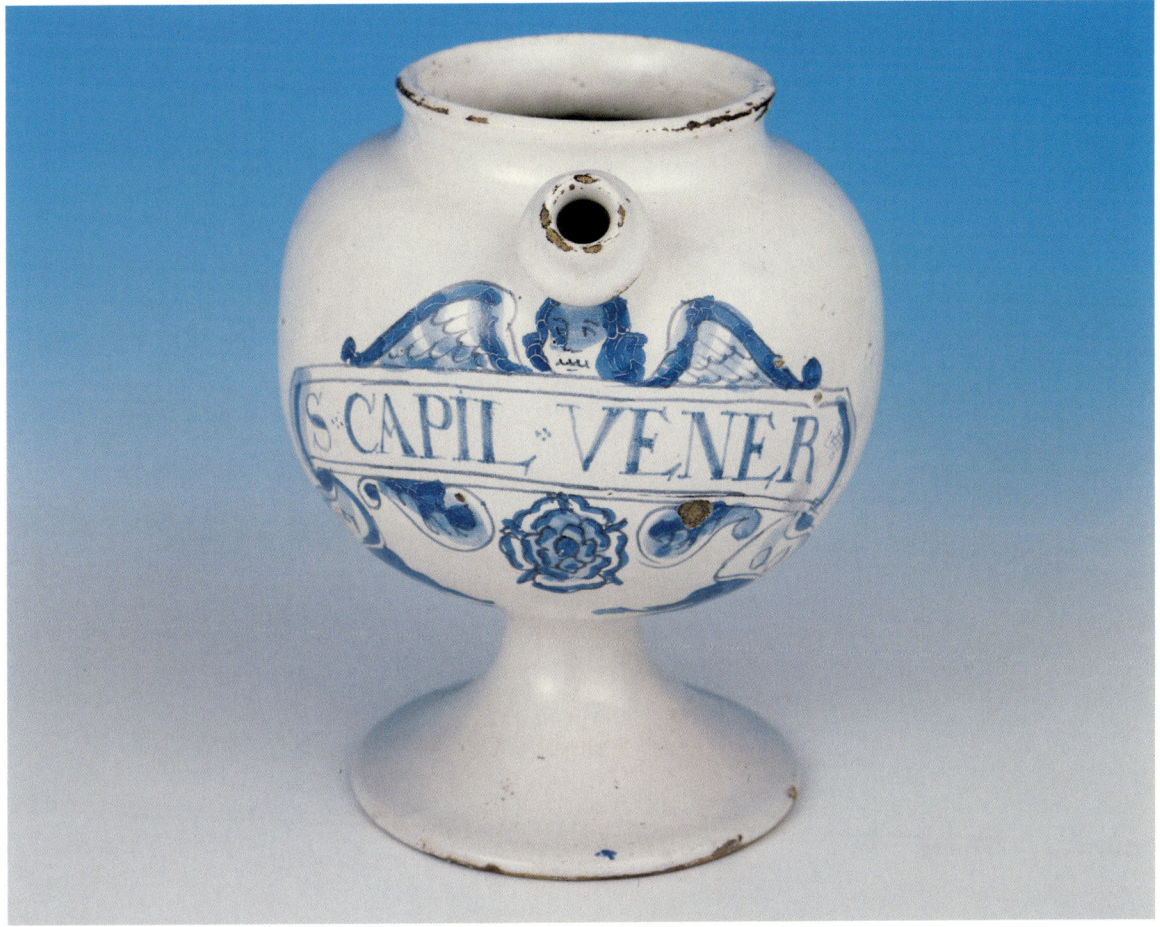

Wet drug jar (Cat.118)

ACCESSION NUMBER: KBG10

DESCRIPTION: Bulbous jar on spreading foot, with spout and fluted strap-like looped handle. White glaze with pinkish tinge and design in blue. Label panel curved slightly upwards, framed in two thin even lines. Neck ridged with glazed rim, flanged spout, hollowed and glazed base with unglazed edge.

DESIGN: Angel with outspread wings and rose

INSCRIPTION: 17 S CAPIL VENER 00

MEANING OF INSCRIPTION: *Syrupus capillorum veneris*, syrup of maidenhair fern (*Adiantum capillus-Veneris*), made from small pieces of maidenhair fern, boiled with water, the whites of two eggs and sugar. Orange flower water was added for flavour.

CONTEMPORARY ACCOUNT: (White): "This is very plentiful about *Narbon* in *France*. It grows likewise in many places in *England*, chiefly on rocky Ground. It is used in Decays of the lungs; and therefore enters much into the Composition of *Pectorals*, both in the Shops and common Prescription. It is also esteem'd as an *Epatick*, and a Remover of Obstructions in the Kidneys, and likewise a Promoter of the *Menses*; but it is not much used in those Intentions."

(Black): "This is also used in the same Intentions as the former, and is reckon'd good in Coughs, Asthma's, Pleurisies, Jaundice, and Obstructions of the Spleen and Kidneys; tho not greatly used for those purposes..." (J. Quincy, *A Compleat English Dispensatory*, 1718, p. 115)

DATE OF MANUFACTURE: 1700

PLACE OF MANUFACTURE: London

DIMENSIONS: Height 190 mm, maximum width 165 mm

PROVENANCE: Bought in 1957, Howard Collection. Published by J. E. Hodgkin (see below), which suggests that the jar was part of his collection in 1891. Sold from the collection of Mrs Radford by Sotheby's, 3/11/1943 (part lot 10).

CONDITION: Good; 1 cm of glaze flaked from below label, glaze flaked from handle and spout and neck and base rims.

REFERENCES: Hodgkin, Examples of Early English Pottery.
Lipski and Archer, Dated English Delftware, No. 1662.

Angel with outspread wings

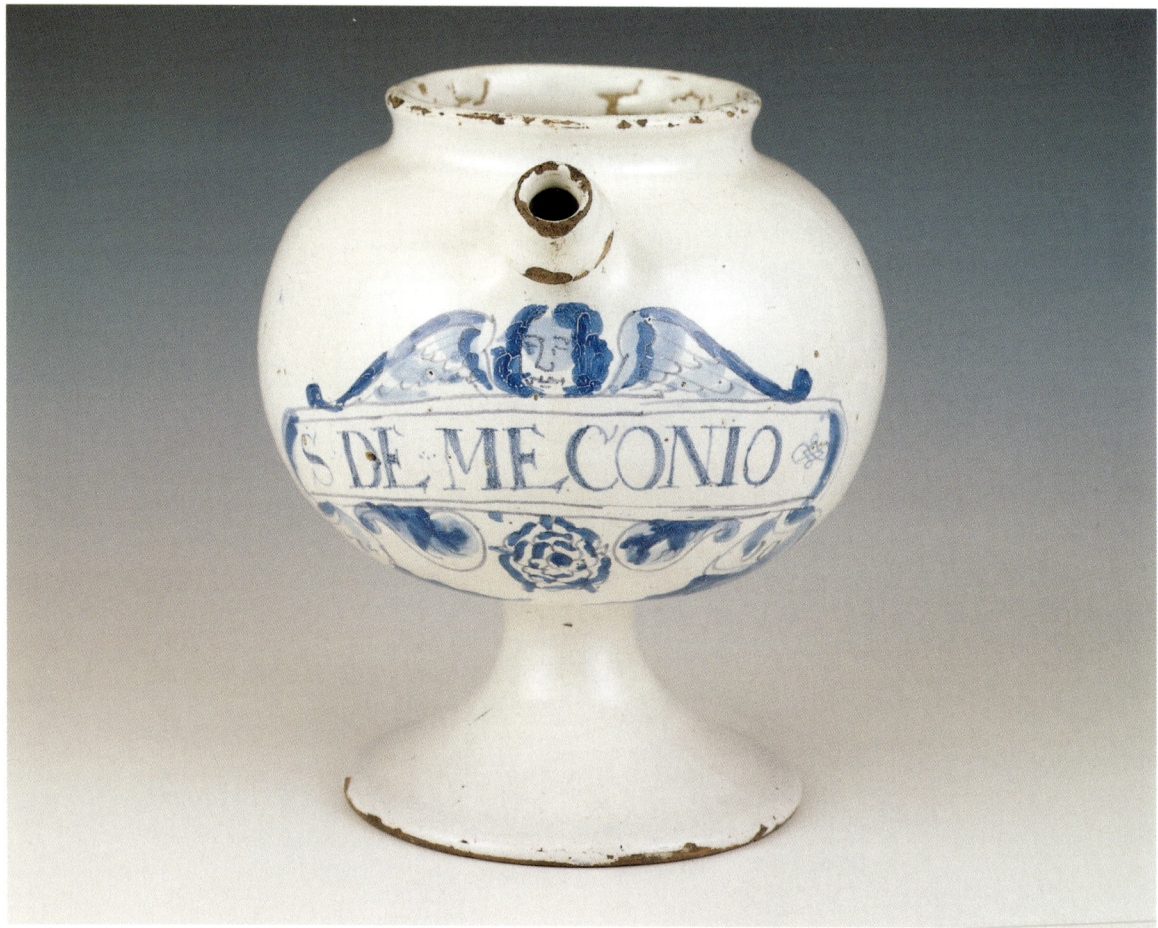

Wet drug jar (Cat. 119)

ACCESSION NUMBER: KBG9
DESCRIPTION: Bulbous jar on spreading foot, with spout and fluted strap-like handle. White glaze with pinkish tinge and design in blue. Label panel straight, framed in two thin even lines. Neck ridged with glazed rim, flanged spout, hollowed glazed base with unglazed edge.
DESIGN: Angel with outspread wings and rose
INSCRIPTION: 17 S DE MECONIO 00
MEANING OF INSCRIPTION: *Syrupus de meconio*, weak syrup of poppy (*Papaver somniferum*)
CONTEMPORARY ACCOUNT: "'Take Garden white Poppy-Heads with their Seeds ℔ ss. Heads of black Poppies ℨ vi. Steep them well bruised in ℔ viii. of Water 24 hours, and then boil it to ℔ iii. Press the Liquor out hard, and boil it up to a Syrup with ℔ iss. of white Sugar.'

"This, considering the Importance of its Intention, and the Certainty with which it answers it, is a better Medicine, and does more good than all under this Division besides put together. This ought by no means to be clarify'd, because it robs it of its chief Properties… This is used to procure Sleep, in which it acts as any other *Opiate*… It also, better than many other Forms of this kind, stops *Defluxions* and *Catarrhs*, with all Coughs from thin Rheum. It may be given from ℨ i. to ℨ iii. to Children, and from ℨ iii. to ℥ i. to grown Persons. In making this, more Sugar is generally used than what is order'd in the *Recipe*."
(J. Quincy, *A Compleat English Dispensatory*, 1718, pp. 377–378)
DATE OF MANUFACTURE: 1700
PLACE OF MANUFACTURE: London
DIMENSIONS: Height 190 mm, maximum width 170 mm
PROVENANCE: Bought in 1957, Howard Collection. Label found on jar reads: Fenton & Sons, 11, New Oxford Street, London. Published by J. E. Hodgkin (see below), which suggests that the jar was part of his collection in 1891. Sold from the collection of Mrs Radford by Sotheby's, 3/11/1943 (part lot 10).
CONDITION: Good; two cracks encircling handle, glaze flaked on spout and handle and rims of neck and base.
REFERENCES: Hodgkin, Examples of Early English Pottery.
Lipski and Archer, Dated English Delftware, No. 1662A.

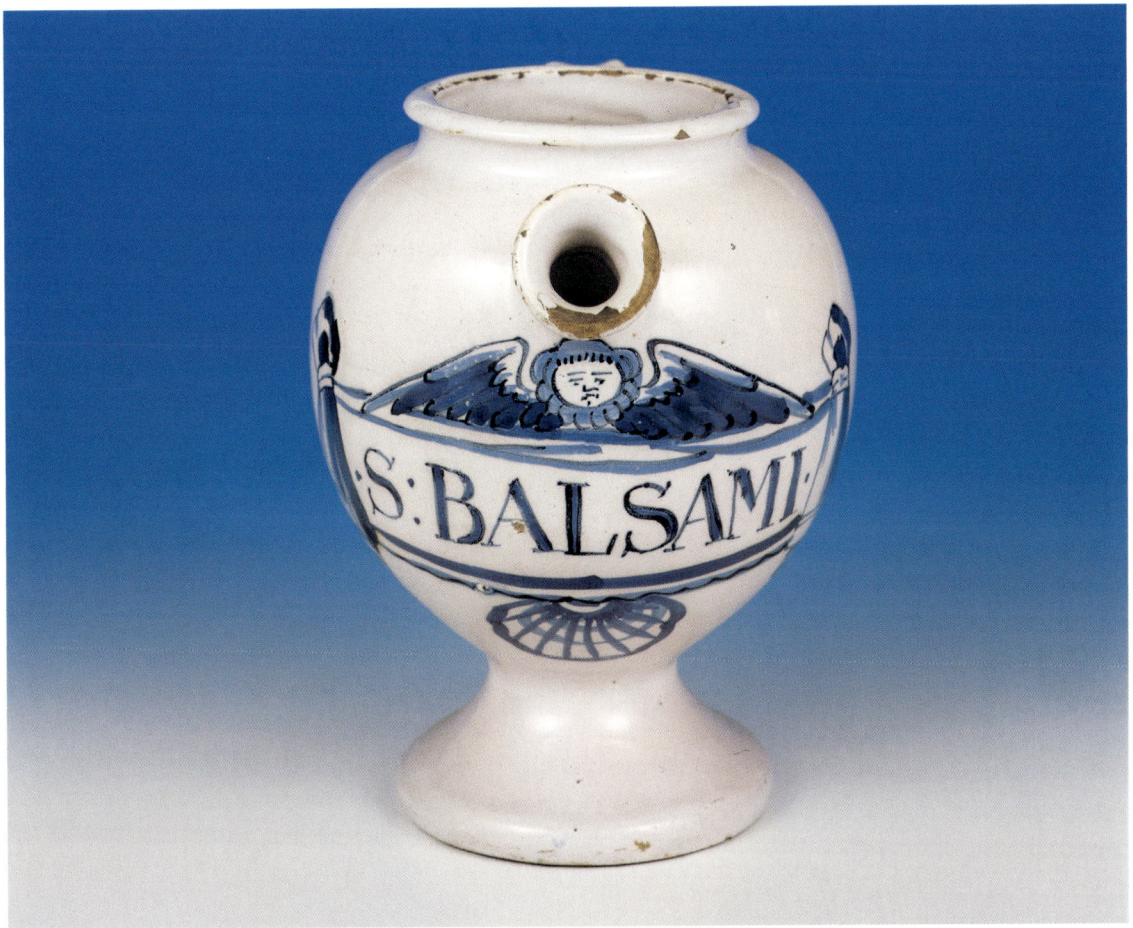

Wet drug jar (Cat.120)

ACCESSION NUMBER: KDG3

DESCRIPTION: Bulbous jar on spreading foot, with spout and fluted strap-like looped handle. White glaze with pinkish tinge and design in blue. Label panel straight, outlined with two thick lines. Neck everted with flat glazed rim, flared spout, hollowed base with unglazed edge.

DESIGN: Angel with outspread wings and with shell

INSCRIPTION: S:BALSAMI

MEANING OF INSCRIPTION: *Syrupus balsamicus*, balsamic syrup

CONTEMPORARY ACCOUNT: "'Take Balsam of *Tolu* ℥ ii. Colts-Foot-Water ℥ xii. Boil them in a circulatory Vessel with the Juncture well luted, in a Sand-Heat three hours. When it is cold, in the strain'd Water by degrees dissolve ℥ xx. of Sugar without any heat.'

"This is very judiciously contriv'd yet many neglect the Care here enjoin'd, and boil in an open Vessel, by which they lose the finer parts of the Balsam. As for the Water here order'd, common Water will do as well. But if it be done with Rose or Orange-Water, it will be a most delightful Medicine, and much more of a Cordial..." (J. Quincy, *A Compleat English Dispensatory*, 1718, pp. 384–385)

DATE OF MANUFACTURE: 1700–1725

PLACE OF MANUFACTURE: London

DIMENSIONS: Height 180 mm, maximum width 143 mm

PROVENANCE: Bought in 1957, Howard Collection.

CONDITION: Good; several hair cracks on bowl, spout chipped, glaze crazed and flaked on neck, spout and handle.

COMMENT: Howard notes that this is a pair with KDG4 (Cat. 121). Only 13 jars survive with this specific design, plus one more crudely painted jar which is probably later.

REFERENCE: Howard, English Delftware Drug Jars, pp. 19–20 and No. 32.

Angel with outspread wings

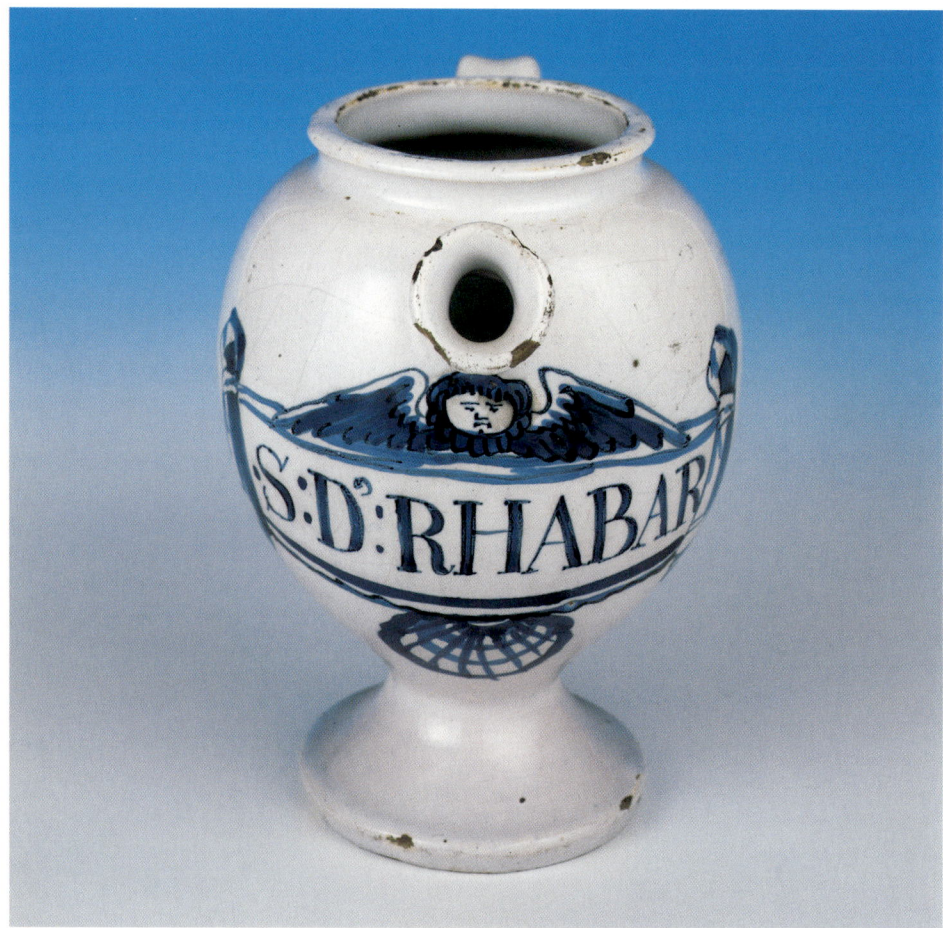

Wet drug jar (Cat.121)

ACCESSION NUMBER: KDG4

DESCRIPTION: Bulbous jar on spreading foot, with spout and fluted strap-like looped handle. White glaze with pinkish tinge and design in blue and black. Label panel straight, outlined with two thick lines. Neck everted with flat glazed rim, flared spout, hollowed and glazed base with unglazed edge.

DESIGN: Angel with outspread wings and shell

INSCRIPTION: S:D':RHABAR

MEANING OF INSCRIPTION: *Syrupus de rhabarbarum*, syrup of rhubarb

CONTEMPORARY ACCOUNT: "'Take Rhabarb, Sena, ana ʒ iiss. Violet-Flowers m.i. Cinnamon ʒ iss. Ginger ʒ ss. Waters of Betony, Succory, and Bugloss, ana ℔ iss. Steep together some time, then boil it, and make up the strain'd liquor into a Syrup with fine Sugar ℔ ii. and Syrup of Roses solutive ʒ iv.'

"The Virtues of this may be judg'd by the Rhubar and *Sena*, for the other Ingredients are good for nothing; and even the Spices, as Correctors, in such small quantities, are ridiculous: as likewise are the simple Waters, were they to be had; and therefore the Pump for them is an honest *Succedaneum*. The Dose of this is from ʒ ss to ʒ ii." (J. Quincy, *A Compleat English Dispensatory*, 1718, p. 380)

DATE OF MANUFACTURE: 1700–1725

PLACE OF MANUFACTURE: London

DIMENSIONS: Height 180 mm, maximum width 148 mm

PROVENANCE: Bought in 1957, Howard Collection.

CONDITION: Good; several hair cracks on bowl, spout chipped, glaze crazed and flaked on neck, spout, handle and base.

COMMENT: Howard notes that this is a pair with KDG3 (Cat. 120). Only 13 jars survive with this specific design, plus one more crudely painted jar which is probably later.

REFERENCE: Howard, English Delftware Drug Jars, pp. 19–20, referred to in Plate IX, but not illustrated.

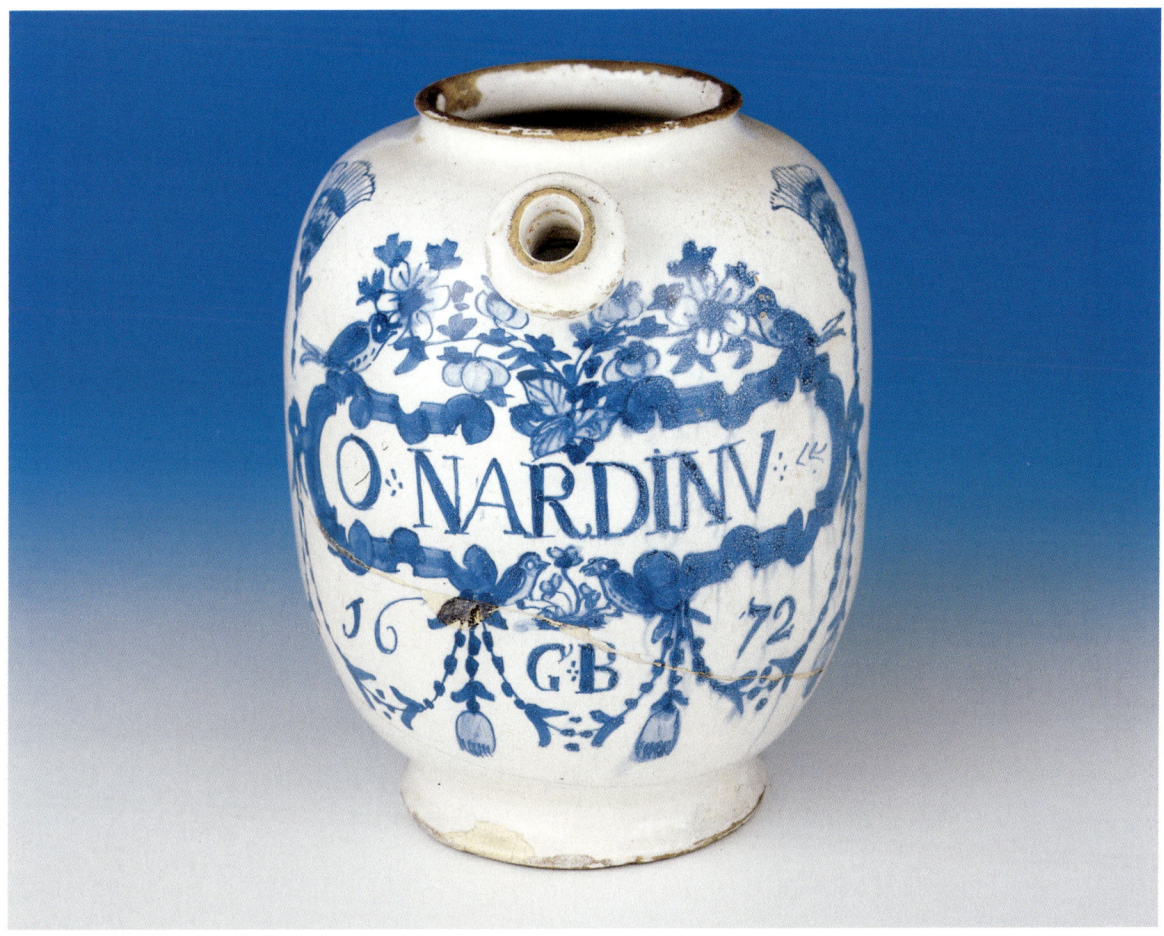

Wet drug jar (Cat.122)

ACCESSION NUMBER: KBY1

DESCRIPTION: Ovoid jar, tapering slightly towards splayed base, with spout and strap-like looped handle. White glaze with pinkish tinge and design in blue. Label panel straight with wavy strap-work frame. Neck everted with unglazed rim, flanged spout, flat unglazed base.

DESIGN: Early songbirds

INSCRIPTION: O NARDINV 16 G:B 72

MEANING OF INSCRIPTION: *Oleum nardinum*, oil of *Nardus indica*, root of Indian nard or spikenard. 'G:B' are the initials of the apothecary who commissioned the jar.

CONTEMPORARY ACCOUNT: "This is reckon'd of kin to our Lavender, both by *Family* as the *Botanists* term it, and *Virtues*. It grows in many parts of *Germany* and *Italy*, and particularly on the Mountains of *Tyrol*. It is esteem'd as an *Alexipharmick*, being warm and spicy, and helpful to promote Sweating... It is likewise reckon'd a good *Stomachick*, a Strengthener of the Fibres, and a Dispeller of Wind and crude Flatulencies."
(J. Quincy, *A Compleat English Dispensatory*, 1718, p. 169)

DATE OF MANUFACTURE: 1672

PLACE OF MANUFACTURE: London

DIMENSIONS: Height 200 mm, maximum width 170 mm

PROVENANCE: Bought in 1954 from the collection of Mrs Robert Sargeant. Previously in C. Hemming's collection and sold by Sotheby's 1/7/1947 (lot 42).

CONDITION: Poor; large cracks encircling bowl, has been repaired, base and handle chipped and cracked, glaze flaked off from handle, spout and base and neck rims.

COMMENT: The apothecary who commissioned the jar could have been George Bearcroft (Hoffbrand and Cook, p. 33). There is a second jar from this set in a private collection in London.

REFERENCES: Hoffbrand and Cook. The Victor Hoffbrand Collection p. 33.
   Lipski and Archer, Dated English Delftware, No. 1629.
   Hemming. Lambeth Delft. p. 195, Pl.II, centre.

Apollo

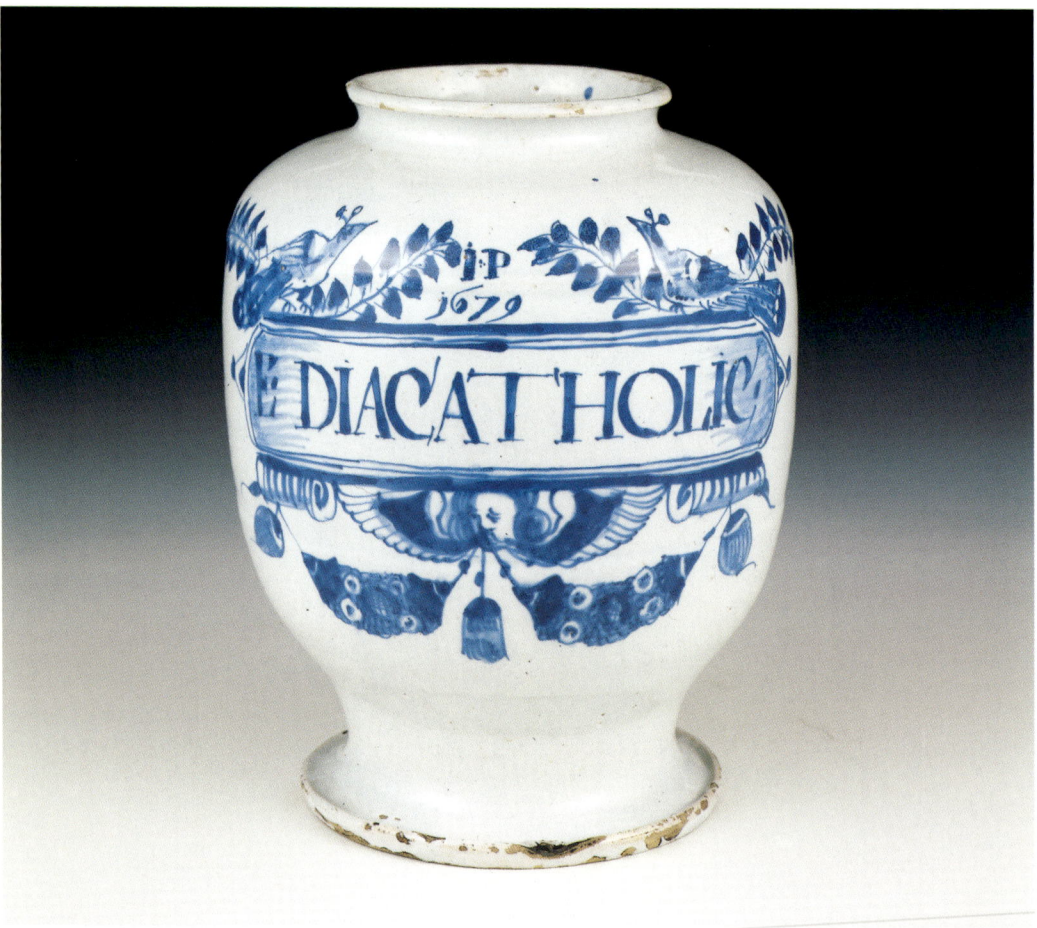

Dry drug jar (Cat.123)

ACCESSION NUMBER: KAY1

DESCRIPTION: Ovoid jar, tapering slightly towards splayed and ridged base, with two narrow ridges encircling bowl, one below the neck and the other below the label. White glaze with bluish tinge and design in blue. Label panel straight, framed with two thin even lines and thicker (outer) third line. Neck everted with glazed rim, flat unglazed base.

DESIGN: Apollo and peacocks, with initials and date in place of Apollo.

INSCRIPTION: E.DIACATHOLIC. I:P 1679

MEANING OF INSCRIPTION: *Electuarium diacatholicon*, a purgative electuary. 'I:P' are the initials of the apothecary who commissioned the jar.

CONTEMPORARY ACCOUNT: "'Take Polypody of the Oak ℥ iii. Sweet Fennel-Seeds ℥ vi. Boil in a sufficient quantity of Water to ℔ ii. To the strain'd Liquor put Sugar ℔ ii. and boil to the Consistence of a thick Syrup, to which add Sena in Powder ℥ ii. Violets, Polypody, Rhubarb, ana ℥ i. Aniseeds, Penydates, Sugar-Candy, Liquorice, and of the four greater cold Seeds, ana ℥ ii.

Pulps of Cassia and Tamarinds, ana ℥ ii. and stir them all together.'

"This is used as a gentle Lenitive, but wears much out of practice, and is now seldom order'd." (J. Quincy, *A Compleat English Dispensatory*, 1718, p. 402)

DATE OF MANUFACTURE: 1679

PLACE OF MANUFACTURE: London

DIMENSIONS: Height 195 mm, maximum width 160 mm

PROVENANCE: Bought in 1957, Howard Collection.

CONDITION: Good; neck and base chipped, glaze flaked from neck and base rims.

COMMENT: There are four jars from this set known: this jar, one in the Greg Collection, City Art Gallery, Manchester, and two whose current whereabouts are unknown (C. LVIVLAE illustrated in 'The Queen', May 1907, later sold at Sotheby's (lot 3) on 3/11/1943 from Mrs Radford's collection, and DIASCORDIV Illustrated Horne XV 1995, No. 417).

REFERENCES: Lipski and Archer, Dated English Delftware, No. 1645A.

Lothian. Vessels for Apothecaries. p. x and Plate No. XXVIII.

'The Queen', Vol. III, May 1907, Fig. 3, collection of Mr B. Butler of Reading.

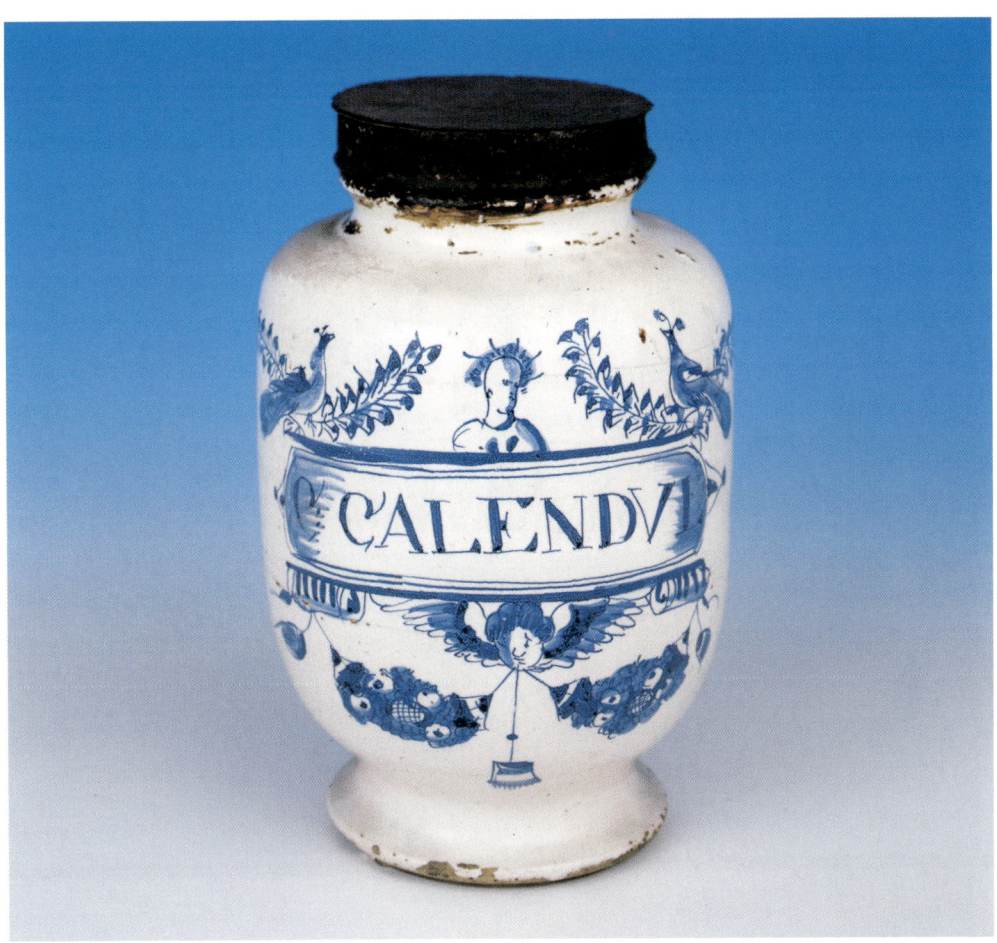

Dry drug jar (Cat.124)

ACCESSION NUMBER: KCI6
DESCRIPTION: Ovoid jar, tapering slightly towards splayed base, with two faint narrow ridges encircling bowl, one below the neck and the other below the label. White glaze with pinkish tinge and design in blue. Label panel straight, framed in two thin even lines and thicker (outer) third line. Neck ridged with glazed rim, slightly concave unglazed base. Metal lid.
DESIGN: Apollo and peacocks.
INSCRIPTION: C:CALENDVL
MEANING OF INSCRIPTION: *Conserva calendula*, conserve of marigold flower (*Calendula officinalis*)
CONTEMPORARY ACCOUNT: "These blow almost all the Summer. They are well known in the Kitchin as well as the Shops. Amongst Physical Writers they pass for *Alexipharmicks*, tho in a much inferior degree to *Saffron*, which it is compar'd to. Many also speak of them as *Hystericks*… They are an Ingredient in the *Plague-Water*… The *Conserve* … is hardly ever made, or to be met with in Prescription." (J. Quincy, *A Compleat English Dispensatory*, 1718, p. 163)

DATE OF MANUFACTURE: 1675–1700
PLACE OF MANUFACTURE: Probably Southwark, London
COMMENT: Howard notes that this is one of a set of 14 jars (p. 21). These are KCI1-13 and KDI1 (Cat. 124–137).
DIMENSIONS: Height 198 mm, maximum width 143 mm
PROVENANCE: Bought in 1957, Howard Collection.
CONDITION: Good; base chipped, some glaze missing from shoulder, glaze flaked on rim of base, some pitting.
REFERENCE: Howard, English Delftware Drug Jars, p. 21, referred to in Plate XII, but not illustrated.

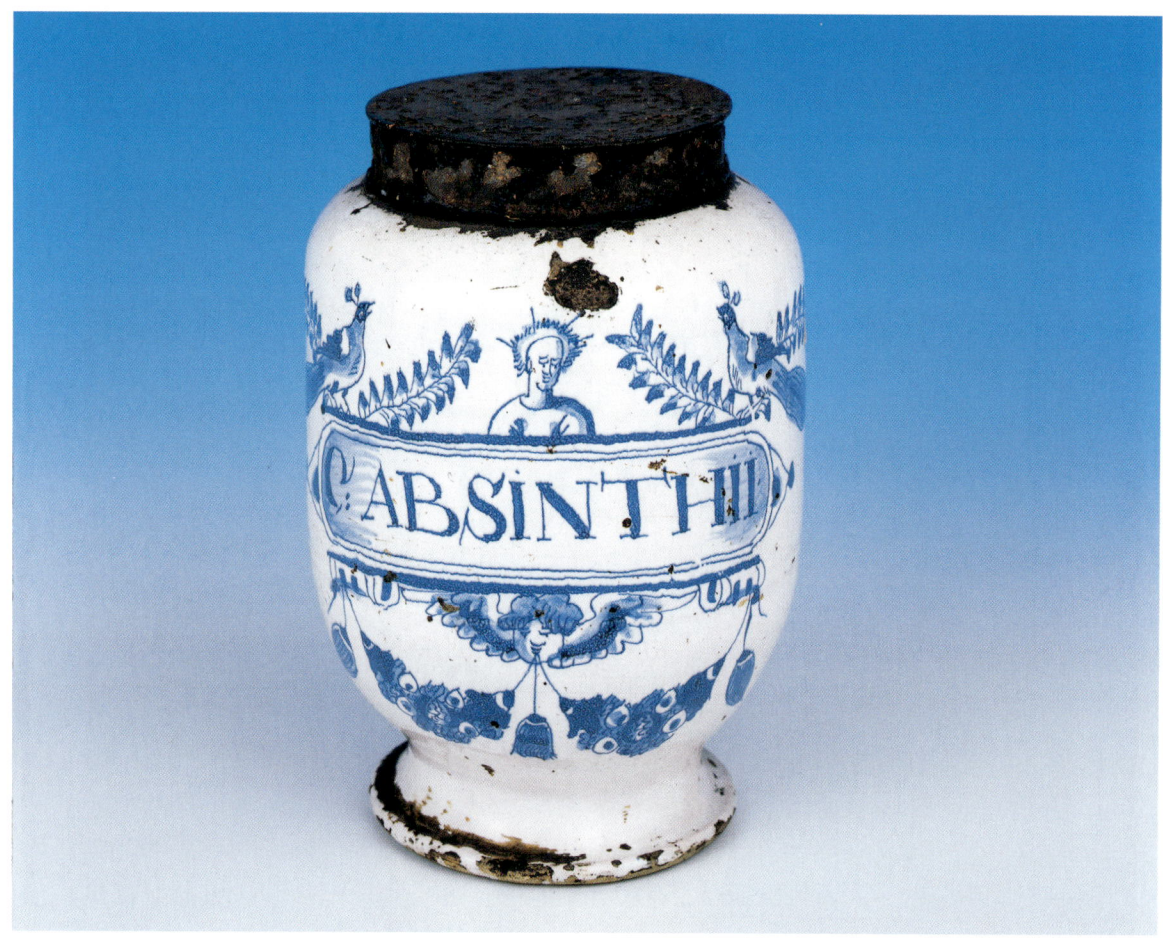

Dry drug jar (Cat.127)

ACCESSION NUMBER: KCI13
DESCRIPTION: Ovoid jar, tapering slightly towards splayed base, and with two faint ridges encircling bowl, one below the neck and the other below the label. White glaze with pinkish tinge and design in blue. Label panel straight, framed in two thin even lines and thicker (outer) third line. Neck has fixed metal lid, slightly concave unglazed base.
DESIGN: Apollo and peacocks.
INSCRIPTION: C:ABSINTHII
MEANING OF INSCRIPTION: *Conserva absinthii*, conserve of wormwood (*Artemisia absinthium*)
CONTEMPORARY ACCOUNT: "It is not by much so bitter as the *common Wormwood*, but is a much more grateful *Stomatick*. It astringes, incides, discusses, prevents Putrefaction, and carries off *Choler* by *Urine*; whereupon it is good in all Disorders of the *Liver*, and abates Pains and Wind in the Stomach and Bowels... A Conserve made of it, is now much in use in the Shops." (J. Quincy, *A Compleat English Dispensatory*, 1718, p. 109)
DATE OF MANUFACTURE: 1675–1700

PLACE OF MANUFACTURE: Probably Southwark, London
DIMENSIONS: Height 200 mm, maximum width 145 mm
PROVENANCE: Bought in 1957, Howard Collection.
CONDITION: Good; glaze flaked on body and rim of base.
COMMENT: Howard notes that this is one of a set of 14 jars (p. 21). These are KCI1-13 and KDI1 (Cat. 124–137).
REFERENCE: Howard, English Delftware Drug Jars, p. 21, referred to in Plate XII, but not illustrated.

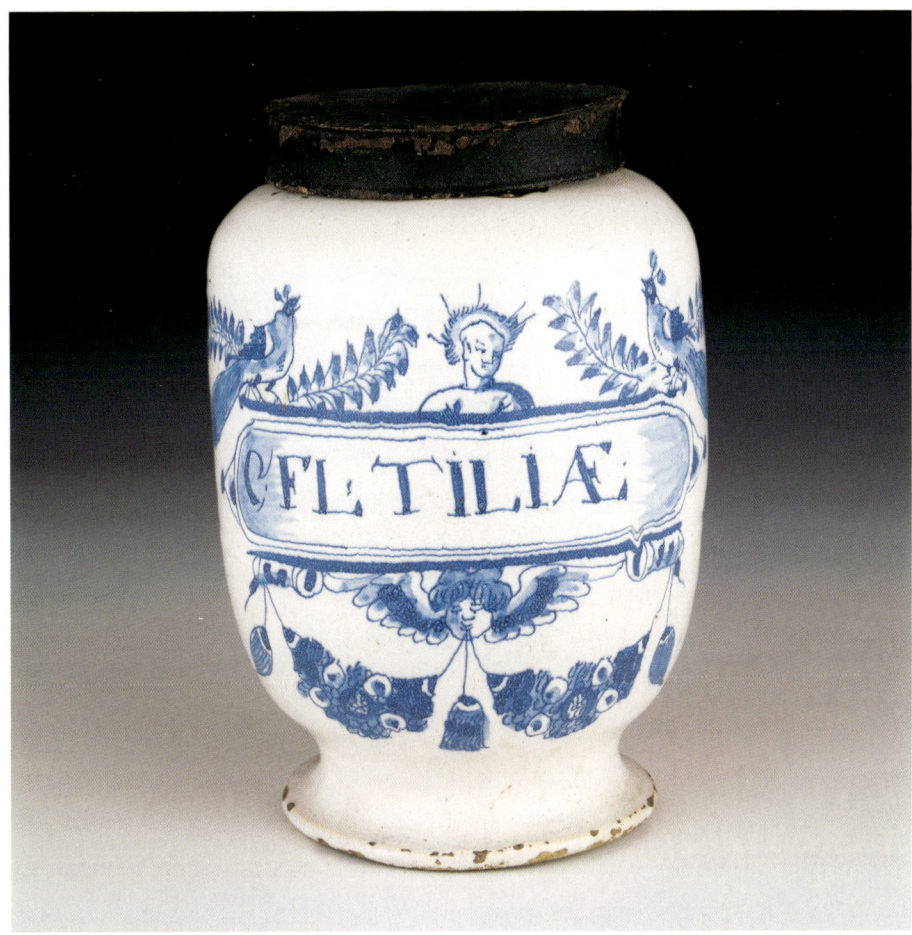

Dry drug jar (Cat.128)

ACCESSION NUMBER: KCI5
DESCRIPTION: Ovoid jar, tapering slightly towards splayed base, with two faint narrow lines encircling bowl, one below the neck and the other below the label. White glaze with pinkish tinge and design in blue. Label panel straight, framed in two thin even lines and thicker (outer) third line. Neck ridged with glazed rim, slightly concave unglazed base. Metal lid.
DESIGN: Apollo and peacocks.
INSCRIPTION: C FL TILIAE
MEANING OF INSCRIPTION: *Conserva de floribus tiliae*, conserve of lime flowers. It was prepared by boiling fresh lime flowers with sugar and water.
CONTEMPORARY ACCOUNT: "They are universally recommended in Epilepsies, and all nervous Distempers." (J. Quincy, *A Compleat English Dispensatory*, 1718, p. 82)
DATE OF MANUFACTURE: 1675–1700
PLACE OF MANUFACTURE: Southwark, London
DIMENSIONS: Height 200 mm, maximum width 140 mm
PROVENANCE: Bought in 1957, Howard Collection.

CONDITION: Good; rim of base chipped, glaze flaked from rim of base, some pitting.
COMMENT: Howard notes that this is one of a set of 14 jars (p. 21). These are KCI1-13 and KDI1 (Cat. 124–137).
REFERENCE: Howard, English Delftware Drug Jars, p. 21, referred to in Plate XII, but not illustrated.

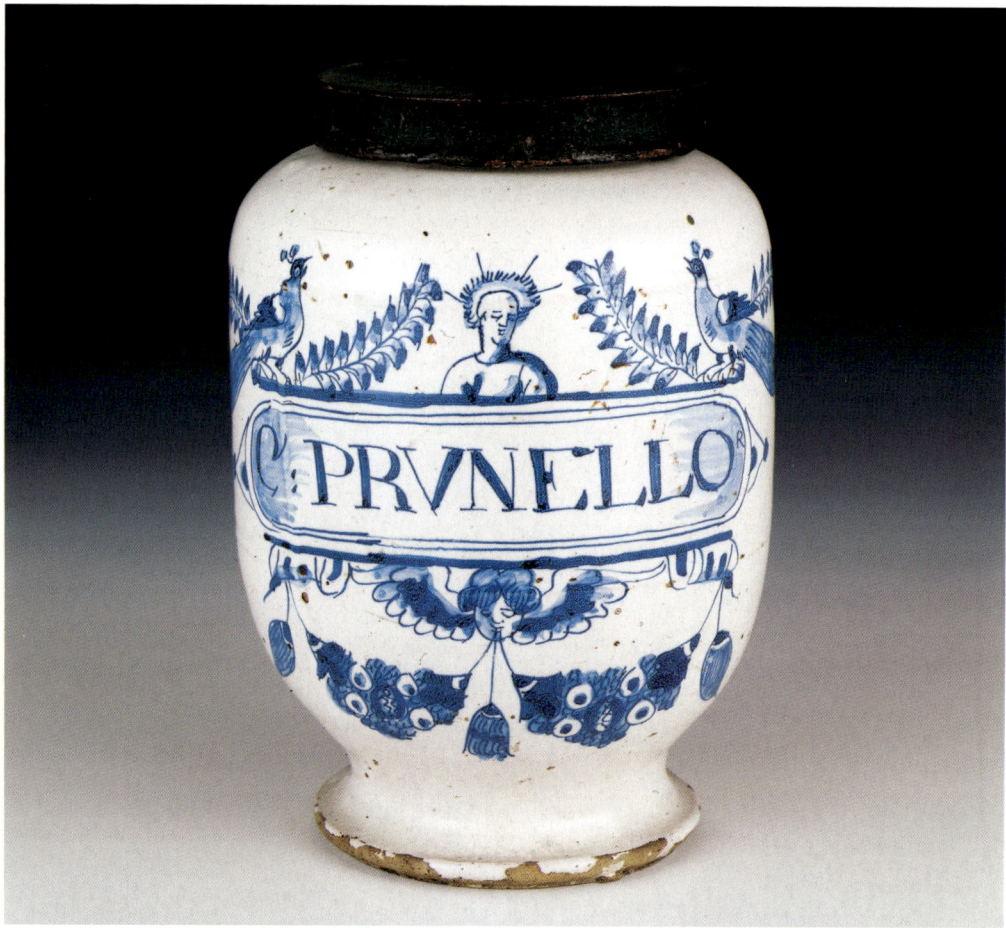

Dry drug jar (Cat.129)

ACCESSION NUMBER: KCI3

DESCRIPTION: Ovoid jar, tapering slightly towards splayed base, with two narrow ridges encircling bowl, one below the neck and the other below the label. White glaze with pinkish tinge and design in blue. Label straight, framed in two thin even lines and thicker (outer) third line. Neck ridged with glazed rim, slightly concave unglazed base. Metal lid.

DESIGN: Apollo and peacocks.

INSCRIPTION: C:PRVNELLOR

MEANING OF INSCRIPTION: *Conserva prunellorum*, conserve of sloes (*Prunellorum sylvestris*)

CONTEMPORARY ACCOUNT: "We have in the Shops a Conserve made with them, which with care is a very good one. For this purpose they are to be gather'd before they begin to wither and mellow upon the Trees; for after they are frostbit, as the Country-People call it, to make them fit for eating, they are not so rough, and consequently not so suitable for this Intention in Medicine. In Looseness of the Belly they are effectual in stopping it; but sometimes they tye the Bowels up so much as to throw the Patient into the contrary Extreme. Caution therefore is to be taken in their Prescription; and generally some Aromatick Mixtures are necessary to prevent those Gripings, which otherwise their Coldness and Roughness are apt to occasion." (J. Quincy, *A Compleat English Dispensatory*, 1718, pp. 100–101)

DATE OF MANUFACTURE: 1675–1700

PLACE OF MANUFACTURE: Probably Southwark, London

DIMENSIONS: Height 200 mm, maximum width 145 mm

PROVENANCE: Bought in 1957, Howard Collection.

CONDITION: Good; several hair cracks on bowl, glaze crazed and flaked on rim of base, some pitting.

COMMENT: Howard notes that this is one of a set of 14 jars (p. 21). These are KCI1-13 and KDI1 (Cat. 124–137). Note that the final letter (R) of the inscription has been added, presumably as an afterthought due to lack of space.

REFERENCE: Howard, English Delftware Drug Jars, p. 21, referred to in Plate XII, but not illustrated.

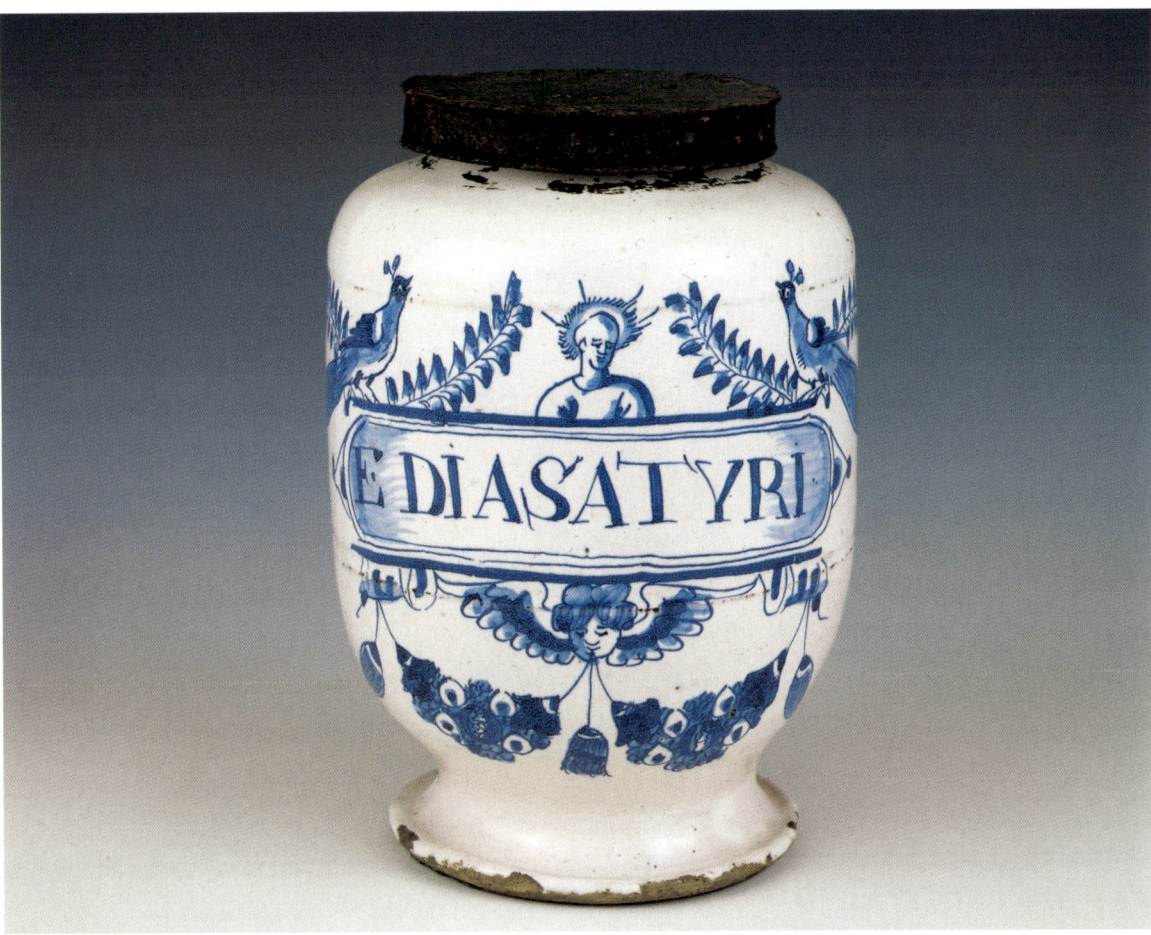

Dry drug jar (Cat.130)

ACCESSION NUMBER: KCI4

DESCRIPTION: Ovoid jar, tapering slightly towards splayed base, with two narrow ridges encircling bowl, one below the neck and the other below the label. White glaze with pinkish tinge and design in blue. Label panel straight, framed in two thin lines and thicker (outer) third line. Neck ridges with glazed rim, slightly concave unglazed base. Metal lid.

DESIGN: Apollo and peacocks.

INSCRIPTION: E DIASATYRI

MEANING OF INSCRIPTION: *Electuarium diasatyrion*, electuary of satyrion (*Orchis mascula*).

CONTEMPORARY ACCOUNT: "The *Electuarium Diasatyrion*, which is in many Dispensatories, and which takes its name from this Root [satyrion], is certainly with good reason commended for a great Strengthener; and it wonderfully warms and titillates the Nerves, whereby such Desires are excited: and on the like account in many Constitutions may cure Barrenness, and promote Conception. But as there are some warm *Aromaticks* in that Compositions besides, it is to be doubted whether they do not come in for the greatest share in these Effects." (J. Quincy, *A Compleat English Dispensatory*, 1718, p. 86)

DATE OF MANUFACTURE: 1675–1700

PLACE OF MANUFACTURE: Southwark, London

DIMENSIONS: Height 198 mm, maximum width 145 mm

PROVENANCE: Bought in 1957, Howard Collection.

CONDITION: Good; glaze flaked from rim of base, some pitting.

COMMENT: Howard notes that this is one of a set of 14 jars (p. 21). These are KCI1-13 and KDI1 (Cat. 124–137).

REFERENCE: Howard, *English Delftware Drug Jars*, p. 21 and No. 41.

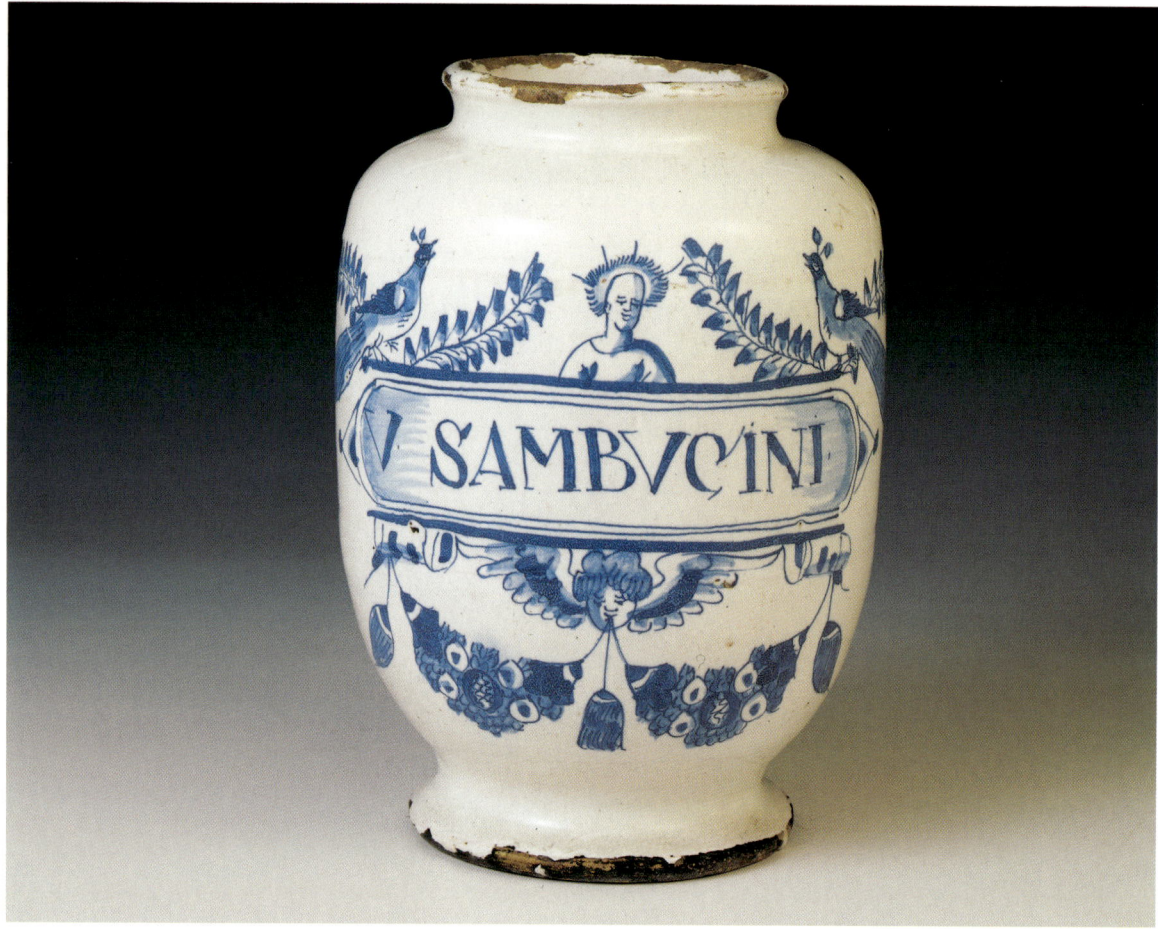

Dry drug jar (Cat.131)

ACCESSION NUMBER: KCI8

DESCRIPTION: Ovoid jar, tapering slightly towards splayed base, with two narrow ridges encircling bowl, one below the neck and the other below the label. White glaze with pinkish tinge and design in blue. Label panel straight, framed in two thin even lines and thicker (outer) third line. Neck ridged with glazed rim, slightly concave unglazed base.

DESIGN: Apollo and peacocks

INSCRIPTION: V SAMBVCINI

MEANING OF INSCRIPTION: *Unguentum Sambucinum*, ointment of bark, flowers and berries of the elder (*Sambucus nigra*)

CONTEMPORARY ACCOUNT: "A good Ingredient for all those Compositions which are intended against Distempers from Obstructions of the *Viscera*, and particularly of the *Liver* and *Kidneys*; for it mightily cleanses the former, and promotes the Passage and Separation of *Urine* through the latter. It is likewise accounted a good *Antiscorbutick*, and given in many Compositions of that Intention." (J. Quincy, *A Compleat English Dispensatory*, 1718, p. 139)

DATE OF MANUFACTURE: 1675–1700

PLACE OF MANUFACTURE: Southwark, London

DIMENSIONS: Height 195 mm, maximum width 145 mm

PROVENANCE: Bought in 1957, Howard Collection.

CONDITION: Good; rims of base and neck chipped, glaze flaked on rim of neck and base, some pitting.

COMMENT: Howard notes that this is one of a set of 14 jars (p. 21). These are KCI1-13 and KDI1 (Cat. 124–137).

REFERENCE: Howard, English Delftware Drug Jars, p. 21, referred to in Plate XII, but not illustrated.

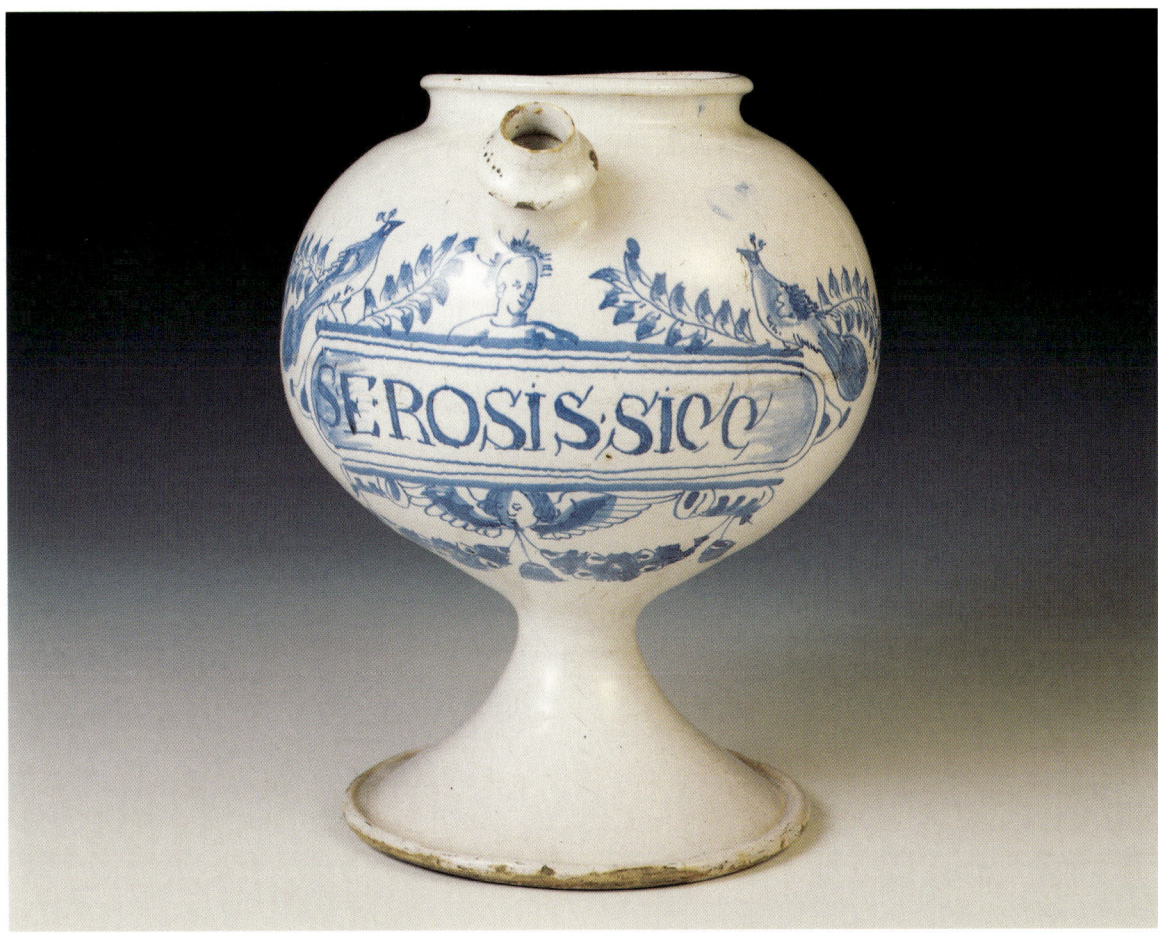

Wet drug jar (Cat.132)

ACCESSION NUMBER: KDI1
DESCRIPTION: Bulbous jar on spreading foot, with spout and
fluted strap-like looped handle. White glaze with pinkish tinge
and design in blue. Label panel straight, framed in two thin even
lines and thicker outer line. Neck ridged with glazed rim, flanged
spout, ridged, hollowed and unglazed base.
DESIGN: Apollo and peacocks
INSCRIPTION: S E ROSIS SICC
MEANING OF INSCRIPTION: *Syrupus e rosis siccis*, syrup of
dried roses
CONTEMPORARY ACCOUNT: "'Take ℔ iv of hot Spring
Water, and in it infuse ℔ ss of Rose Leaves hastily dried in the
Sun; the next day press out the Liquor, and with ℔ ii of Sugar
boil it up to a Syrup, S. A.'

"This stands ordered so antiently as by Mesue, and has been
retained the same, in all the Dispensatories of the College: but it
is very rarely made or prescribed." (J. Quincy, *A Compleat
English Dispensatory*, 1718, p. 400)
DATE OF MANUFACTURE: 1675–1700

PLACE OF MANUFACTURE: Southwark, London
DIMENSIONS: Height 200 mm, maximum width 165 mm
PROVENANCE: Bought in 1957, Howard Collection.
CONDITION: Good; base chipped, glaze crazed and flaked from
handle, spout, neck and base rims.
COMMENT: Howard notes that this is one of a set of 14 jars
(p. 21). These are KCI1-13 and KDI1 (Cat. 124–137).
REFERENCE: Howard, *English Delftware Drug Jars*, p. 21,
referred to in Plate XII, but not illustrated.

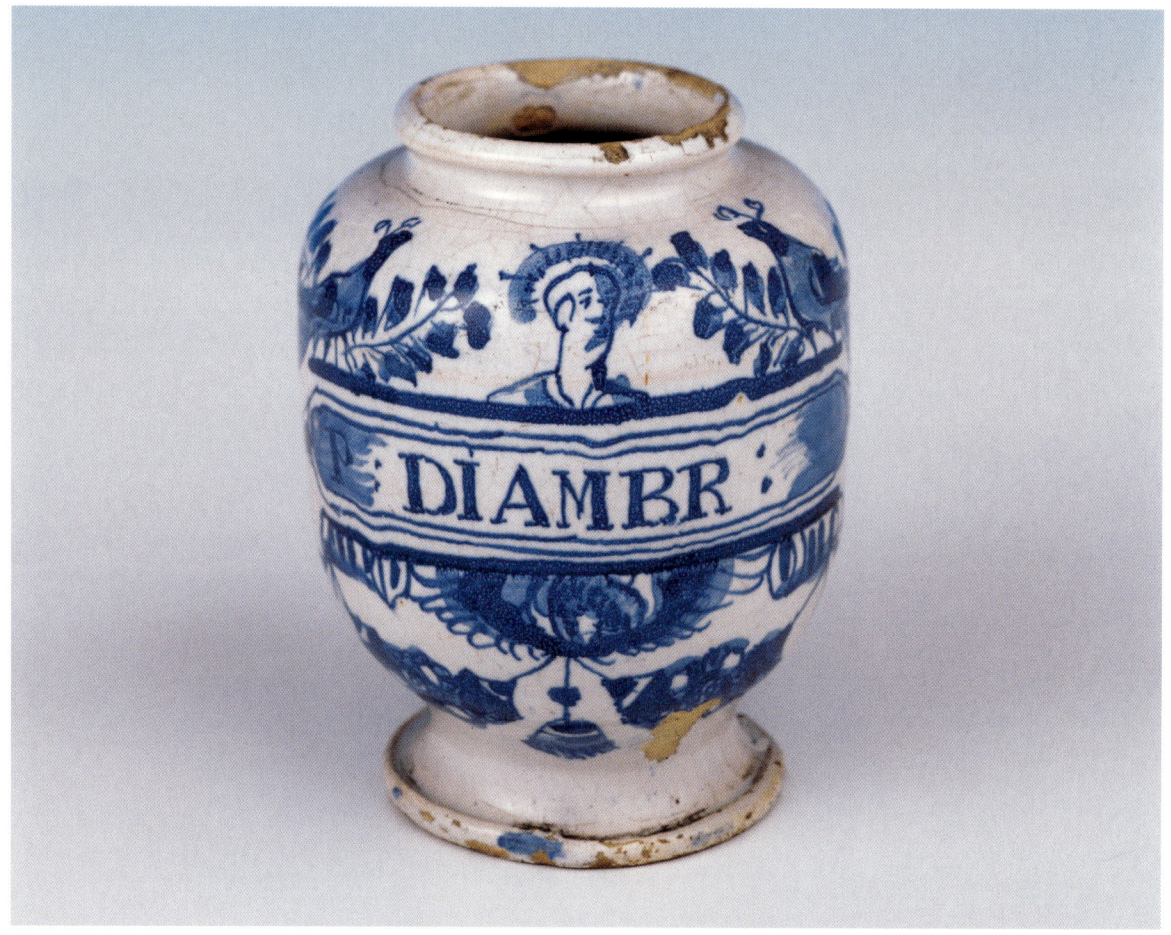

Dry drug jar (Cat.133)

ACCESSION NUMBER: KCI11

DESCRIPTION: Ovoid jar, tapering slightly towards splayed base, and with two faint narrow ridges encircling bowl, one below the neck and the other below the label. White glaze with pinkish tinge and design in blue. Label panel straight, framed in two thin even lines and thicker (outer) third line. Neck everted with glazed rim, slightly concave and partly glazed base.

DESIGN: Apollo and peacocks

INSCRIPTION: P:DIAMBR:

MEANING OF INSCRIPTION: *Pilulae diambrae*, diambra pills

CONTEMPORARY ACCOUNT: "Take of new Gum Guaiacum and the Rosated Aloes, ana ℈ iii, of the Simile Hiera Picra ℈ iss, of Mastich ℈ i, of the Species Diambrae, without the perfumes ℈ ss. Let all these be reduced to a fine Powder, and with a sufficient quantity of Peruvian Balsam, be made into a Mass of due Consistence for Pills.

"I do not find this in any Dispensatory ...; nor have I ever met with it in extemporaneous Prescription, or seen it yet in the Shops." (J. Quincy, *A Compleat English Dispensatory*, 1728, p. 459)

DATE OF MANUFACTURE: 1675–1700

PLACE OF MANUFACTURE: Probably Southwark, London

DIMENSIONS: Height 95 mm, maximum width 80 mm

PROVENANCE: Bought in 1957, Howard Collection.

CONDITION: Good; large chip on base, glaze flaked on bowl neck and base rims.

COMMENT: Howard notes that this is one of a set of 14 jars (p. 21). These are KCI1-13 and KDI1 (Cat. 124–137).

REFERENCE: Howard, English Delftware Drug Jars, p. 21, referred to in Plate XII, but not illustrated.

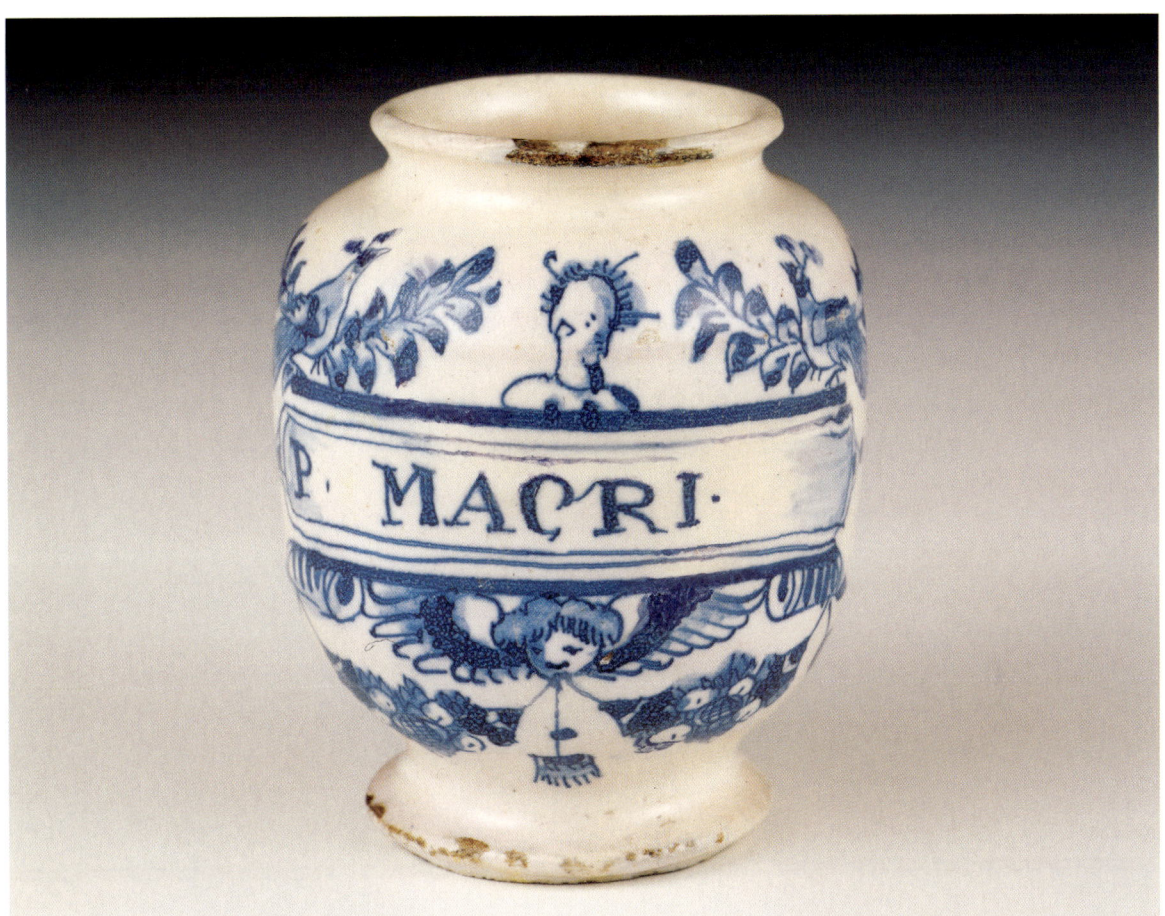

Dry drug jar (Cat.134)

ACCESSION NUMBER: KCI2

DESCRIPTION: Ovoid jar, tapering slightly towards splayed base, and with two narrow ridges encircling bowl, one below the neck and the other below the label. White glaze with pinkish tinge and design in blue. Label panel straight, framed in two even lines and thicker (outer) third line. Neck everted, with partly glazed rim, slightly concave glazed base.

DESIGN: Apollo and peacocks

INSCRIPTION: P MACRI

MEANING OF INSCRIPTION: *Pilulae Macri*, Macer's pills. Named after Aemilius Macer (first century BC), a Roman author whose works included writings on drugs.

CONTEMPORARY ACCOUNT: "Colledg. *Take of Aloes two ounces, Mastich half an ounce, dried Marjoram two drams, salt of wormwood one dram: make them all, being in powder, into a mass according to art with juyce of Colworts and sugar so much as is sufficient.*"

Culpeper: "It is a gallant composed pill, whoever was the Author of it, I have not time to search, it strengthens both Stomach and Brain, especially the Nerves and Muscles...and easeth them of such humors as afflict them; and hinder the motion of the body: they open Obstructions of the Liver and Spleen, and take away diseases thence coming. Your best way is to take them often going to bed, you may take a scruple or half a dram at a time. I commend it to such people as have had hurts or bruises, whereby the use of their Limbs is impaired; and I desire them to take it often, because diseases in remote parts of the body cannot be taken away at a time, it will not hinder their following of their business at all, and therefore is the fittest for poor people." (N. Culpeper, *The Physicians Library*, 1667, p. 184)

DATE OF MANUFACTURE: 1675–1700

PLACE OF MANUFACTURE: Probably Southwark, London.

DIMENSIONS: Height 95 mm, maximum width 80 mm

PROVENANCE: Bought in 1957, Howard Collection.

CONDITION: Fair; has been restored, large chip at foot, glaze chipped and partly flaked at rim and base.

COMMENT: Howard notes that this is one of a set of 14 jars (p. 21). These are KCI1-13 and KDI1 (Cat. 124–137).

REFERENCE: Howard, English Delftware Drug Jars, p. 21 and No. 42.

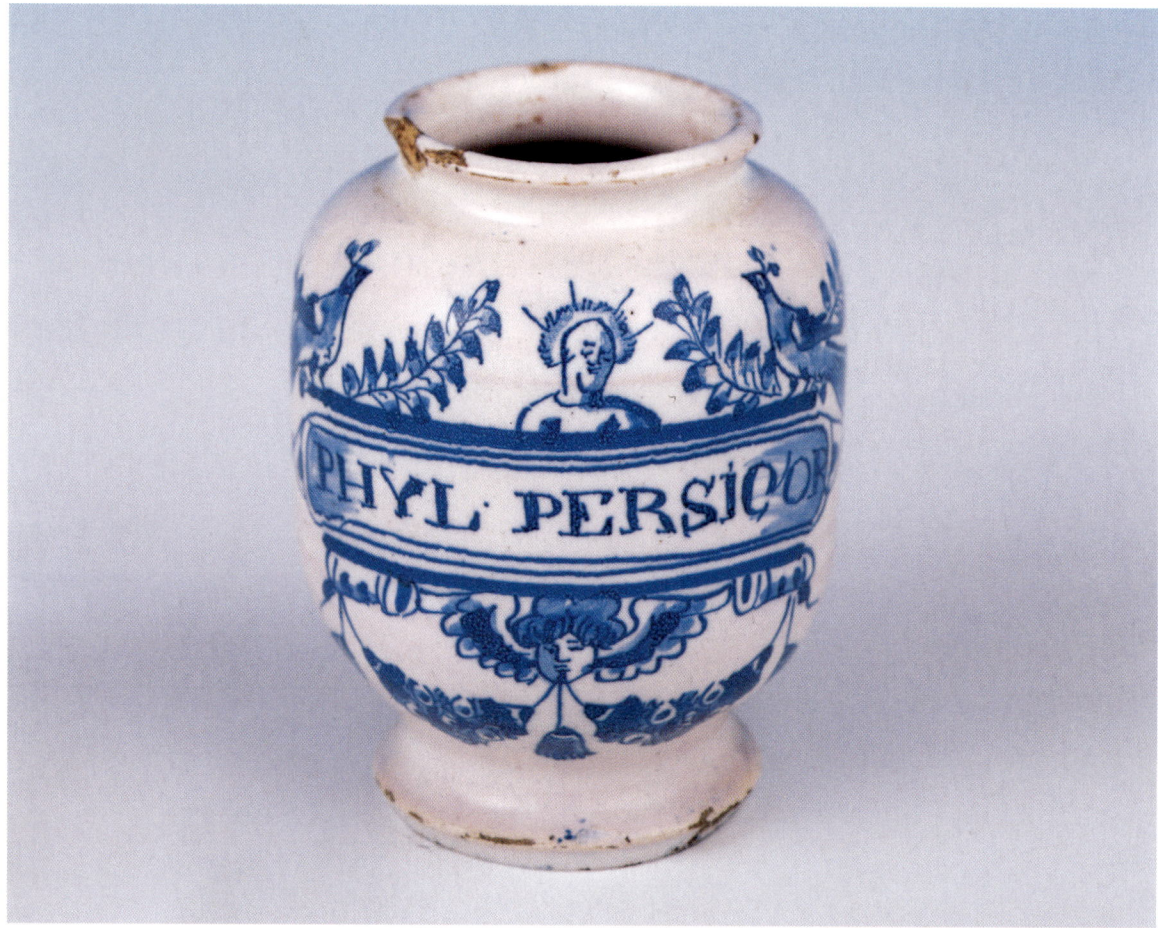

Dry drug jar (Cat.135)

ACCESSION NUMBER: KCI10

DESCRIPTION: Ovoid jar, tapering slightly towards splayed base, and with two faint narrow ridges encircling bowl, one below the neck and the other below the label. White glaze with pinkish tinge and design in blue. Label panel straight, framed in two thin even lines and thicker (outer) third line. Neck everted with glazed rim, slightly concave and partly glazed base.

DESIGN: Apollo and peacocks

INSCRIPTION: PHYL PERSICOR

MEANING OF INSCRIPTION: *Philonium Persicum*, Persian medicine. Philon of Tarsus (first century BC) was a physician.

CONTEMPORARY ACCOUNT: "Take of white Pepper, the seeds of White Henbane of each two drachms, Opium Earth of Lemnos of each ten drachms, Lap. Hematitis, Saffron of each five drachms, Castorium, Indian Spicknard, Euphorbium prepared, Pellitary of Spain, Pearls, Amber, Zeodary, Alicampane, Troch Ramach, of each a drachm, Camphire, a scruple, with their treble weight in Honey-Roses make it into an Electuary according to art.

"...It stops blood flowing from any part of the body, the immoderate flowing of the terms in women, the hemorrhoyds in men, spitting of blood, bloody fluxes, and it is profitable for such women as are subject to miscarry ..." (Culpeper, *London Pharmacopoeia*, 1653, p. 131)

DATE OF MANUFACTURE: 1675–1700

PLACE OF MANUFACTURE: Probably Southwark, London.

DIMENSIONS: Height 93 mm, maximum width 80 mm

PROVENANCE: Bought in 1957, Howard Collection.

CONDITION: Good; large chip on neck, glaze flaked on rim of neck and base.

COMMENT: Howard notes that this is one of a set of 14 jars (p. 21). These are KCI1-13 and KDI1 (Cat. 124–137).

REFERENCE: Howard, *English Delftware Drug Jars*, p. 21, referred to in Plate XII, but not illustrated.

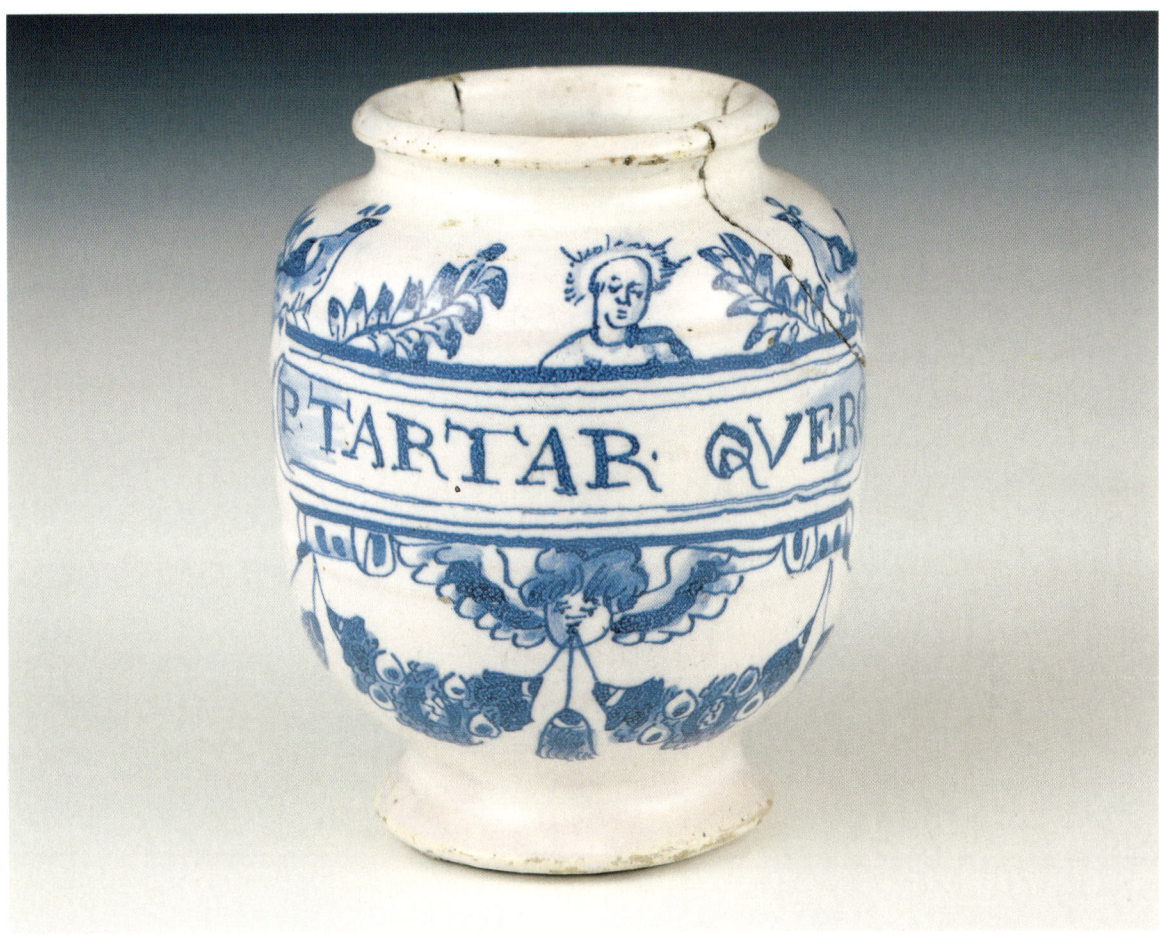

Dry drug jar (Cat. 136)

ACCESSION NUMBER: KCI9
DESCRIPTION: Ovoid jar, tapering slightly towards splayed base, with two narrow ridges encircling bowl, one below the neck and the other below the label. White glaze with pinkish tinge and design in blue. Label panel straight, framed in two thin even lines and thicker (outer) third line. Neck ridged with glazed rim, slightly concave and partly glazed base.
DESIGN: Apollo and peacocks
INSCRIPTION: P TARTAR QVERC
MEANING OF INSCRIPTION: *Pilulae tartareae quercetanus*, tartar pills of Quercetanus. This is the Latinised form of Joseph du Chesne, a French chemist (1544–1609).
CONTEMPORARY ACCOUNT: "'Take Aloes ʒ iii. Gum Ammoniacum strain'd with Vinegar of Squills ʒ iss. Tartar of Vitriol ʒ iss. Extract of Rhubarb ʒ ss. Mix S.A.'

"...This is a Prescript of *Bontius*, and is much better than that of *Quercetan*, which our *College* retains. This makes a good Purge in all Cases that are attended with a *Lentor* in the Blood, or viscid pituitous Juices in the Glands and Capillaries. It is

therefore good in hypocondriacal and splenetick Disorders, and of service, with continuance, in the Gout, Rheumatism, and scrophulous Indurations upon the Glands. It may be given from Ɔ i. to ʒ i. at a Dose. But such Medicines are better in small quantities, and frequently repeated; otherwise what is *Cathartick*, and forcing in the first Passages, will carry the rest through before they get into the Blood, and have any effect where they are chiefly intended." (J. Quincy, *A Compleat English Dispensatory*, 1718, p. 427)
DATE OF MANUFACTURE: 1675–1700
PLACE OF MANUFACTURE: Probably Southwark, London.
DIMENSIONS: Height 95 mm, maximum width 80 mm
PROVENANCE: Bought in 1957, Howard Collection.
CONDITION: Poor; three large cracks descending from neck and joining round bowl (has been stuck together), glaze chipped on bowl.
COMMENT: Howard notes that this is one of a set of 14 jars (p. 21). These are KCI1-13 and KDI1 (Cat. 124–137).
REFERENCE: Howard, English Delftware Drug Jars, p. 21, referred to in Plate XII, but not illustrated.

Apollo

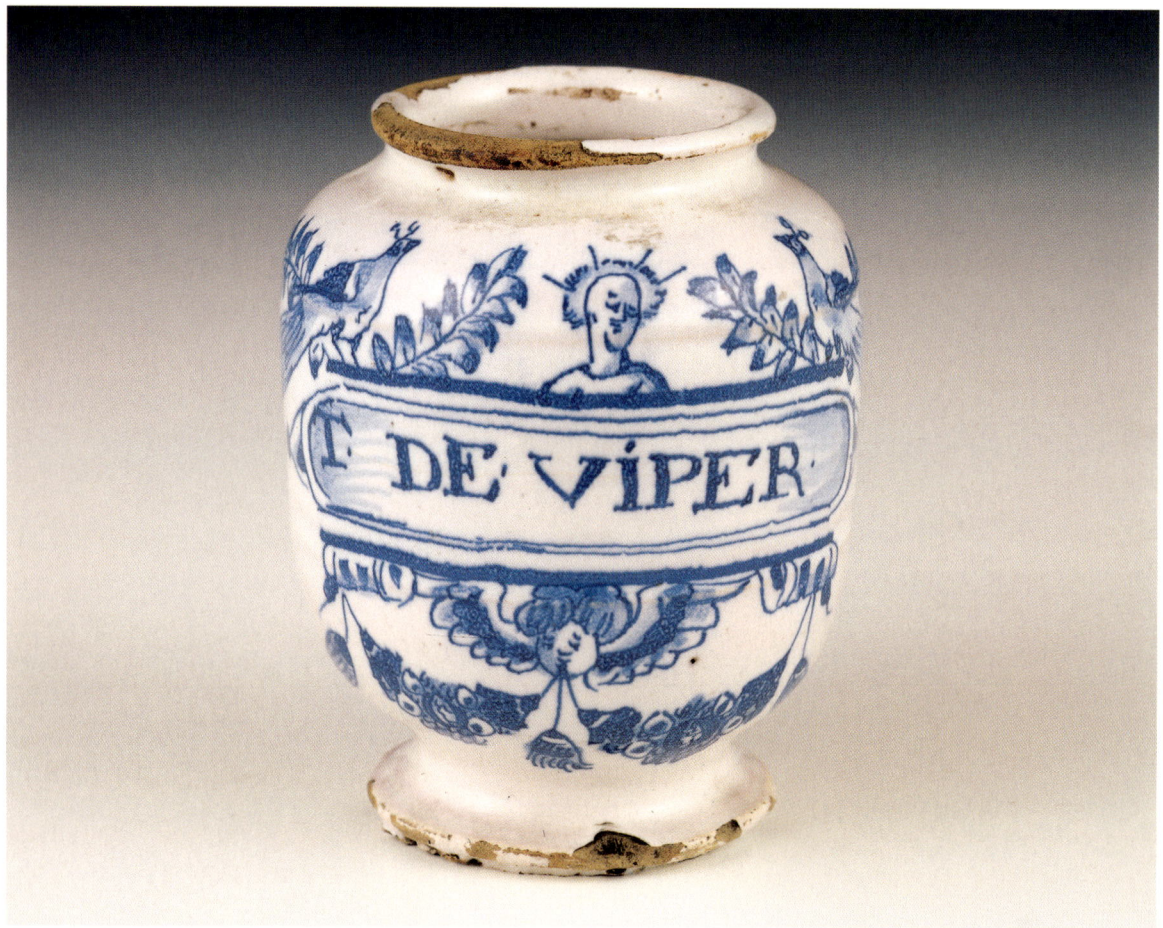

Dry drug jar (Cat.137)

ACCESSION NUMBER: KCI1
DESCRIPTION: Ovoid jar, tapering slightly towards splayed base, and with two narrow ridges encircling bowl, one below the neck and the other below the label. White glaze with pinkish tinge and design in blue. Label panel straight, framed in two thin even lines and thicker (outer) third line. Neck everted, with glazed rim, slightly concave glazed base.
DESIGN: Apollo and peacocks
INSCRIPTION: T DE VIPER
MEANING OF INSCRIPTION: *Trochisci de Vipera*, viper lozenges. Viper lozenges of Venice were renowned throughout Europe in the 1600s to prevent the plague and as an antidote to poisons. Their main use was as one of the many ingredients in the various theriacs.
CONTEMPORARY ACCOUNT: "Take the Flesh of Vipers without Skin, Head, Bones, or Entrails, and boil'd with a little Salt and Dill-Seed in the Water ℔ ss. White Bread ℨ ii. and knead them into a Paste, with Hands greas'd over with Oil of Nutmegs by Expression, or Opobalsam; and cut it out into Troches."

(J. Quincy, *A Compleat English Dispensatory*, 1718, p. 418)
DATE OF MANUFACTURE: 1675–1700
PLACE OF MANUFACTURE: Southwark, London
DIMENSIONS: Height 95 mm, maximum width 78 mm
PROVENANCE: Bought in 1957, Howard Collection.
CONDITION: Good; glaze chipped at neck and base and partly removed.
COMMENT: Howard notes that this is one of a set of 14 jars (p. 21). These are KCI1-13 and KDI1 (Cat. 124–137).
REFERENCE: Howard, English Delftware Drug Jars, p. 21 and No. 40.

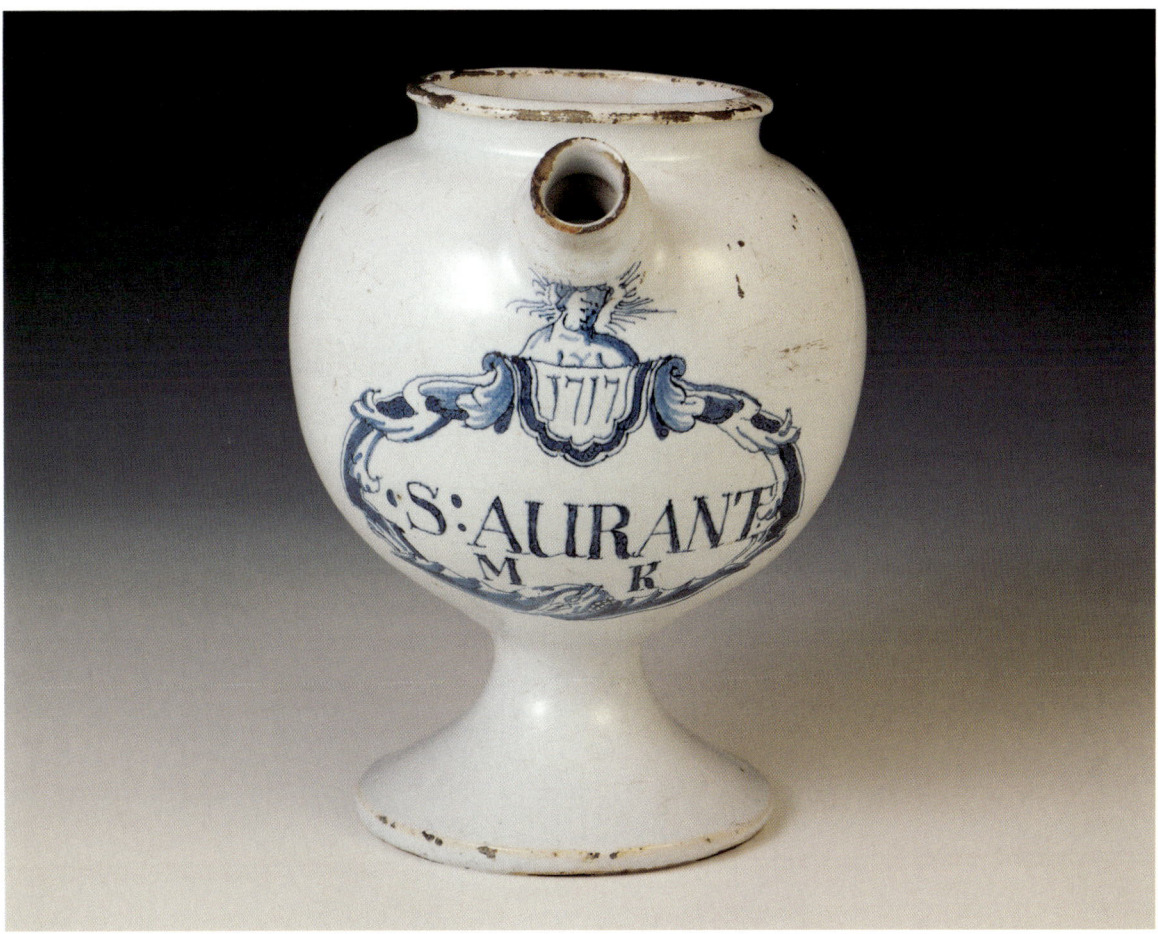

Wet drug jar (Cat.138)

ACCESSION NUMBER: KBH1

DESCRIPTION: Bulbous jar on spreading foot, with spout and fluted strap-like looped handle. White glaze with pinkish tinge and design in blue. Label panel straight, outlined with leaf design and body of a sea-serpent. Neck everted with glazed rim, flanged spout, hollowed, glazed base.

DESIGN: Apollo and serpents

INSCRIPTION: S:AURANT MK 1717

MEANING OF INSCRIPTION: *Syrupus aurantiorum*, syrup of oranges. 'MK' are the initials of the apothecary who commissioned the jar.

CONTEMPORARY ACCOUNT: "'Dissolve in ℔ i. of the Juice of Oranges, which has stood till settled fine, Loaf-Sugar ℔ ii. with a gentle Heat.'

"This is a grateful Syrup, and proper to dulcify any refrigerating Juleps; and agrees sometimes with those which are intended for *Alexipharmicks*, because it astringes the Solids... By its pleasant Acidity too, it is grateful to the Stomach, and helps in such Compositions as are intended to stop Vomitings, and remove Nauseas: for which purposes it is frequently prescrib'd as also to promote Expectoration, for the same reason as that of Vinegar; which is to cut the Phlegm, as it is commonly call'd, and make it come up the easier." (J. Quincy, *A Compleat English Dispensatory*, 1718, p. 374)

DATE OF MANUFACTURE: 1717

PLACE OF MANUFACTURE: London

DIMENSIONS: Height 190 mm, maximum width 150 mm

PROVENANCE: Bought in 1957, Howard Collection.

CONDITION: Good; rims of neck and spout chipped, glaze crazed and flaked on neck, handle and spout.

COMMENT: Eleven jars and one fragmentary jar of this type have survived. Three of them are dated 1717, including this one. The undated jars include KCH1 (Cat. 139), and the fragmentary pill pot is in the Cuming Museum, London.

REFERENCES: Austin, British Delft at Williamsburg, 1994, p. 215, No. 463.

Grigsby, The Longridge Collection of English Slipware and Delftware. catalogue number D407.

Howard, English Delftware Drug Jars, p. 21 and No. 44.

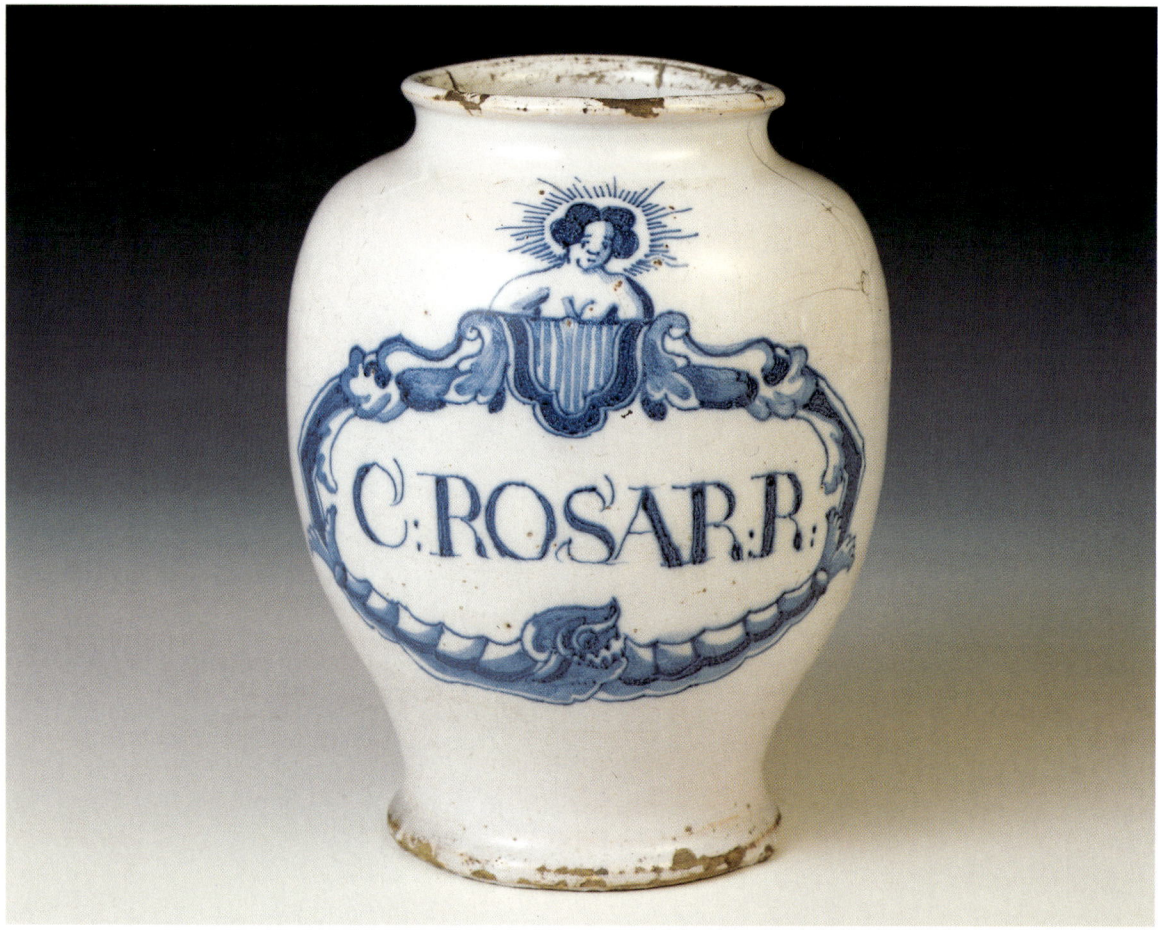

Dry drug jar (Cat.139)

ACCESSION NUMBER: KCH1

DESCRIPTION: Ovoid jar, tapering slightly towards splayed base. White glaze with pinkish tinge and design in blue. Label panel straight, outlined with leaf design and sea-serpent. Neck everted with uneven glazed rim, slightly concave glazed base.

DESIGN: Apollo and serpents

INSCRIPTION: C:ROSAR:R:

MEANING OF INSCRIPTION: *Conserva rosarum rubrarum,* conserve of red roses

CONTEMPORARY ACCOUNT: "These blow in *May* and *June.* They are sufficiently known to all Persons. What are used in the Shops, unless for the distill'd Water, are the Buds before they quite blow; because then they are much rougher and more astringent. The Conserve made of them is deservedly in great esteem, but the common Notion of its being the better for Age, is an Error: for their Astringency, which arises from the Solidity and Asperity of their component Parts, by long lying in the Sugar, which mellows and softens them, very much decays... The Conserve is judg'd useful in Inflammations of the Eyes, apply'd

outwardly: And the Leaves steep'd in Vinegar are accounted good for the Head-Ach, apply'd to the Temples." (J. Quincy, *A Compleat English Dispensatory,* 1718, p. 99)

DATE OF MANUFACTURE: 1710–1730

PLACE OF MANUFACTURE: London

DIMENSIONS: Height 180 mm, maximum width 143 mm

PROVENANCE: Bought in 1957, Howard Collection.

CONDITION: Fair; two large cracks and one small crack descending from neck, glaze crazed and flaked on rim of neck and base, some pitting.

COMMENT: Eleven jars and one fragmentary jar of this type have survived. Three of them are dated 1717, including KBH1 (Cat. 138). The undated jars include this one, and the fragmentary pill pot is in the Cuming Museum, London.

REFERENCES: Austin, British Delft at Williamsburg, p. 215, No. 463.

Drey, Apothecary Jars. Plate 68C and p. 136.

Grigsby, The Longridge Collection of English Slipware and Delftware. catalogue number D407.

Howard, English Delftware Drug Jars, pp. 21–22 and No. 43.

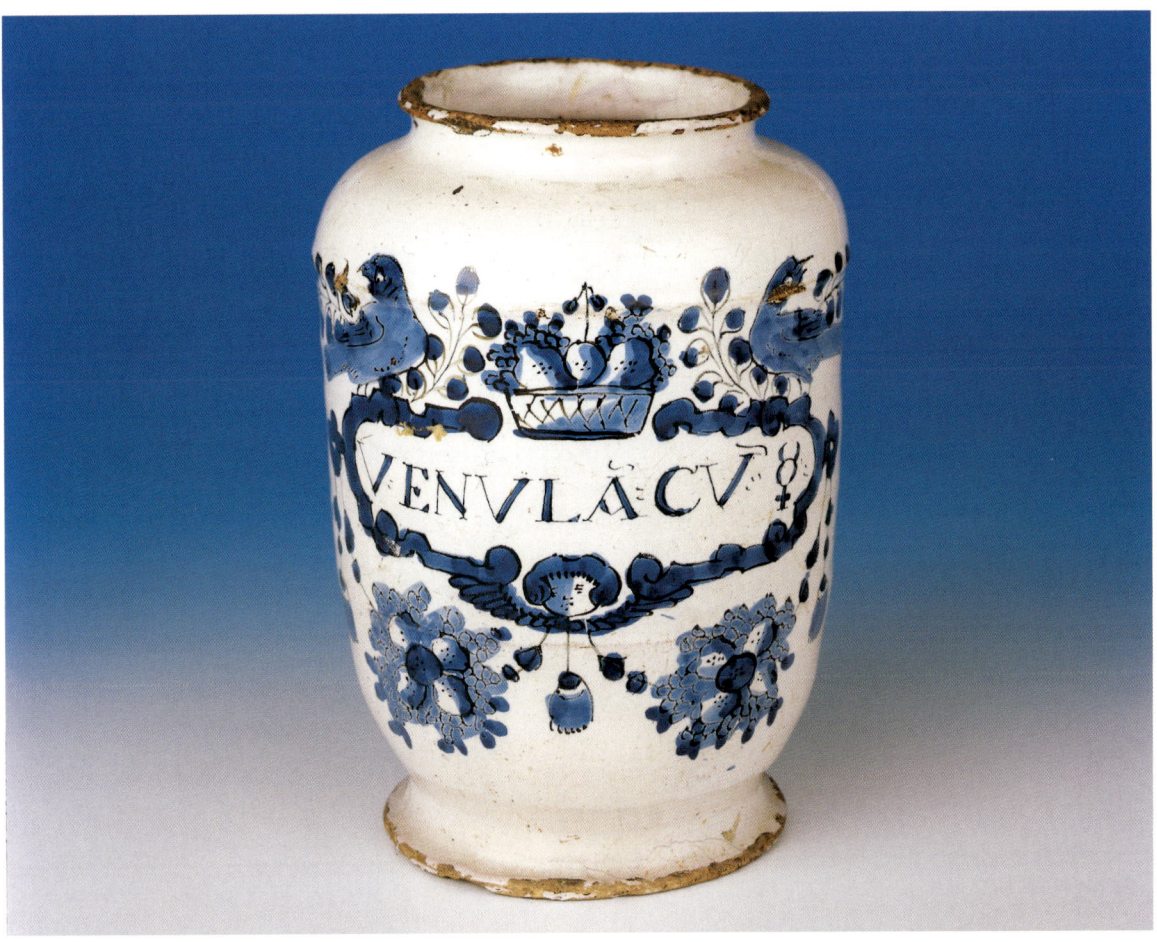

Dry drug jar (Cat.140)

ACCESSION NUMBER: KCK5
DESCRIPTION: Ovoid jar, tapering slightly towards splayed base, with two narrow ridges encircling bowl, one below the neck and the other below the label. White glaze with pinkish tinge and design in blue and black. Label panel straight with wavy strap-work frame. Neck everted with unglazed rim, slightly concave and partly glazed base.
DESIGN: Later songbirds
INSCRIPTION: V:ENVLA:CV ☿
MEANING OF INSCRIPTION: *Unguentum Enulatum cum Mercurio*, made with *Enula campana*, the root of elecampane (*Inula helenium*) with mercury. An ointment to treat itching, an expectorant, diuretic, diaphoretic, cathartic, stomachic and emmenagogue.
CONTEMPORARY ACCOUNT: "This is made of the foregoing Ointment, with the Addition of ℥ ii. of Quick-silver, first very well kill'd, or incorporated with a sufficient Quantity of Turpentine."

"The 'foregoing Ointment' is ointment of Elecampane:

'Take Elecampane Root, boiled in Vinegar, beat and pulped thro' a Sieve, ℔ i. of Turpentine washed in the same Decoction, ℥ ii. of yellow Wax, ℥ i. of Old Hogs Lard salted, and of old Oil, ana ℥ iv, of common Salt, ℥ ss. Let the Lard, Wax, and Oil melt together, and afterwards add the Turpentine, the Pulp of Elecampane, and Salt, finely powdered, so as to make all together into an Ointment, S.A.'

"This is continued in the last, as the former Dispensatories of the *College*, with a very little Alteration in some of the Quantities of the Ingredients; but it is little used except as altered in the following." (J. Quincy, *A Compleat English Dispensatory*, 1718, pp. 502–503)
DATE OF MANUFACTURE: 1700–1720
PLACE OF MANUFACTURE: London
DIMENSIONS: Height 215 mm, maximum width 160 mm
PROVENANCE: Bought in 1964.
CONDITION: Good; neck and base chipped, glaze crazed and flaked on neck and base rims.
REFERENCE: Lothian Short, Apothecary Jar Inscriptions p. 146.

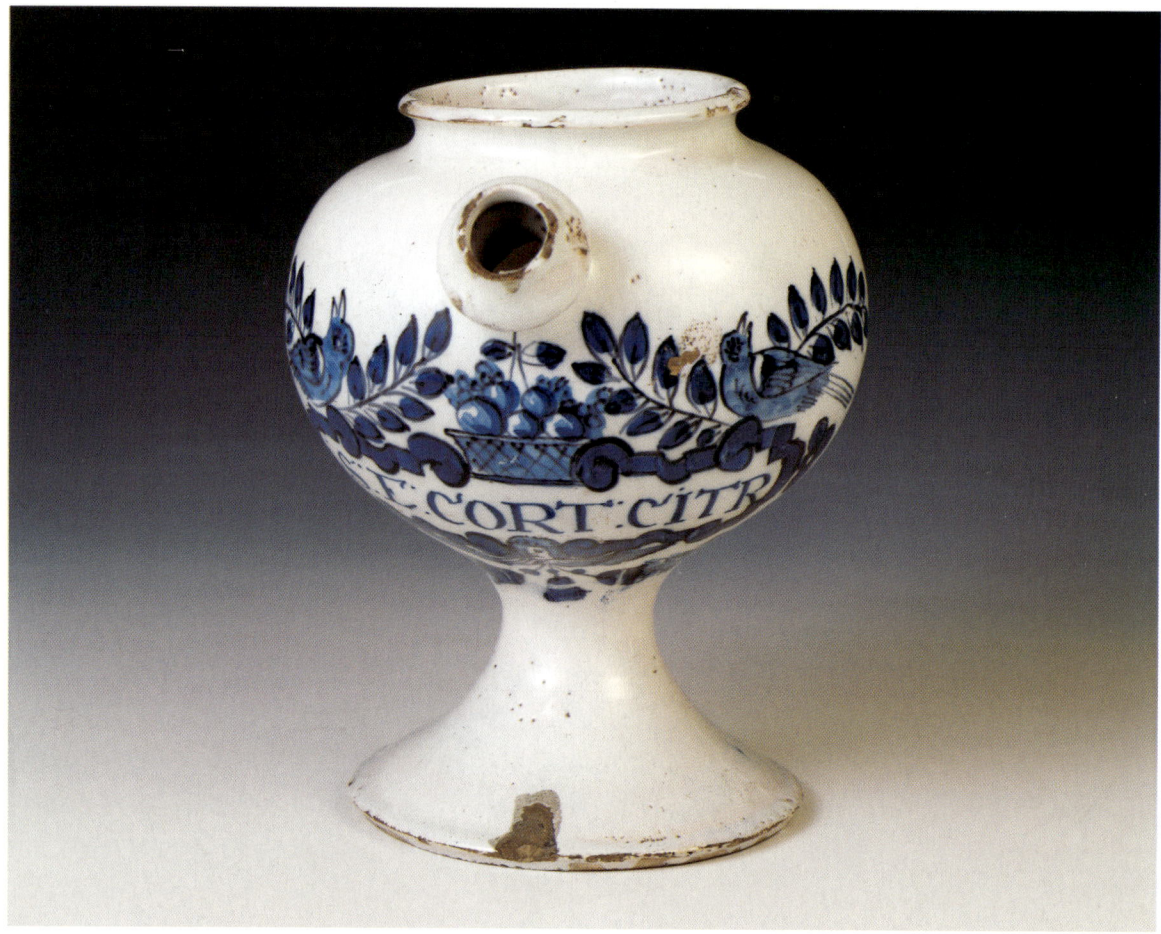

Wet drug jar (Cat.141)

ACCESSION NUMBER: KDK4

DESCRIPTION: Bulbous jar on spreading foot with spout and strap-like looped handle. White glaze with pinkish tinge and design in blue and black. Label panel straight with wavy strap-work frame. Neck everted with glazed rim, flanged spout, hollowed and partly glazed base.

DESIGN: Later songbirds

INSCRIPTION: S:E:CORT:CITR

MEANING OF INSCRIPTION: *Syrupus e corticum citronum*, syrup of lemon peel

CONTEMPORARY ACCOUNT: "Take of yellow, ripe and fresh Citron Peels ℥ v, Berries of Kermes (or their Juices brought over to us) ℥ ii, Spring Water ℔ ii, digest them for a Night in B.M., strain, and with white Sugar ℔ iiss by boiling in B.M. make a Syrup, S.A. ...

"'Tis a good Cephalick, Stomatick and Cordial, good against Apoplexies, Epilepsies, Convulsions, Vertigoes, Palpitation, Fainting or Swooning. It strengthens the Heart, resists Poison, revives the Spirits, and restores in Hectick Fevers and Consumptions. Dose ℥ i or ℥ iss." (W. Salmon, *The New London Dispensatory*, 1716, p. 523)

DATE OF MANUFACTURE: 1700–1730

PLACE OF MANUFACTURE: London

DIMENSIONS: Height 195 mm, maximum width 163 mm

PROVENANCE: Bought in 1950.

CONDITION: Good; hair cracks encircling bowl, base chipped, glaze crazed and pitted and flaked from spout and handle and neck and base rims.

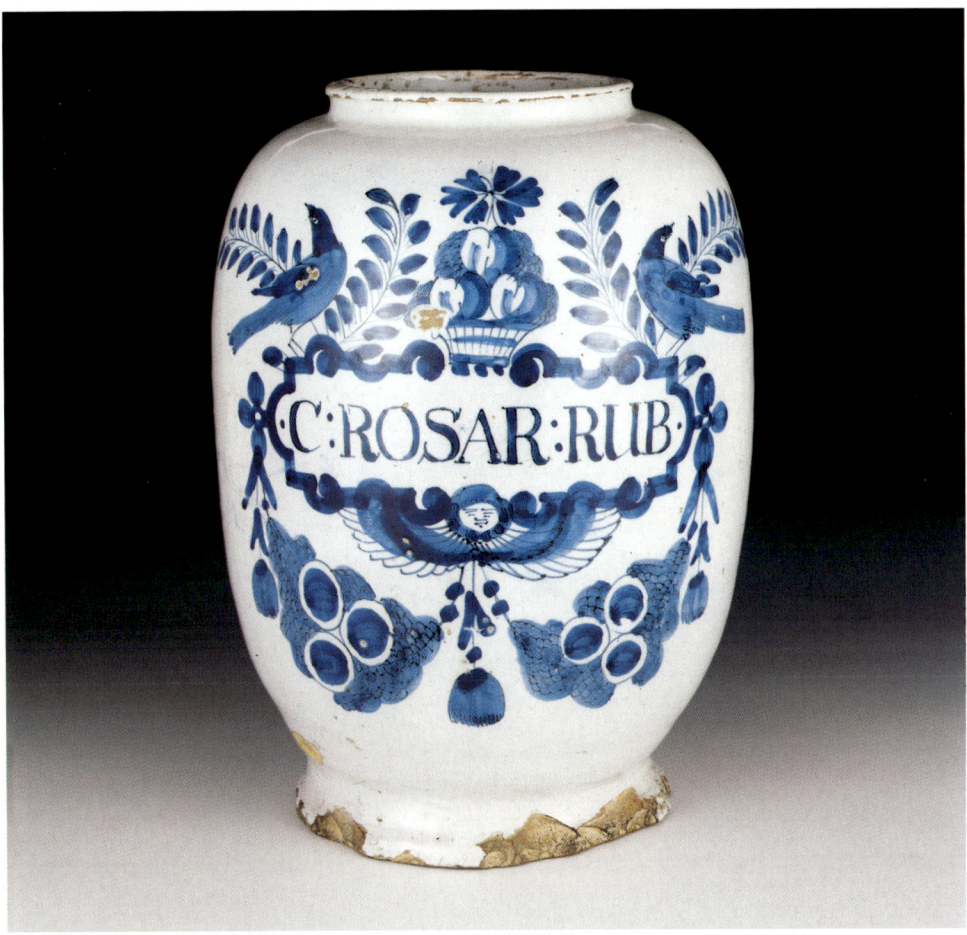

Dry drug jar (Cat.142)

ACCESSION NUMBER: KCK1

DESCRIPTION: Ovoid jar, tapering slightly towards splayed base. White glaze with pinkish tinge and design in blue. Label panel straight, with wavy strap-work frame. Neck ridged, with glazed rim, flat unglazed base.

DESIGN: Later songbirds

INSCRIPTION: C:ROSAR:RUB

MEANING OF INSCRIPTION: *Conserva rosarum rubrum*, conserve of red roses

CONTEMPORARY ACCOUNT: "These blow in *May* and *June*. They are sufficiently known to all Persons. What are used in the Shops, unless for the distill'd Water, are the Buds before they quite blow; because then they are much rougher and more astringent. The Conserve made of them is deservedly in great esteem, but the common Notion of its being the better for Age, is an Error: for their Astringency, which arises from the Solidity and Asperity of their component Parts, by long lying in the Sugar, which mellows and softens them, very much decays. They are good in almost all Distempers of the Lungs, and particularly in Defluxions of Rheum." (J. Quincy, *A Compleat English Dispensatory*, 1718, p. 99)

DATE OF MANUFACTURE: 1700–1740

PLACE OF MANUFACTURE: London

DIMENSIONS: Height 350 mm, maximum width 260 mm

PROVENANCE: Bought in 1954.

CONDITION: Good; large chips at base, glaze crazed and flaked at rim of neck.

Later songbirds

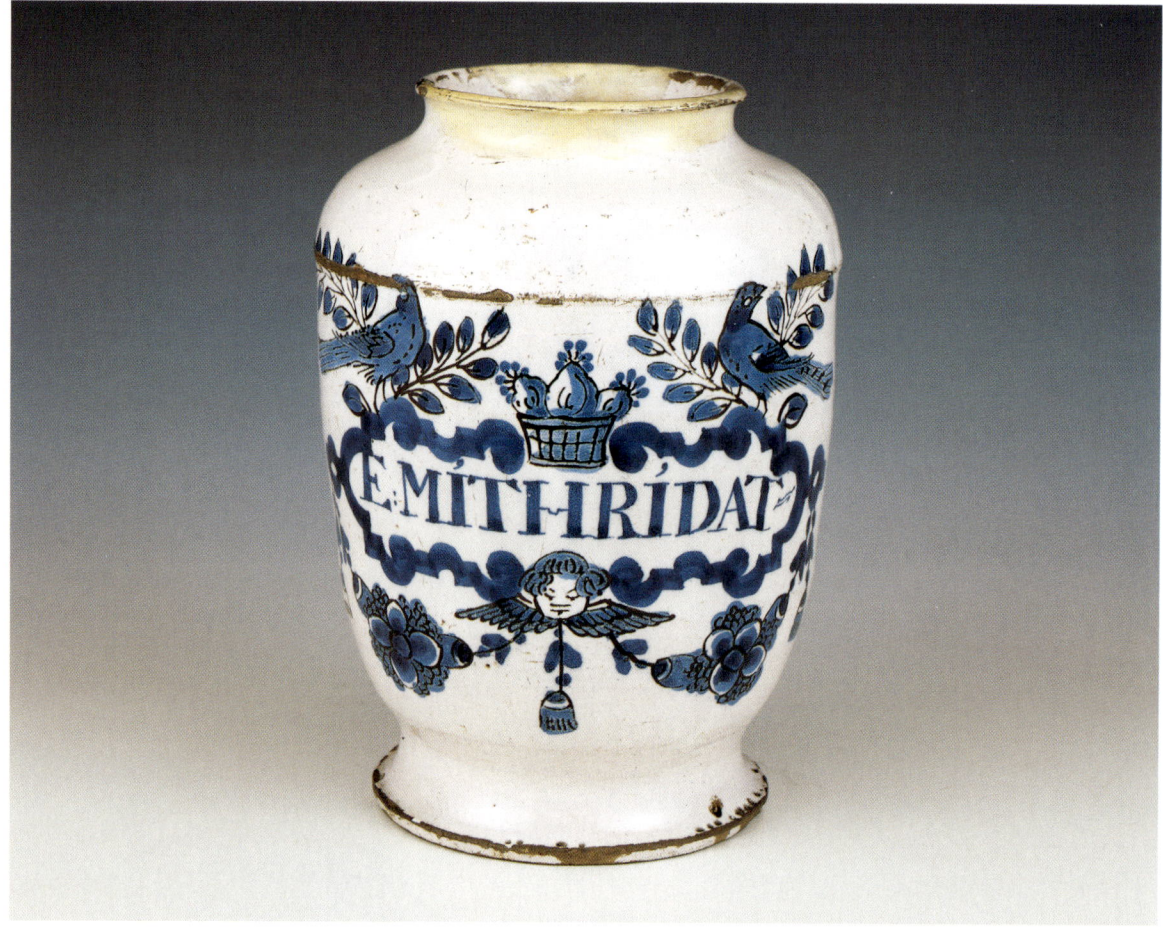

Dry drug jar (Cat.143)

ACCESSION NUMBER: KCK3

DESCRIPTION: Ovoid jar, tapering slightly towards splayed base, with two narrow ridges encircling bowl, one below the neck and the other below the label. White glaze with pinkish tinge and design in blue and black. Label panel straight with wavy strapwork frame. Neck everted with glazed rim, flat and partly glazed base. 'D' in black on base.

DESIGN: Later songbirds

INSCRIPTION: E:MITHRIDAT

MEANING OF INSCRIPTION: *Electuarium Mithridatum*, Mithridates' electuary. One of several forms of theriac (treacle) still popular in the 17th century as a universal antidote against poisons and infectious diseases. The name Mithridate is derived from Mithridates VI, king of Pontus (132–63 BC), who was believed to have rendered himself immune to poisoning by the constant use of antidotes.

CONTEMPORARY ACCOUNT: "Take of Arabian Myrrh, Saffron, Agaric, Ginger, Cinnamon, Spikenard, Frankincense, and Seeds of Treacle-Mustard, ana з x. of the Seeds of Hartwort, Opobalsamum, or in its stead, expressed Oil of Nutmegs, Sweet-Rush, Arabian Stoechas, the true Costus, Galbanum, Cyprus Turpentine, Long Pepper, Castor, Juice of Hypocistis, Styrax, Opoanax, and Indian Leaf, or in its stead Mace, ana з i. of Cassia Bark, Polymountain, white Pepper, Scordium, Seeds of wild Carrot, Carpobalsam, or Cubebs, Troches of Cypheos, and Bdellium, ana з vii. of Spikenard cleansed, Gum Arabic, Macedonian Parsley Seed, Opium, the lesser Cardamoms, Fennel Seeds, Gentian Root, red Rose Flowers, and Dittany of Crete, ana з v. of Aniseeds, Asarum, Acorus or Calamus Aromaticus, Orrice, the greater Valerian, and Sagapenum, ana з iii. of Meum Root, Acacia, Stinks, and the tops of St. John's Wort, ana з iiss. of the best Canary, enough to dissolve the Gums and Juices, which will take up about з xxvi. of clarify'd Honey as much as the Weight of all the Ingredients, except the Wine; and make into an Electuary, S.A."

(J. Quincy, *A Compleat English Dispensatory*, 1718, pp. 431–432)

DATE OF MANUFACTURE: 1700–1770

PLACE OF MANUFACTURE: London

DIMENSIONS: Height 195 mm, maximum width 150 mm

PROVENANCE: Bought in 1949.

CONDITION: Good; glaze crazed and flaked on body, neck and base.

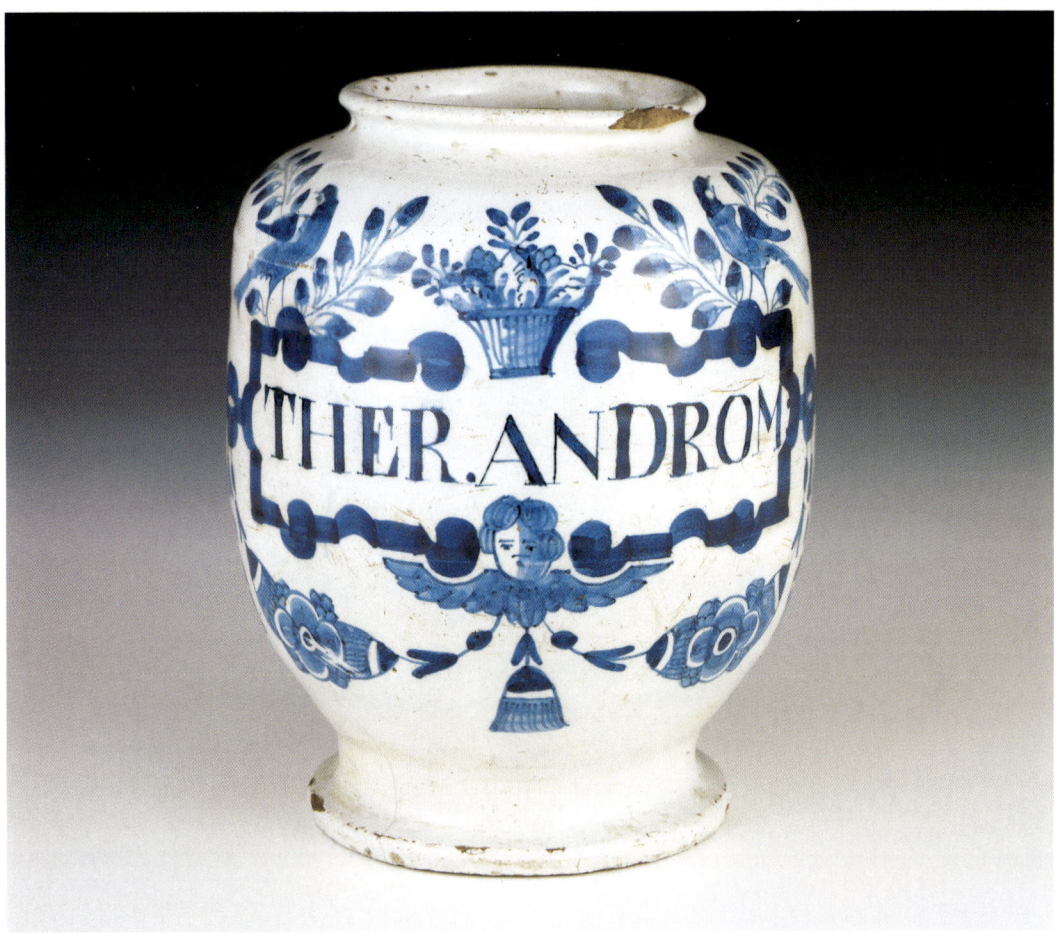

Dry drug jar (Cat.144)

ACCESSION NUMBER: KCK11

DESCRIPTION: Ovoid jar, with splayed base, with two narrow ridges encircling bowl, one below the neck and the other below the label. White glaze with yellowish tinge and design in blue. Label panel straight with wavy strap-work frame. Neck ridged with glazed rim, slightly concave unglazed base.

DESIGN: Later songbirds

INSCRIPTION: THER ANDROM

MEANING OF INSCRIPTION: *Theriaca Andromachi*, the treacle or theriaca of Andromachus, a preparation traced back to Andromachus, physician to the Emperor Nero (AD 37) was supposed to be an antidote to all poisons. It was also used in the 1600s to prevent the plague.

CONTEMPORARY ACCOUNT: "This is not only the Capital Alexipharmick of our Shops, but of all *Europe*; and has a great deal more wrote about it, than could be contain'd in the largest Volume: we shall therefore content our selves with as short Remarks upon this grand Medicine, as is consistent with that Acquaintance every one in the Practice of Physick ought to have of it. This claims for its Author the Person whose Name it bears, and who was Physician to *Nero* the Tyrant: that we frequently call it *Venice*-Treacle, is from the great Quantities made there, and thence transported to most Parts of the World. As this has pass'd through many Ages, and the Hands of many, in their own Opinions, able to alter it for the better, there are abundance of different Recipe's extant in Dispensatory-Writers: and this of our College, seems to be one of the best..." (J. Quincy, *A Compleat English Dispensatory*, 1718, p. 409)

DATE OF MANUFACTURE: 1720–1740

PLACE OF MANUFACTURE: London

DIMENSIONS: Height 170 mm, maximum width 150 mm

PROVENANCE: Donated by Mr Pinchen, 1955.

CONDITION: Fair; crack encircling body, two cracks ascending from foot, 2 cm chip in neck, circular hole (1.5 cm) in base, glaze flaked from base rims.

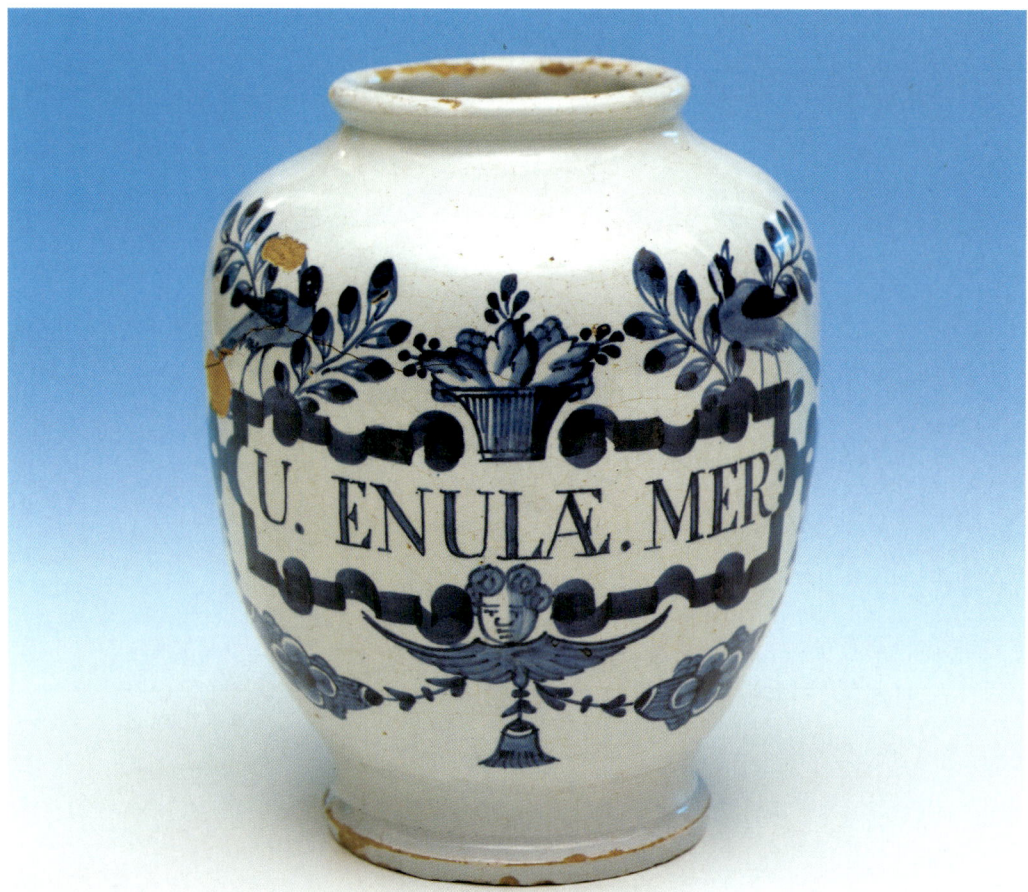

Dry drug jar (Cat.145)

ACCESSION NUMBER: 2002.60.3

DESCRIPTION: Ovoid jar, tapering slightly towards splayed base. White glaze with tinge and design in blue. Label panel straight, with wavy strap-work frame. Neck ridged, with glazed rim, flat unglazed base.

DESIGN: Later songbirds

INSCRIPTION: U. ENULAE.MER:

MEANING OF INSCRIPTION: *Unguentum enulatum cum mercurio*, made with *Enula campana*, the root of elecampane (*Inula helenium*) with mercury. An ointment to treat itching, an expectorant, diuretic, diaphoretic, cathartic, stomachic and emmenagogue.

CONTEMPORARY ACCOUNT: "This is made of the foregoing Ointment, with the Addition of ℥ ii. of Quick-silver, first very well kill'd, or incorporated with a sufficient Quantity of Turpentine."

The "foregoing Ointment" is ointment of Elecampane:

"Take Elecampane Root, boiled in Vinegar, beat and pulped thro' a Sieve, ℔ i. of Turpentine washed in the same Decoction,

℥ ii. of yellow Wax, ℥ i. of Old Hogs Lard salted, and of old Oil, ana ℥ iv, of common Salt, ℥ ss. Let the Lard, Wax, and Oil melt together, and afterwards add the Turpentine, the Pulp of Elecampane, and Salt, finely powdered, so as to make all together into an Ointment, S.A.

This is continued in the last, as the former Dispensatories of the *College*, with a very little Alteration in some of the Quantities of the Ingredients; but it is little used except as altered in the following." (J. Quincy, *A Compleat English Dispensatory*, 1718, pp. 502–503)

DATE OF MANUFACTURE: 1710–1730

PLACE OF MANUFACTURE: Lambeth, London

DIMENSIONS: Height 185 mm, maximum width 50 mm

PROVENANCE: Bequest, 2002. Originally Saville Peck collection.

CONDITION: Good, some large areas of glaze flaked from body, chips to rim and base.

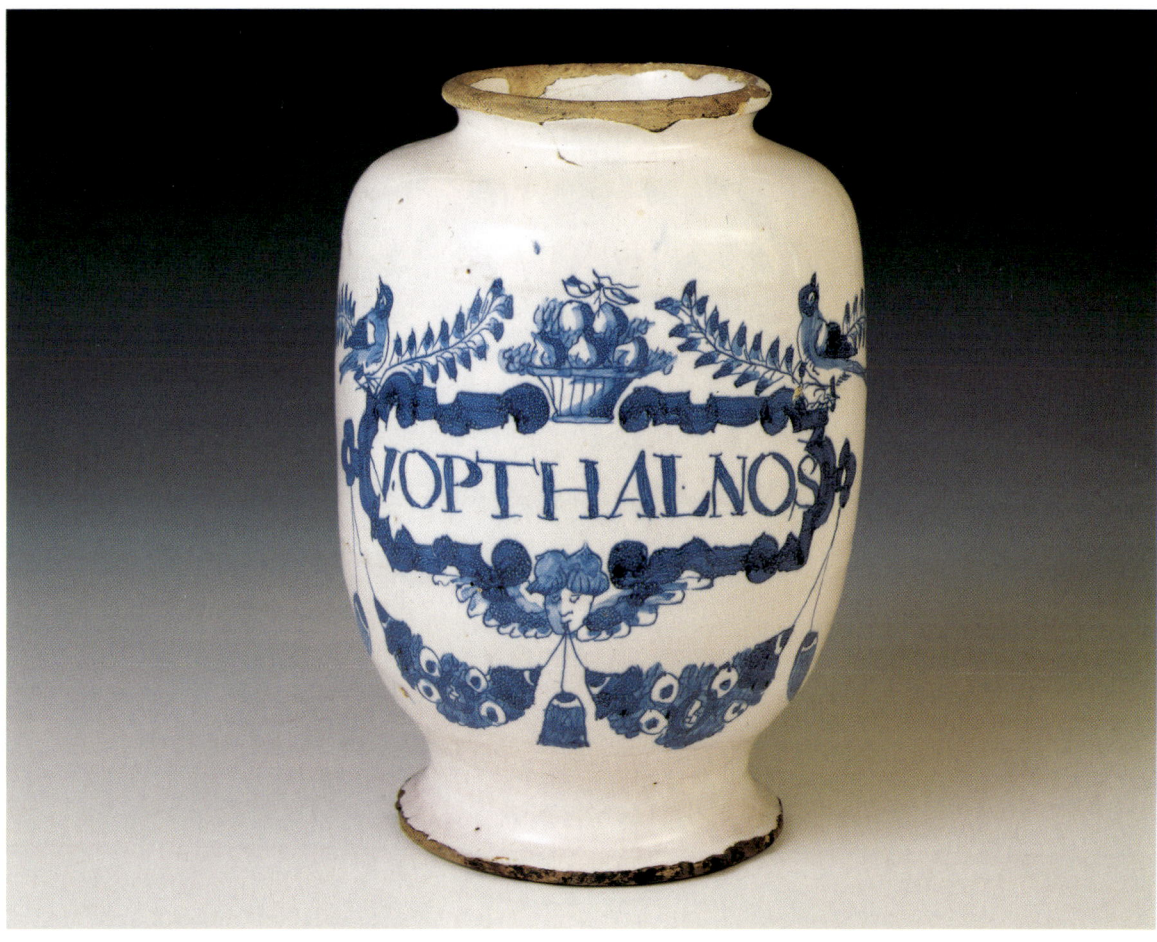

Dry drug jar (Cat.146)

ACCESSION NUMBER: KCK8

DESCRIPTION: Ovoid jar, tapering slightly towards splayed base, with two narrow ridges encircling bowl, one below the neck and the other below the label. White glaze with pinkish tinge and design in blue. Label panel straight with wavy strap-work frame. Neck ridged with unglazed rim, slightly concave unglazed base.

DESIGN: Later songbirds

INSCRIPTION: V OPTHALNOS

MEANING OF INSCRIPTION: *Unguentum ophthalmicum,* ointment for disorders of the eye

CONTEMPORARY ACCOUNT: "Colledg. *Take of Bole Armenick washed in Rose water one ounce, Lapis calaminaris washed in Eyebright water, Tutty prepared, of each two drams; Pearls in very fine powder half a dram, Camphire half a scruple, Opium five grains, fresh Butter washed in Plantane water, as much as is sufficient to make it into an Oyntment according to art.*"

Culpeper: "It is exceeding good to stop hot Rhewms that fall down into the Eyes, the Eyelids being but annointed with it." (N.

Culpeper, *The Physicians Library,* 1667, p. 225)

DATE OF MANUFACTURE: 1700–1720

PLACE OF MANUFACTURE: London

DIMENSIONS: Height 190 mm, maximum width 145 mm

PROVENANCE: Bought in 1957, Howard Collection.

CONDITION: Fair; small hole in base, base chipped, glaze pitted and flaked on body and neck and base rims.

REFERENCE: Howard, English Delftware Drug Jars, p. xx and No. 56.

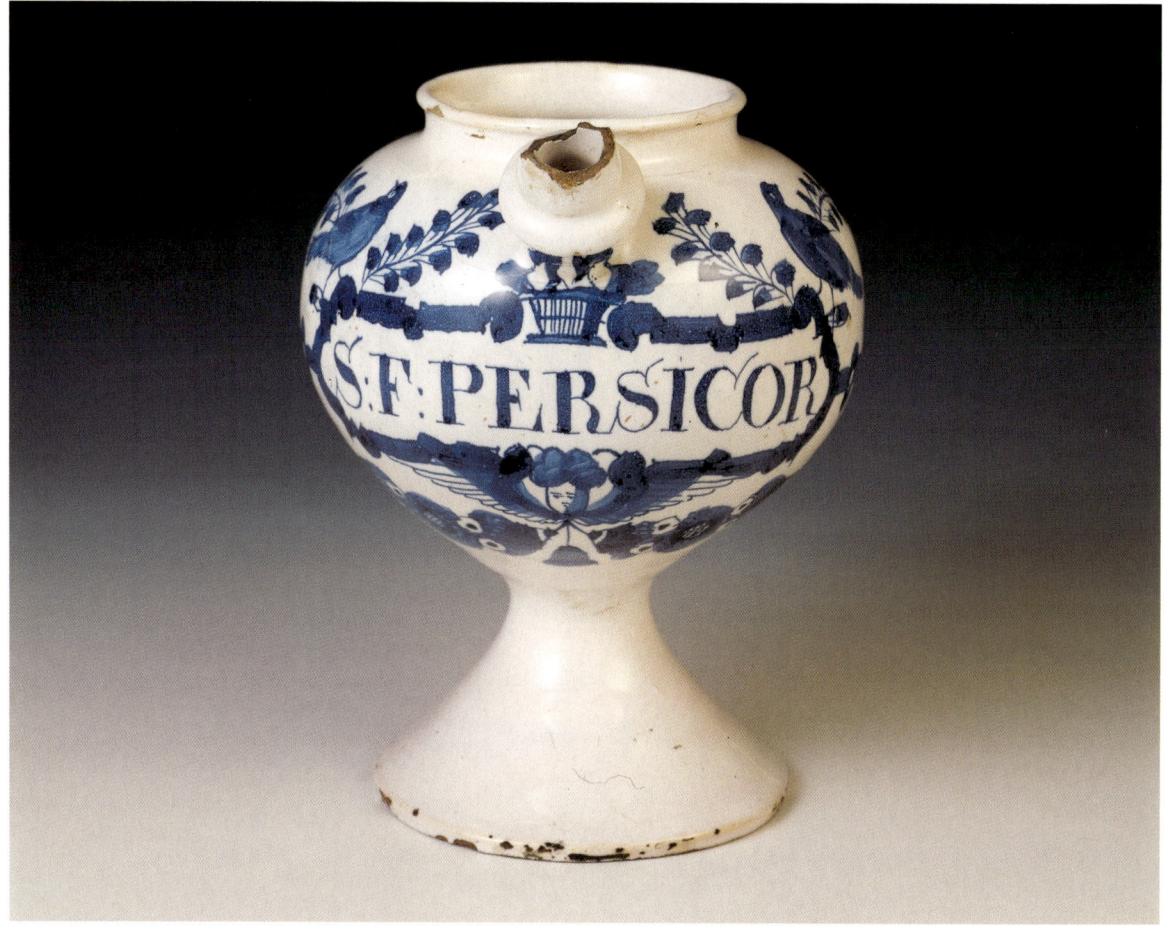

Wet drug jar (Cat.149)

ACCESSION NUMBER: KDK2

DESCRIPTION: Bulbous jar on spreading foot with spout and fluted strap-like handle. White glaze with pinkish tinge and design in blue. Label panel straight with wavy strap-work frame. Neck ridged with glazed rim, flanged spout, hollowed and glazed base with unglazed edge. In blue on base: J.

DESIGN: Later songbirds

INSCRIPTION: S:F:PERSICOR

MEANING OF INSCRIPTION: *Syrupus de floribus persicorum*, syrup of peach blossom (*Prunus persica*)

CONTEMPORARY ACCOUNT: "'Take Flowers of Peaches ℔ i. and pour upon them ℔ iii. of boiling Water: after 24 hours steeping, press out the Liquor, and repeat the Infusion with a fresh quantity of Flowers five times; then in the last straining dissolve ℔ iiss of Sugar, and boil it up to a due Consistence.'

"This is generally made by one Infusion, pouring on only so much as will scald the Flowers. It is a pretty Puke for Children, and opens a little downwards, for which purpose it is much in use. Dose from ℥ ii to ℥ i." (J. Quincy, *A Compleat English*

Dispensatory, 1718, p. 379)

DATE OF MANUFACTURE: 1700–1730

PLACE OF MANUFACTURE: London

DIMENSIONS: Height 190 mm, maximum width 160 mm

PROVENANCE: Bequest, Saville Peck, 1955.

CONDITION: Good; large chip off spout, glaze flaked from spout and handle, and neck and base rims.

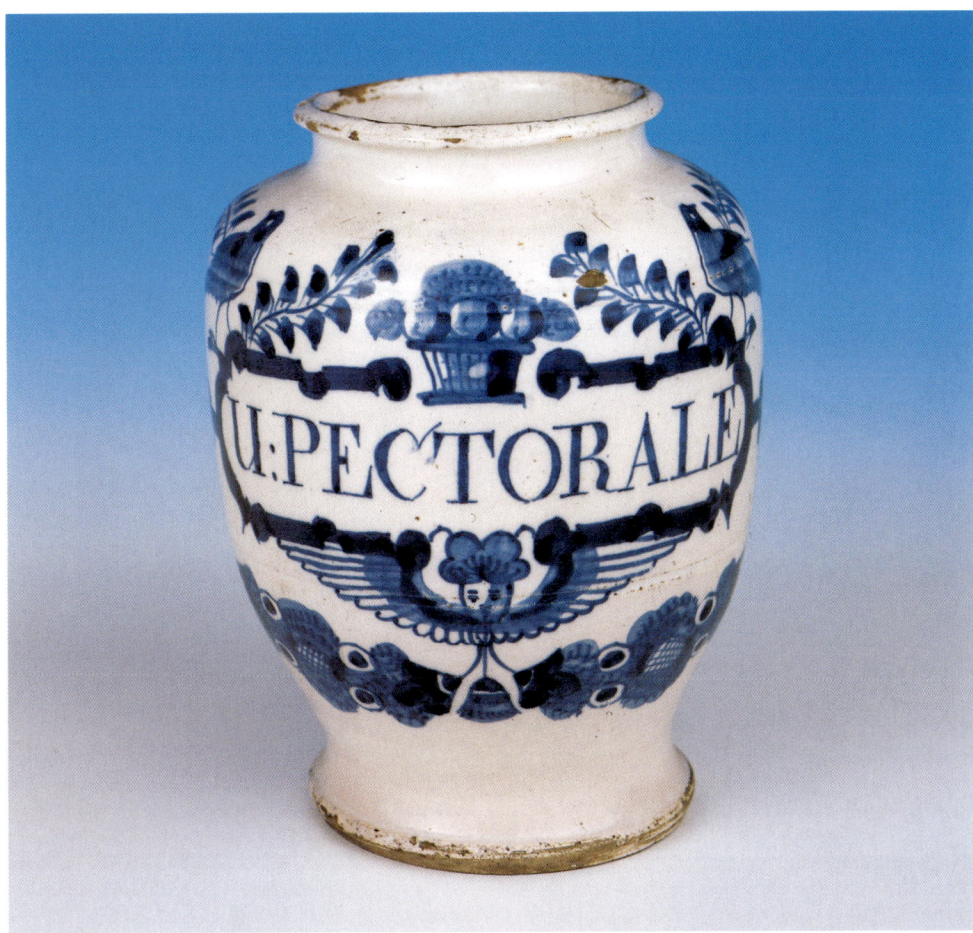

Dry drug jar (Cat.150)

ACCESSION NUMBER: KCK4

DESCRIPTION: Ovoid jar, tapering slightly towards splayed base, with two faint narrow ridges encircling bowl, one below the neck and the other below the label. White glaze with pinkish tinge and design in blue. Label panel straight with wavy strap-work frame. Neck everted with glazed rim, slightly concave glazed base with unglazed edge. In blue on base: 38.

DESIGN: Later songbirds

INSCRIPTION: U:PECTORALE

MEANING OF INSCRIPTION: *Unguentum pectorale*, ointment for disorders of the chest and lungs.

CONTEMPORARY ACCOUNT: "'Take Oil of sweet Almonds ℥ iv. of Camomile and Violets, ana ℥ iii. Fresh Butter wash'd with Violet-Water ℥ vi. Hen's and Duck's-Fat, ana ℥ ii. Orrice –Root ℥ ii. Saffron ℥ ss. Wax ℥ iii. Mix S.A.'

"This is commended to anoint the Breast with, in all Diseases of that Part, as it is suppos'd to open and relax the Vessels, and give more room for their respective Fluids to move in: for which reason it is judg'd of service in Pleurisies, Asthma's, and such-like Ailments. But the present Practice has always recourse to extemporaneous Forms in such Cases, and very rarely takes notice of this. This Medicine likewise will not keep long without turning rancid, and therefore ought to be made but in small quantities by those who have Opinion enough to continue its use. The *Orrice* and *Saffron* are to be finely powder'd, and sifter in, when the other Ingredients have been mix'd, and are almost cold. The Lotion of the Butter...is ridiculous." (J. Quincy, *A Compleat English Dispensatory*, 1718, p. 458)

DATE OF MANUFACTURE: 1700–1750

PLACE OF MANUFACTURE: Probably Lambeth, London

DIMENSIONS: Height 165 mm, maximum width 135 mm

PROVENANCE: Bought in 1957, Howard Collection.

CONDITION: Good; neck chipped, two cracks radiating from a deep pit in back of bowl, glaze flaked on neck and base rims.

COMMENT: Howard suggests that the '38' painted on the base could refer to the individual who painted the jar, but feels that it is unlikely that any Lambeth pottery employed 38 people. Instead, he suggests that this may refer to a production date of 1738 (p. 22).

REFERENCE: Howard, English Delftware Drug Jars, p. 22 and No. 38.

Later songbirds

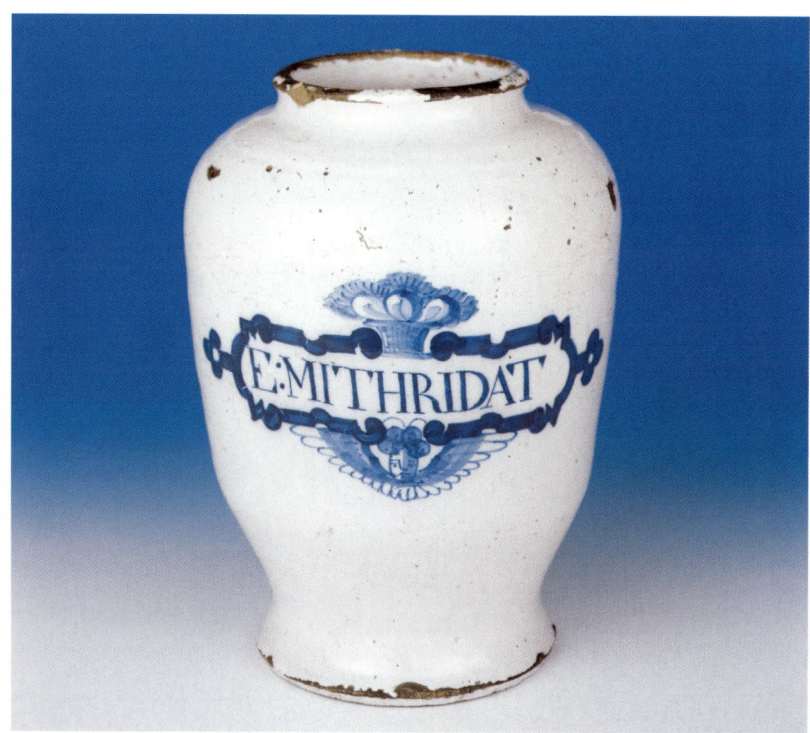

Dry drug jar (Cat.151)

ACCESSION NUMBER: KCY2

DESCRIPTION: Ovoid jar, tapering towards splayed base. White glaze with pinkish tinge and design in blue. Label panel straight with wavy strap-work frame. Neck ridged with partly glazed rim, flat and glazed base, with unglazed edge.

DESIGN: Basket (centred) above label. Angel with outspread wings (centred) below label

INSCRIPTION: E:MITHRIDAT

MEANING OF INSCRIPTION: *Electuarium Mithridatium*, Mithridates' electuary. One of several forms of theriac (treacle) still popular in the 17th century and regarded as a universal antidote against poisons and infectious diseases. The formula given in the London Pharmacopoeia of 1650 had 50 ingredients. The name Mithridate is derived from Mithridates VI, king of Pontus (132–63 BC), who was believed to have rendered himself immune to poisoning by the constant use of antidotes.

CONTEMPORARY ACCOUNT: Quincy has a long and detailed account of this preparation and suggests that the ingredients that have an effect should be increased in quantity, with opium remaining at the same proportion of the whole. The official recipe he provides is as follows:

"Take of Arabian Myrrh, Saffron, Agaric, Ginger, Cinnamon, Spikenard, Frankincense, and Seeds of Treacle-Mustard, ana ℥ x. of the Seeds of Hartwort, Opobalsamum, or in its stead, expressed Oil of Nutmegs, Sweet-Rush, Arabian Stoechas, the true Costus, Galbanum, Cyprus Turpentine, Long Pepper, Castor, Juice of Hypocistis, Styrax, Opoanax, and Indian Leaf, or in its stead Mace, ana ℥ i. of Cassia

Bark, Polymountain, white Pepper, Scordium, Seeds of wild Carrot, Carpobalsam, or Cubebs, Troches of Cypheos, and Bdellium, ana ℥ vii. of Spikenard cleansed, Gum Arabic, Macedonian Parsley Seed, Opium, the lesser Cardamoms, Fennel Seeds, Gentian Root, red Rose Flowers, and Dittany of Crete, ana ℥ v. of Aniseeds, Asarum, Acorus or Calamus Aromaticus, Orrice, the greater Valerian, and Sagapenum, ana ℥ iii. of Meum Root, Acacia, Stinks, and the tops of St. John's Wort, ana ℥ iiss. of the best Canary, enough to dissolve the Gums and Juices, which will take up about ℥ xxvi. of clarify'd Honey as much as the Weight of all the Ingredients, except the Wine, and make into an Electuary, S.A." (J. Quincy, *A Compleat English Dispensatory*, 1718, pp. 431–432)

DATE OF MANUFACTURE: c. 1710–1720

PLACE OF MANUFACTURE: London

DIMENSIONS: Height 250 mm, maximum width 193 mm

PROVENANCE: Bought in 1957, Howard Collection.

CONDITION: Fair; base chipped, large piece of glaze missing at back, glaze badly crazed and pitted and flaked on rims of neck and base.

COMMENT: Howard refers to this jar as having "a distinctly XVIIth century feeling. It is heavy and a little crude." He says that the panel is similar to his number 10 c.1669 (p. 19). However, there are very close parallels on some of the cherub and trumpet jars and some of the later songbird jars, so the date is definitely early 18th century.

There is a second jar of this type inscribed MEL: ANGLIC in the Wilkinson Collection at the Thackray Museum, Leeds. Agnes Lothian's opinion that this was the only other known example (letter from Robert Allbrook 16/8/1962) has not been disproved.

REFERENCE: Howard, G. E. English Delftware Drug Jars, The Medici Society, London, 1931, p. 19 and No. 36.

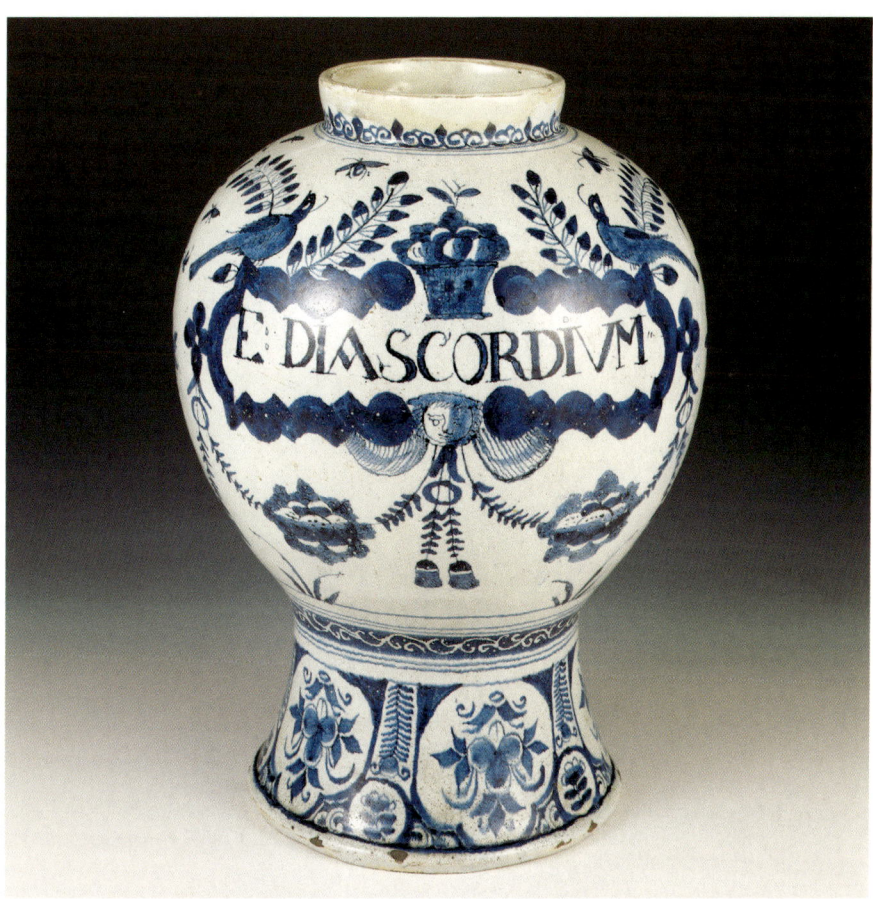

Dry drug jar (Cat.152)

ACCESSION NUMBER: KCK2

DESCRIPTION: Bulbous jar, tapering to a broad, slightly spreading foot. White glaze with bluish tinge and design in dark blue. Label panel straight, with thick wavy strap-work frame. Straight neck with glazed rim. Slightly concave unglazed base.

DESIGN: Later songbirds, with Chinese style design, including a peacock, on reverse

INSCRIPTION: E:DIASCORDIVM

MEANING OF INSCRIPTION: *Electuarium diascordium*, electuary of scordium. The formula for this medicine is traced back to Frascatorius in the 1500s. It was chiefly used for the plague.

CONTEMPORARY ACCOUNT: Quincy includes a substantial entry on this preparation, with the official recipe given and then a long commentary with suggestions of alterations in ingredients and method.

"'Diascordium. *A Composition of Scordium.* Take of Cinnamon, and Cassia Wood, ana ℥ ss. of true Scordium ℥ i. of *Cretan* Dittany, Tormentil, Bistort, Galbanum, and Gum Arabic, ana ℥ iss. of Storax ℥ ivss. of Opium and Seeds of Sorrel, ana ℥ iss. of Gentian ℥ ss. of *Armenian* Bole ℥ iss. of *Lemnian* Sealed Earth ℥ ss. of long Pepper and Ginger, ana ℥ ii. of clarif'd Honey lb iiss. of Sugar of Roses lb i. of generous Canary ℥ viii. Take it into an Electuary, S.A....'

"Everyone knows how much this is of use, and for what purposes, and indeed if the several Ingredients be nicely selected, and the Medicine fresh made, it is excellent in all Fluxes whatsoever, and a great Strengthener both of the Stomach and Bowels. In its influence on the Fluxes, the Opium has no small share, as may be well conceiv'd from the Virtues of that Drug... A very mischievous way some Nurses have got, of giving their Children this Medicine to make them sleep, more for their own Ease than any thing else..." (J. Quincy, *A Compleat English Dispensatory*, 1718, p. 429)

DATE OF MANUFACTURE: 1690–1720

PLACE OF MANUFACTURE: London

DIMENSIONS: Height 360 mm, maximum width 265 mm

PROVENANCE: Bought in 1956.

CONDITION: Good; glaze chipped at rim of base.

COMMENT: It is probable that this highly decorative jar was only used for display purposes.

REFERENCE: Drey, Apothecary Jars. Plate 69A and 69B, and pp. 130 and 136.

Later songbirds

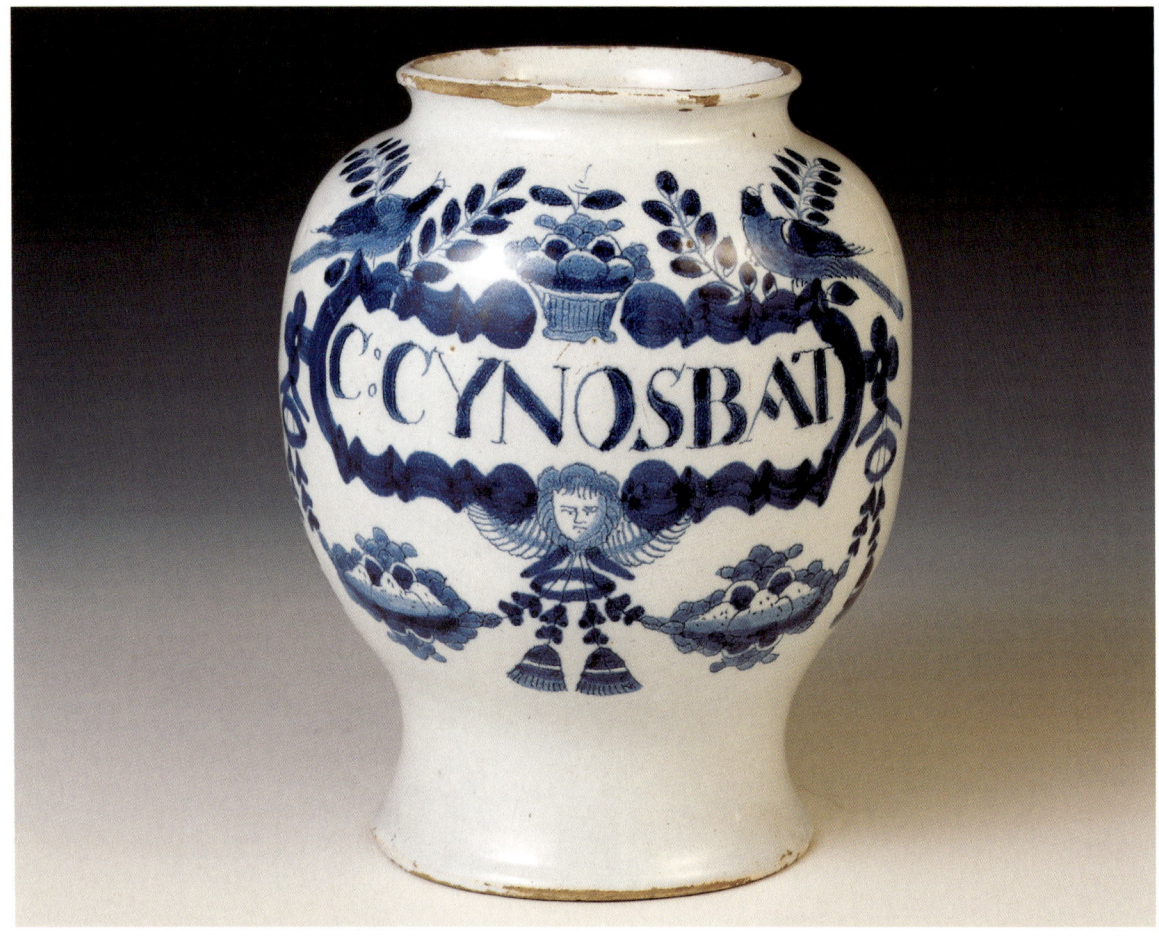

Dry drug jar (Cat.153)

ACCESSION NUMBER: KCK12

DESCRIPTION: Ovoid jar, tapering towards splayed base. White glaze with pinkish tinge and design in blue. Label panel straight with wavy strap-work frame. Neck everted with glazed rim, concave and partly glazed base.

DESIGN: Later songbirds

INSCRIPTION: C:CYNOSBAT

MEANING OF INSCRIPTION: *Conservus cynobastus*, conserve of rosehips from the dog rose (*Rosa caninus*)

CONTEMPORARY ACCOUNT: "Take of the pulp of ripe hips one pound, of double refined sugar twenty ounces; and mix them into a conserve." (H. Pemberton, *The Dispensatory*, 1746, p. 157)

DATE OF MANUFACTURE: 1720–1740

PLACE OF MANUFACTURE: Southwark, London

DIMENSIONS: Height 180 mm, maximum width 158 mm

PROVENANCE: Donated by Mr Hammond, date unknown.

CONDITION: Good; base chipped, glaze flaked from rim of neck.

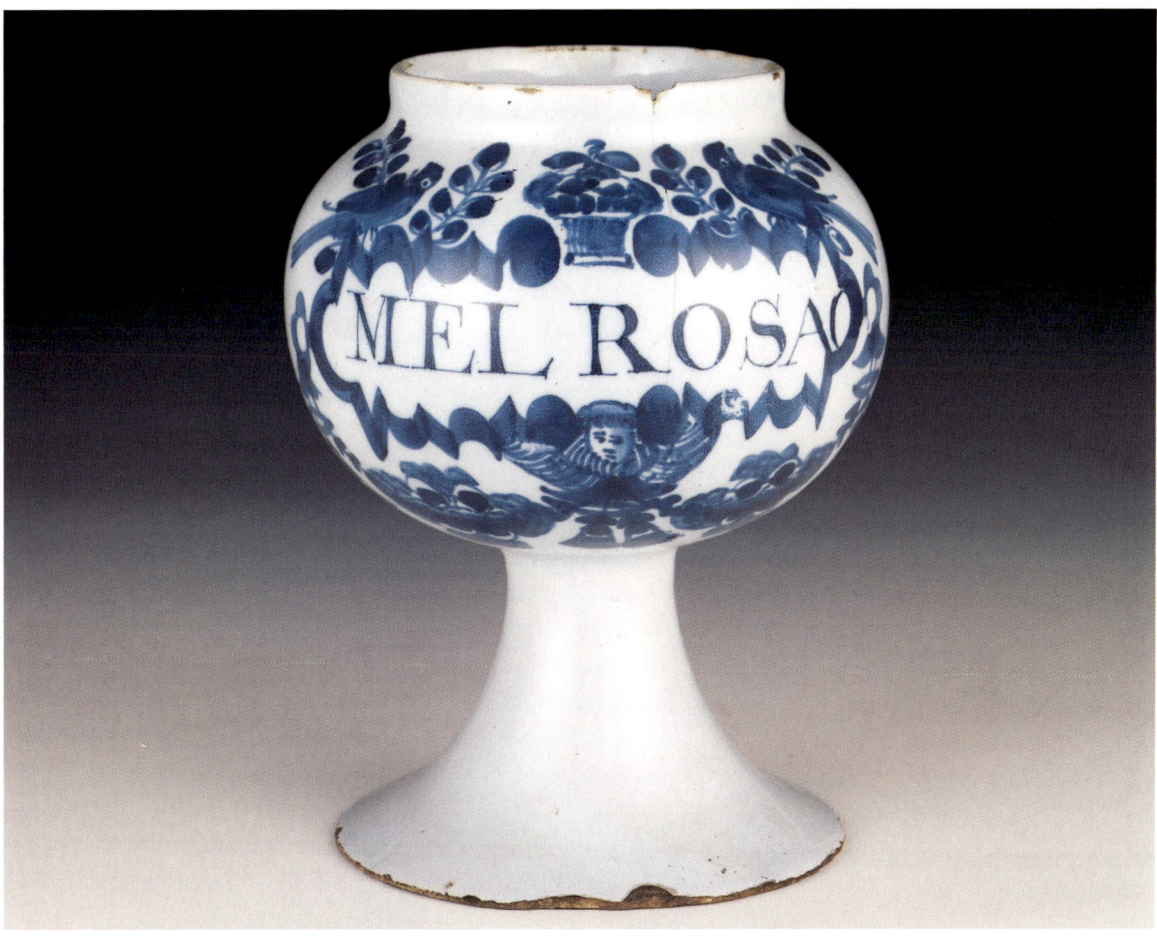

Wet drug jar (Cat.154)

ACCESSION NUMBER: KDK5
DESCRIPTION: Bulbous jar on spreading foot, with spout (on opposite side to label) and no handle. White glaze with bluish tinge and design in blue. Label panel straight with wavy strapwork frame. Neck straight with glazed rim, spout very slightly flared, hollowed and glazed base with unglazed edge.
DESIGN: Later songbirds
INSCRIPTION: MEL ROSAC
MEANING OF INSCRIPTION: *Mel Rosaceum*, honey of roses
CONTEMPORARY ACCOUNT: "Take of red-rose buds quick dried, and their heels cut off, four ounces, of boiling water three pints, of clarified honey five pounds. Steep the roses some hours in water; then to the strained liquor add the honey, and boil to a proper consistence." (H. Pemberton, *The Dispensatory*, 1746, p. 306)
DATE OF MANUFACTURE: 1700–1740
PLACE OF MANUFACTURE: Bristol, London and Dublin have all been proposed
DIMENSIONS: Height 190 mm, maximum width 150 mm

PROVENANCE: Bought in 1957, Howard Collection.
CONDITION: Good; crack descending from chip in neck, base chipped, glaze flaked from neck, spout and base rims.
REFERENCE: Howard, English Delftware Drug Jars, p. 22 and No. 45

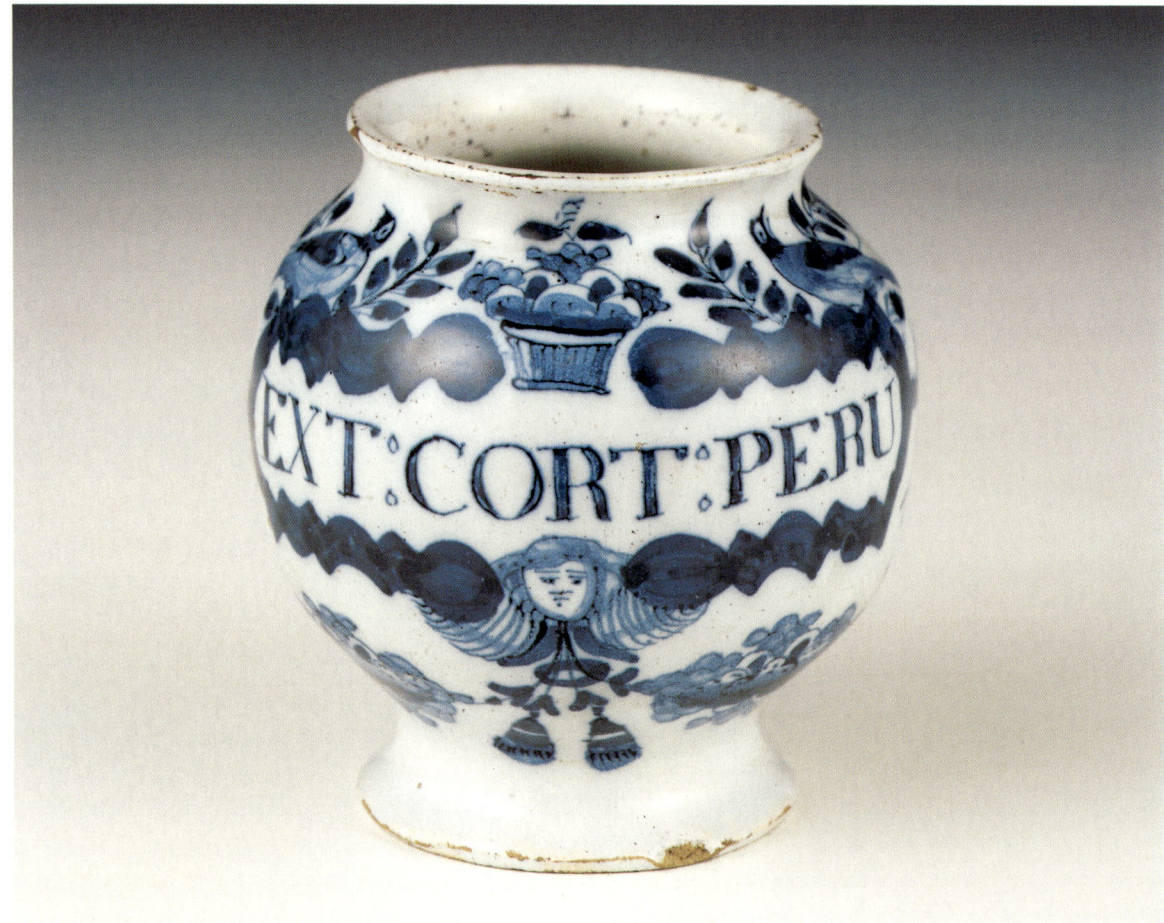

Dry drug jar (Cat.155)

ACCESSION NUMBER: KCK9

DESCRIPTION: Bulbous jar, tapering slightly towards splayed base. White glaze with pinkish tinge and design in blue. Label panel straight with wavy strap-work frame. Neck everted with glazed rim, slightly concave unglazed base.

DESIGN: Later songbirds

INSCRIPTION: EXT:CORT:PERU

MEANING OF INSCRIPTION: *Extractum corticis peruviani*, extract of bark from Peru – cinchona bark

CONTEMPORARY ACCOUNT: "This comes to us from *Peru* in the *West – Indies*; whence the Romish Missionaries first brought it into *Europe*, and gave occasion for its being call'd *Jesuits Bark*. This *Simple* is so lately brought into Medicine, that there is little to be met with in Authors about it; and People's Notions seem yet so confus'd and undetermin'd concerning its Virtues and Efficacy..." (J. Quincy, *A Compleat English Dispensatory*, 1718, pp. 166)

DATE OF MANUFACTURE: 1700–1770

PLACE OF MANUFACTURE: Southwark, London

DIMENSIONS: Height 85 mm, maximum width 83 mm

PROVENANCE: Bought in 1957, Howard Collection.

CONDITION: Good; neck and base chipped, glaze flaked from neck and base rims.

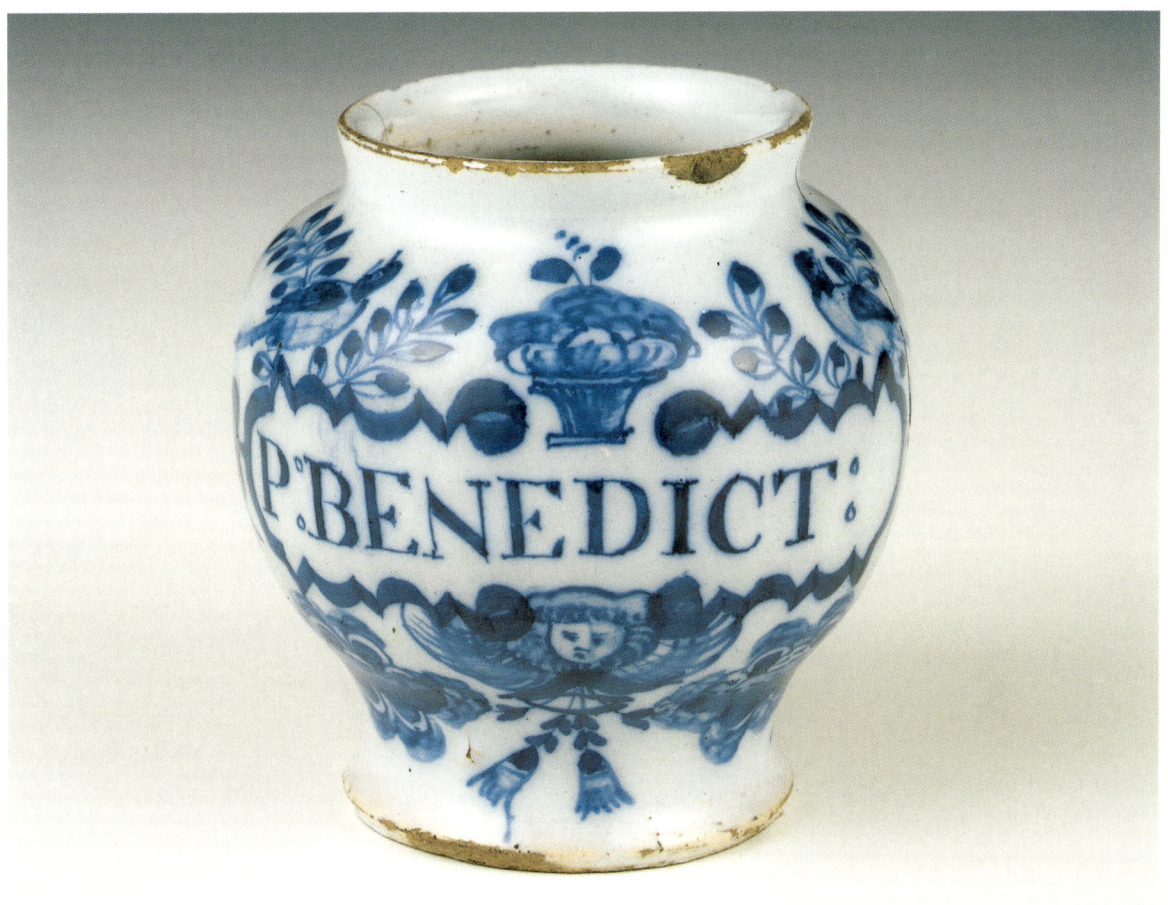

Dry drug jar (Cat.156)

ACCESSION NUMBER: KCK10
DESCRIPTION: Bulbous jar, tapering slightly towards splayed base. White glaze with pinkish tinge and design in blue. Label panel straight with wavy strap-work frame. Neck slightly flared with unglazed rim, glazed base with unglazed edge.
DESIGN: Later songbirds
INSCRIPTION: P:BENEDICT:
MEANING OF INSCRIPTION: *Pilulae Benedictae*, blessed pills
CONTEMPORARY ACCOUNT: "Take Aloes lb ss, Gum Ammoniacum in fine Drops ℥ ii, Juice of Carduus inspissated ℥ i, with Rhenish wine and Carduus Water, make a Mass…

"They purge Choler and Melancholy, all gross and tartarous humours, salt and mucilaginous, from the very profound parts; cure Madness, Frenzy, Melancholy, Quartans, Scabs, Itch, Cancers, Leprosies, Scurvy, Dropsy, Gout, French Pox, and purify the whole Mass of Blood." (W. Salmon, *The New London Dispensatory*, 1716, pp. 606 and 612)
DATE OF MANUFACTURE: 1720–1740
PLACE OF MANUFACTURE: London

DIMENSIONS: Height 75 mm, maximum width 78 mm
PROVENANCE: Bought in 1956.
CONDITION: Fair; two large cracks descending from neck and joining on bowl, base and neck rims chipped, glaze flaked on base and neck rims.

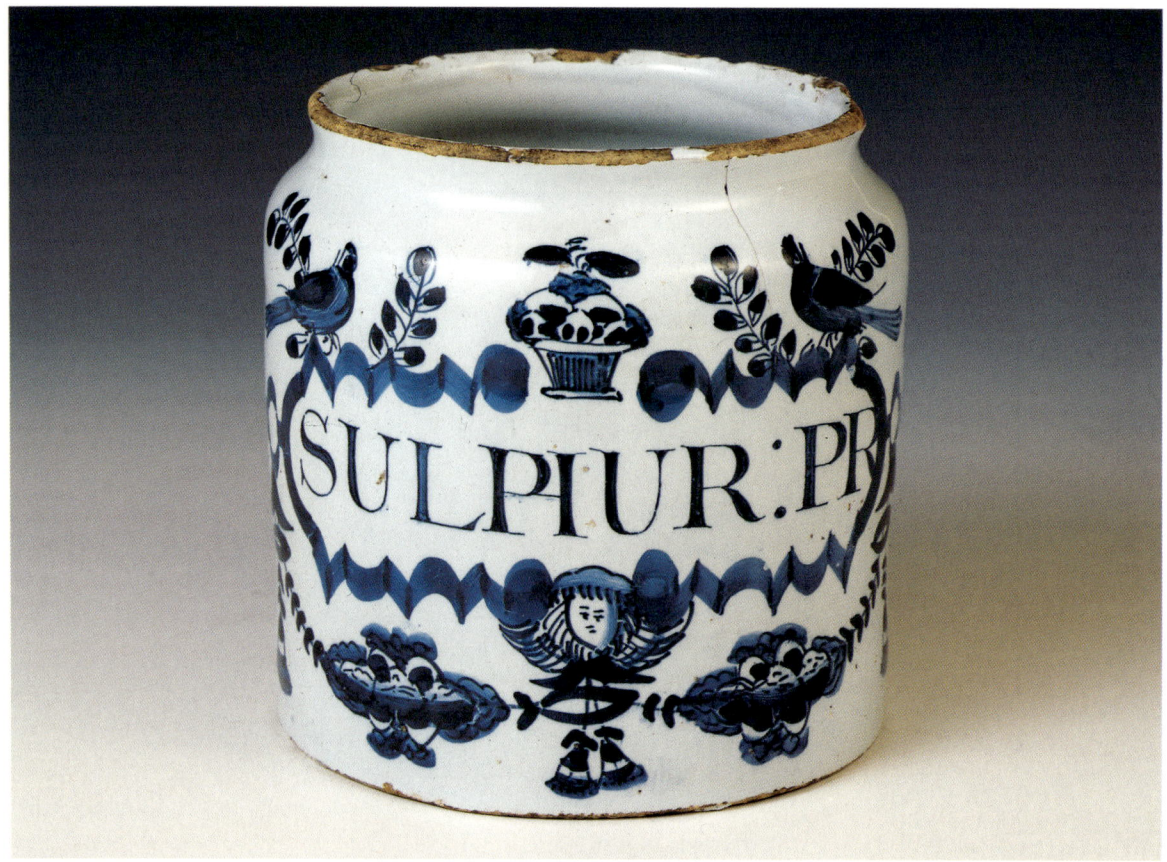

Dry drug jar (Cat.157)

ACCESSION NUMBER: KCK7

DESCRIPTION: Cylindrical jar. White glaze with pinkish tinge and design in blue. Label panel straight with wavy strap-work frame. Neck slightly everted with glazed rim, slightly concave and partly glazed base.

DESIGN: Later songbirds

INSCRIPTION: SULPHUR:PR

MEANING OF INSCRIPTION: *Sulphur praecipitatum*, precipitated sulphur

CONTEMPORARY ACCOUNT: "Boil flowers of sulphur with thrice their weight of quick lime, till the sulphur is dissolved, and filtre the solution through paper; then with weak spirit of vitriol make a precipitation, which is to be often washed, till it is become quite insipid." (H. Pemberton, *The Dispensatory*, 1746 p. 210)

DATE OF MANUFACTURE: 1740–1760

PLACE OF MANUFACTURE: London

DIMENSIONS: Height 125 mm, maximum width 135 mm

PROVENANCE: Bought in 1961.

CONDITION: Good; neck chipped, three cracks descending from neck, glaze flaked on body and neck and base rims.

COMMENT: This is part of the same group as KCK6 (Cat. 158). Note the ligated PH, and the overlap of the final R on the cartouche. It seems that the painter made the letters too big and ran out of space.

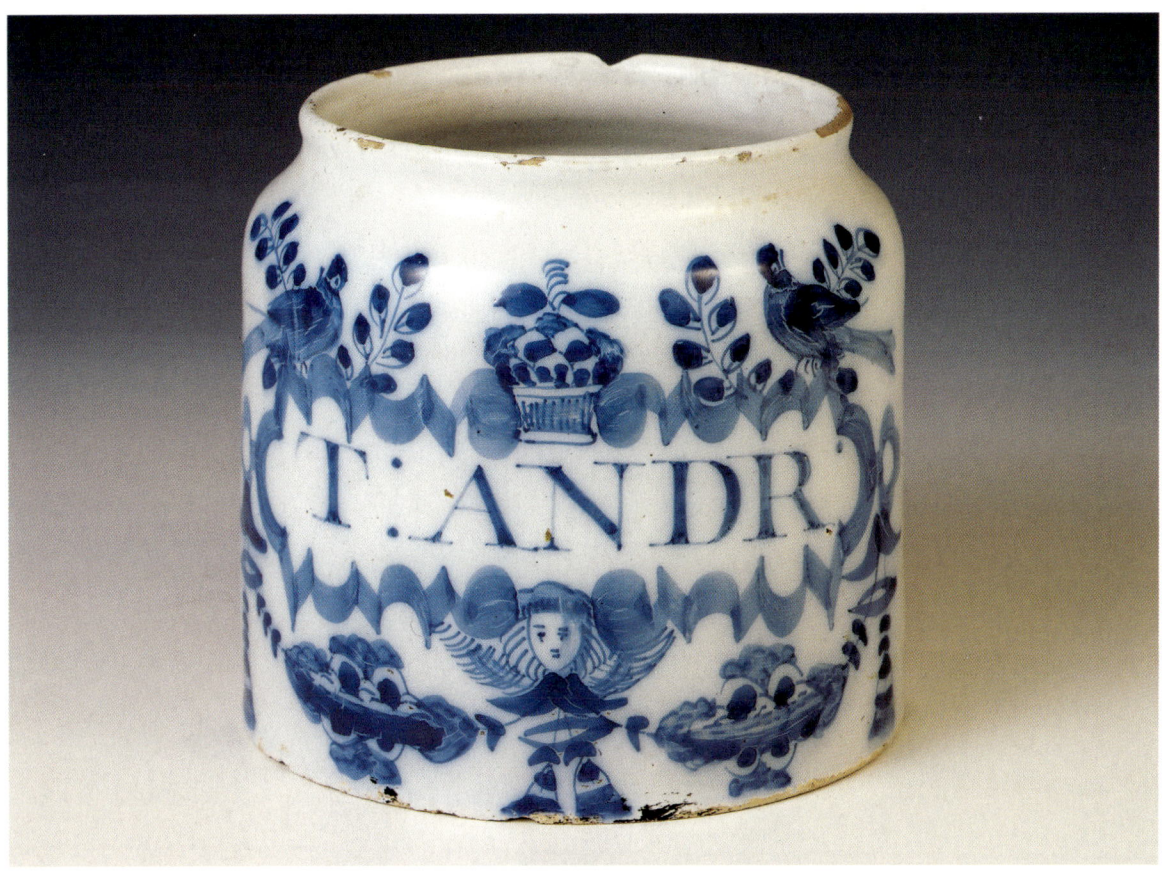

Dry drug jar (Cat.158)

ACCESSION NUMBER: KCK6

DESCRIPTION: Cylindrical jar. White glaze with pinkish tinge and design in blue. Label panel straight with wavy strap-work frame. Neck ridged with glazed rim, slightly concave glazed base with unglazed edge.

DESIGN: Later songbirds

INSCRIPTION: T:ANDR

MEANING OF INSCRIPTION: *Theriaca Andromachi*, the treacle or theriaca of Andromachus, a preparation traced back to Andromachus, physician to the Emperor Nero (AD 37). This extraordinary preparation was supposed to be an antidote to all poisons. It was also used in the 1600s to prevent the plague.

CONTEMPORARY ACCOUNT: "Take *Troches of Squills* ℥ vi. Troches of Vipers, long Pepper, *Opium*, and Troches of Hedycroi, ana ℥ iii. *Red Rose Buds dry'd, Orrice, Juice of Liquorice, Seeds of Sweet Navew*, Tops of Scordium, Opobalsam, *Troches of Agarick*, Cinnamon, ana ℥ iss. Myrrh, Zedoary, Saffron, *Cassia-Bark*, Spikenard, Schoenanth, white and black Pepper, *Frankincense, Dittany of Crete, Rhapontick*, Staecha's, *Hore-Hound, Parsley-Seeds*, Calaminth, *Cyprus* Turpentine, *Roots of Cinque-foil*, and Ginger, ana ℥ vi. *Tops of Polymountain*, Ground-Pine, *Celtick* Spikenard, *Amomus*, Styrax, Meum-Root, Tops of Germander, *Phu-Root, Earth of* Lemnos, Indian Leaf, *Calcanthum, Gentian Root, Gum-Arabick, Juice of Hypocistis*, Cubebs, Seeds of Anise, Cardomoms, Fennel, of *Hartwort, German Acacia*, Seeds of Treacle-Mustard, Tops of St John's-wort, *Seeds of Bishop's-weed*, Sagapenum, ana ℥ iv. Castor, *long Birthwort, Amber*, or *Bitumen Judaicum, Seeds of Daucus*, Opoponax, *Centaury the lesser*, and Galbanum, ana ℥ ii. Canary ℥ xl. Honey, three times the weight of the whole Species when powder'd; and mix all into an Electuary.

This is not only the Capital Alexipharmick of our Shops, but of all *Europe*; and has a great deal more wrote about it, than could be contain'd in the largest Volume" (J. Quincy, *A Compleat English Dispensatory*, 1718, p. 409)

DATE OF MANUFACTURE: 1740–1760

PLACE OF MANUFACTURE: London

DIMENSIONS: Height 125 mm, maximum width 140 mm

PROVENANCE: Bought in 1957, Howard Collection.

CONDITION: Good; neck and base chipped, glaze flaked from neck and base rims.

COMMENT: Howard suspected that this "unusual shape...a questionable specimen" was Dutch (p. 22). This is part of the same group as KCK7 (Cat. 157).

REFERENCE: Howard, English Delftware Drug Jars, p. 22 and No. 52.

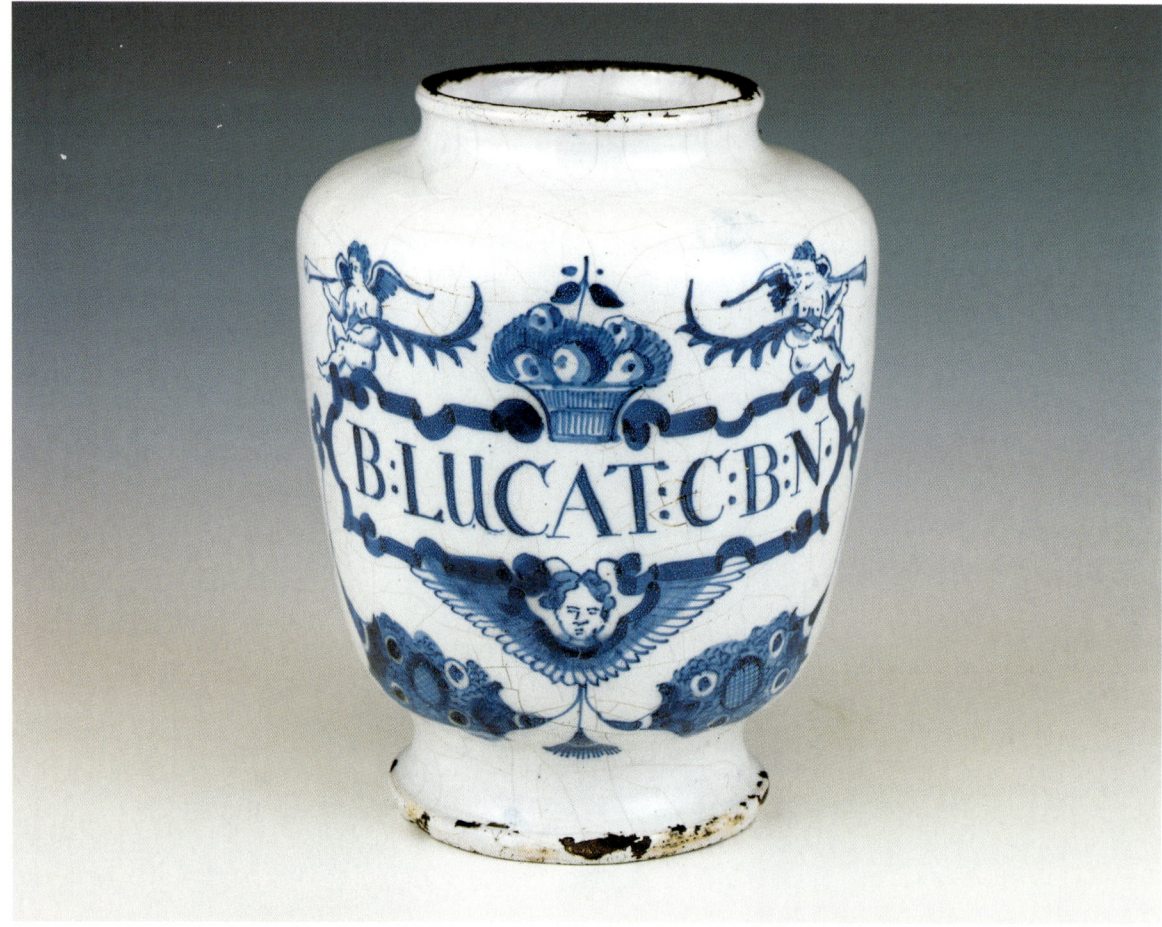

Dry drug jar (Cat.159)

ACCESSION NUMBER: KCM2

DESCRIPTION: Ovoid jar, tapering slightly towards splayed base. White glaze with pinkish tinge and design in blue. Label panel straight with wavy strap-work frame. Neck ridged with unglazed rim, slightly concave and partly glazed base.

DESIGN: Cherubs with trumpets (design of right-hand cherub incomplete)

INSCRIPTION: B:LUCAT:C:B:N

MEANING OF INSCRIPTION: *Balsamum locatelli*, ointment formulated by Lodovico Locatelli (d.1657), an Italian physician.

CONTEMPORARY ACCOUNT: "'From the College. Take yellow Wax melted in a little Canary-Wine ℔ i. Oil of Olives, *Venice* – Turpentine wash'd in Rose-water, ana ℔ iss. Boil them till the Wine is evaporated, and when almost cold, stir in of red Sanders, finely powder'd ℥ ii. and preserve it for use... This Composition stands recommended for an internal *Vulnerary*, and is prescribed in such Coughs as give suspicion of *Tubercules* and *Ulcerations* in the Lungs; and also in all internal Decays from the like Causes, whether the Seat be in the Breast, or any other part.

It is given likewise upon accidental Bruises and inward Bleeding. Externally it is used to deterge and incarnate green Wounds and Ulcers that are not of too long standing."
(J. Quincy, *A Compleat English Dispensatory*, 1718, p. 445)

DATE OF MANUFACTURE: 1700–1725

PLACE OF MANUFACTURE: London, or possibly Bristol.

DIMENSIONS: Height 180 mm, maximum width 150 mm

PROVENANCE: Donation, 1953, Austen Collection.

CONDITION: Good; glaze crazed and flaked on neck and base rims.

COMMENT: The significance of C:B:N: in the inscription remains a mystery.

REFERENCE: Lothian, 'The John Austen Collection' Figure 10 and pp. 97 and 99.

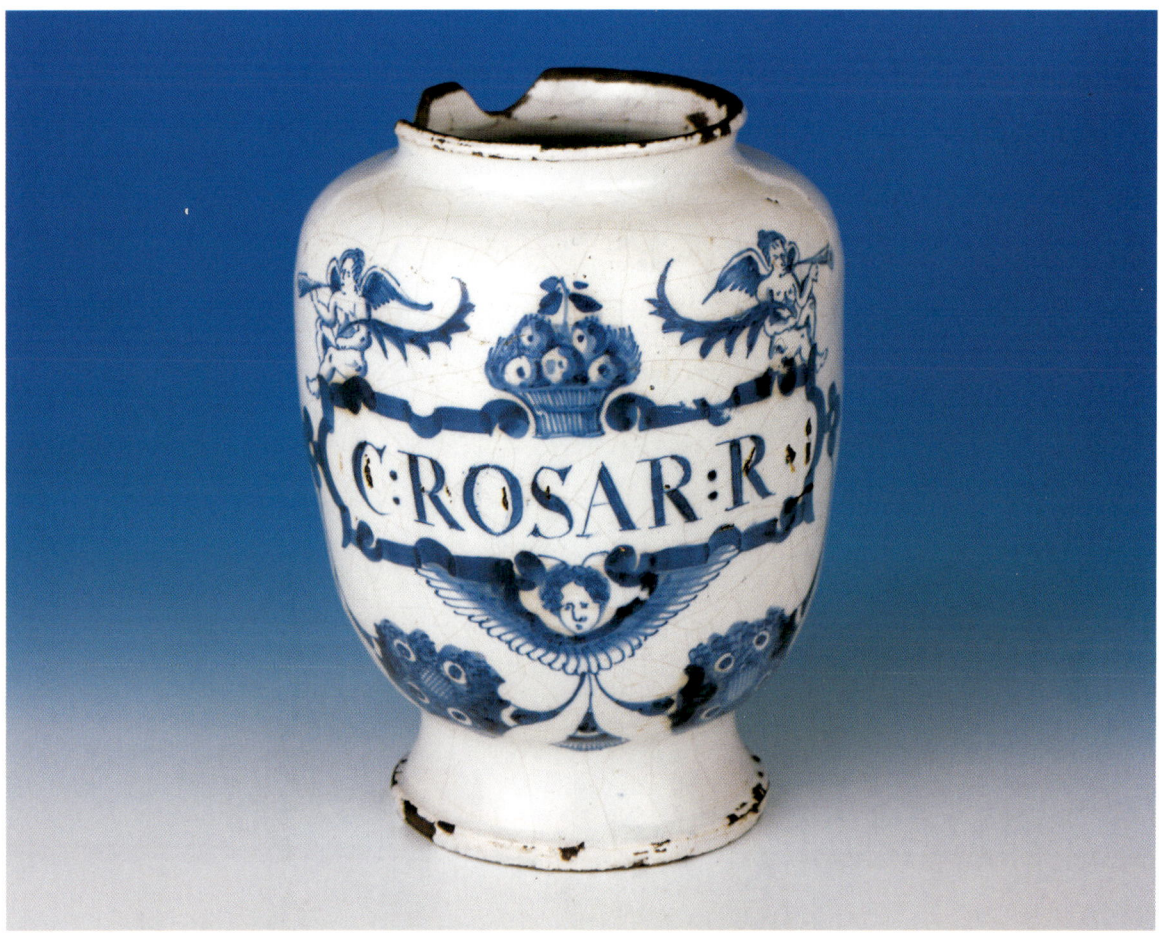

Dry drug jar (Cat.160)

ACCESSION NUMBER: KCM3
DESCRIPTION: Ovoid jar, tapering slightly towards splayed base. White glaze with pinkish tinge and design in blue. Label panel straight with wavy strap-work frame. Neck everted with unglazed rim, slightly concave and partly glazed base.
DESIGN: Cherubs with trumpets
INSCRIPTION: C:ROSAR:R
MEANING OF INSCRIPTION: *Conserva rosarum rubrum*, conserve of red roses.
CONTEMPORARY ACCOUNT: "'These blow in *May* and *June*. They are sufficiently known to all Persons. What are used in the Shops, unless for the distill'd Water, are the Buds before they quite blow; because then they are much rougher and more astringent. The Conserve made of them is deservedly in great esteem, but the common Notion of its being the better for Age, is an Error: for their Astringency, which arises from the Solidity and Asperity of their component Parts, by long lying in the Sugar, which mellows and softens them, very much decays. They are good in almost all Distempers of the Lungs, and particularly in Defluxions of *Rheum*." (J. Quincy, *A Compleat English Dispensatory*, 1718, p. 99)
DATE OF MANUFACTURE: 1700–1725
PLACE OF MANUFACTURE: London, or possibly Bristol.
DIMENSIONS: Height 175 mm, maximum width 143 mm
PROVENANCE: Donation, 1953, Austen Collection.
CONDITION: Fair; two large chips from neck, glaze crazed and flaked on neck and base rims.
REFERENCE: Lothian, 'The John Austen Collection' Figure 10 and p. 97.

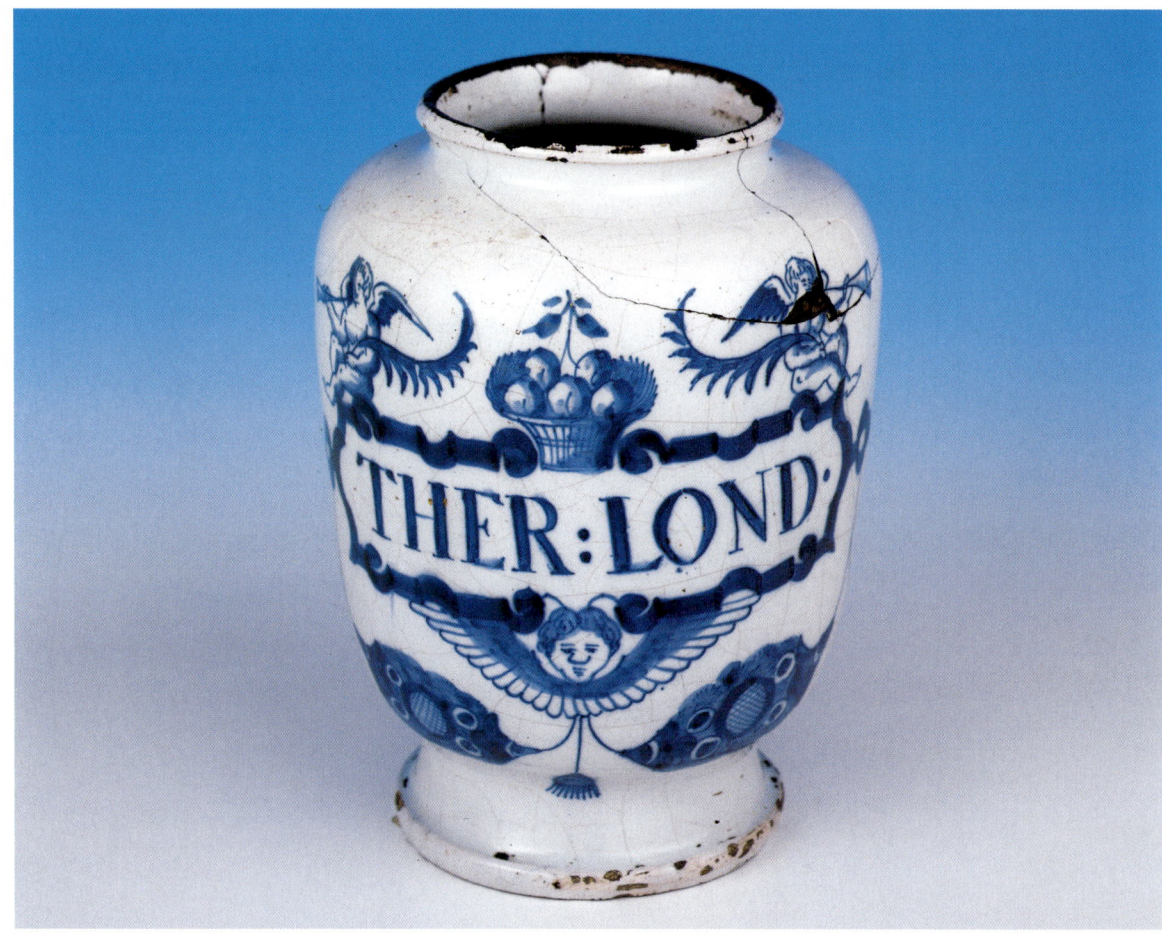

Dry drug jar (Cat. 161)

ACCESSION NUMBER: KCM1

DESCRIPTION: Ovoid jar, tapering slightly towards splayed base. White glaze with pinkish tinge and design in blue. Label panel straight with wavy strap-work frame. Neck everted with unglazed rim, slightly concave glazed base with unglazed edge.

DESIGN: Cherubs with trumpets

INSCRIPTION: THER:LOND

MEANING OF INSCRIPTION: *Theriaca Londinensis*, London treacle

CONTEMPORARY ACCOUNT: "'Take Raspings of Harts-horn ℨ ii. Seeds of Citrons, Sorrel, Piony, and Basil, ana ℨ i. Corallina, Scordium, ana ℨ vi. Roots of Angelica, Tormentils, Piony, Leaves of Dittany, Berries of Juniper and Laurel, ana ℨ ss. Flowers of Marigolds, Clove-Gillyflowers, of Rosemary, Tops of St. John's-wort, Nutmegs, Saffron, ana ℨ iii. Roots of Gentian, Zedoary, Ginger, Mace, Myrrh, Leaves of Carduus, Scabious, Devil's-bit, ana ℨ ii. Cloves, Opium, ana ℨ i. Honey, three times the quantity of the whole; Canary, sufficient to make an Electuary.'

"This is so indifferent a Composition, that even *Salmon* has much mended it, tho his is a very odd Medley with which he pretended to cure so many in the last great *Sickness* 1665, and in the use of which he affirms none miscarry'd. This is now so much out of practice, that it is not worth our particular Animadversion: we shall only therefore observe, that it has but gr. i. of *Opium* to each Ounce of *Theriaca*; and that it is sometimes used amongst the Surgeons as a warm Discutient, externally apply'd in *Cataplasms*." (J. Quincy, *A Compleat English Dispensatory*, 1718, p. 412)

DATE OF MANUFACTURE: 1700–1725

PLACE OF MANUFACTURE: London, or possibly Bristol

DIMENSIONS: Height 180 mm, maximum width 145 mm

PROVENANCE: Donation, 1953, Austen Collection.

CONDITION: Poor; has been repaired, three large cracks descending from neck, large chip missing from right-hand cherub, glaze crazed and flaked on neck and base rims.

REFERENCE: Lothian, 'The John Austen Collection' Figure 10 and pp. 97–98.

Cherubs with trumpets

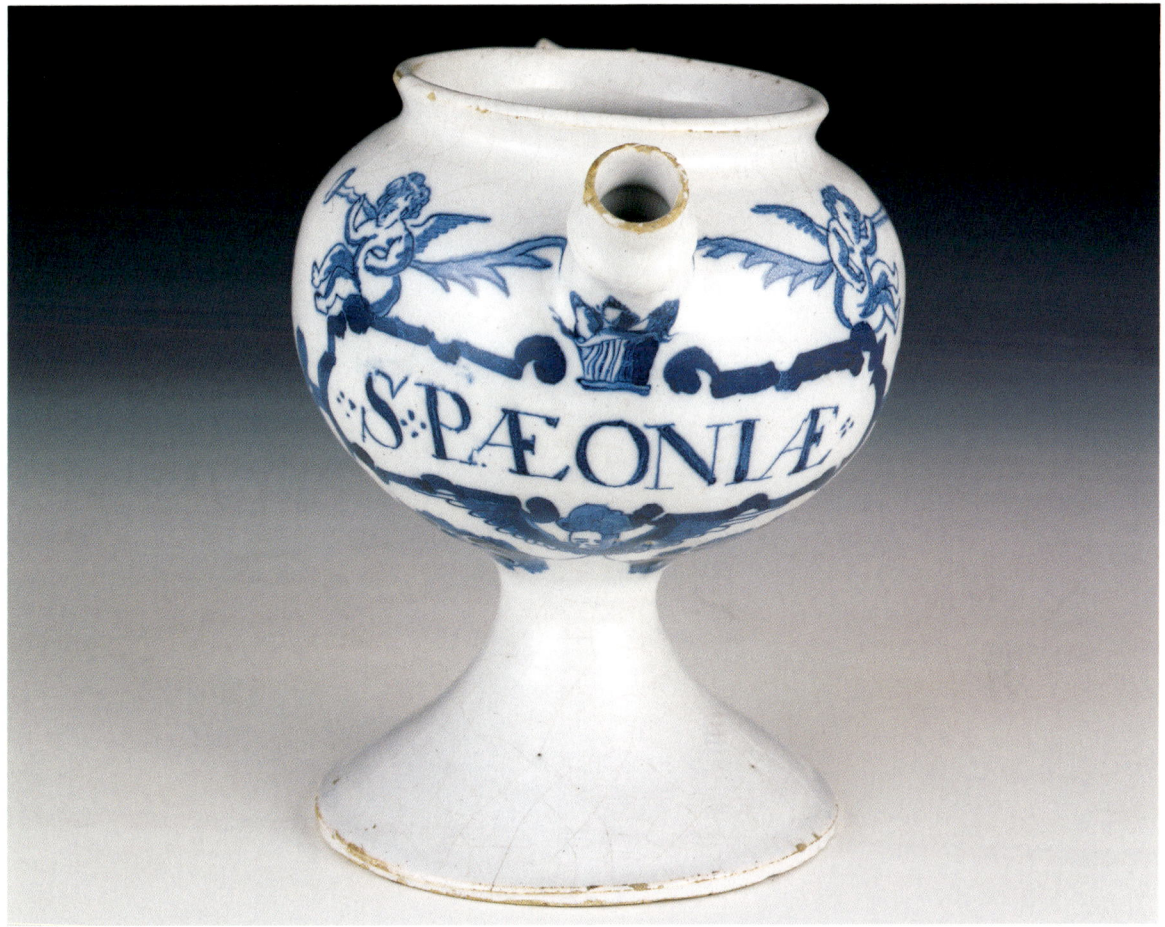

Wet drug jar (Cat.162)

ACCESSION NUMBER: KDM2

DESCRIPTION: Bulbous jar on spreading foot with spout and fluted strap-like looped handle. White glaze with pinkish tinge and design in blue. Label panel straight with wavy strap-work frame. Neck everted with glazed rim, flanged spout, glazed base with unglazed edge.

DESIGN: Cherubs with trumpets

INSCRIPTION: S PAEONIAE

MEANING OF INSCRIPTION: *Syrupus paeonia*, syrup of peonies (*Peonia officinalis*)

CONTEMPORARY ACCOUNT: "'Take Roots of fresh Pioney, Male and Female, ana ℥ iss. infused in White-Wine; of Contrayerva ℥ ss. Bastard-Lovage ℥ vi. Elks-Hoof ℥ i. Rosemary with the Flowers m.i. Betony, Origanum, Hyssop, Ground-Pine, and Rue ana ℥ iii. Wood of Aloes, Cloves and the lesser Cardamoms, ana ℥ ii. Ginger and Spikenard, ana ℥ ii. Staechas and Nutmegs, ana ℥ iiss. Water of Pioney-Root ℔ vi. Digest them together some hours, and boil to ℔ iv. To the straining add ℔ ivss. of Sugar, and make into a Syrup.' This is much prescribed in extemporaneous Forms, either to sweeten Liquors, or to give due Consistence, in all nervous Intentions; but very little good can be expected from it."

(J. Quincy, *A Compleat English Dispensatory*, 1718, p. 379)

DATE OF MANUFACTURE: 1700–1725

PLACE OF MANUFACTURE: London, or possibly Bristol.

DIMENSIONS: Height 170 mm, maximum width 143 mm

PROVENANCE: Bought in 1962. Museum records suggest that this jar was obtained in part exchange with another jar.

CONDITION: Good; spout chipped, glaze crazed and flaked on handle, spout and base rims.

COMMENT: The cherubs in this design appear to have only one wing, and their trumpets are a different design to others of this type.

Cherubs with trumpets

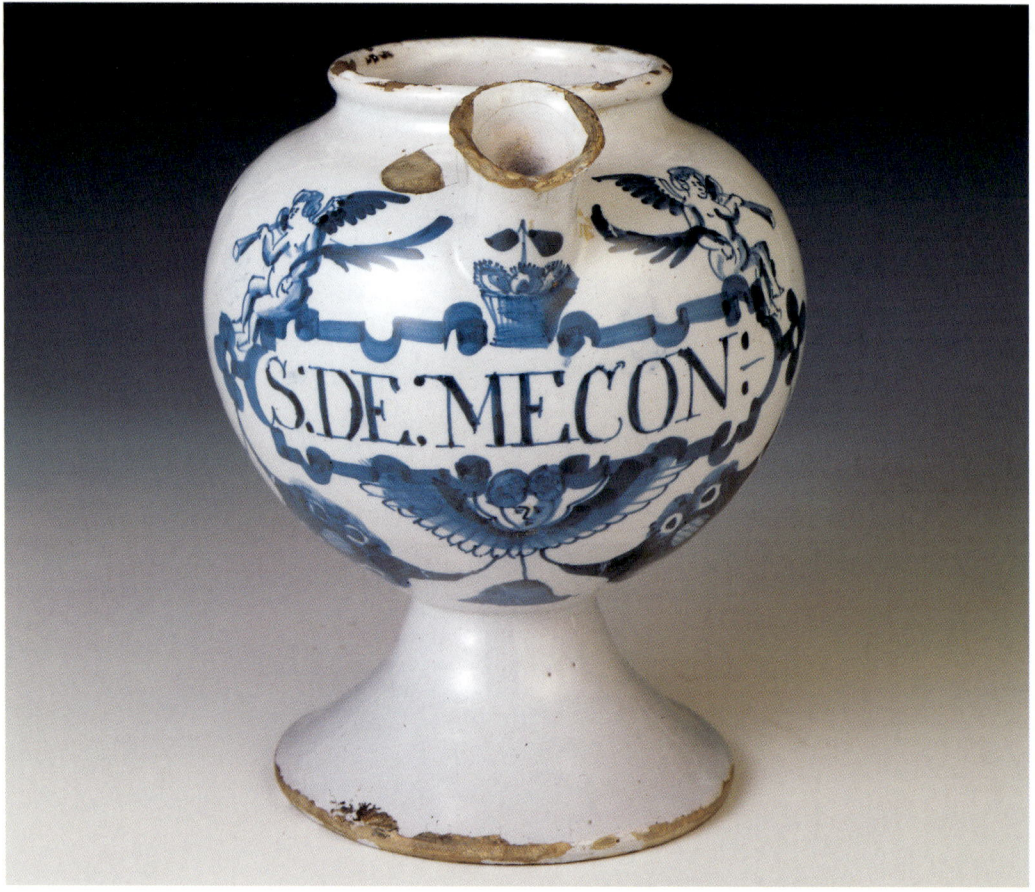

Wet drug jar (Cat.163)

ACCESSION NUMBER: KDM1

DESCRIPTION: Bulbous jar on spreading foot, with spout and fluted strap-like handle. White glaze with bluish tinge and design in blue. Label panel straight, with wavy strap-work frame. Neck ridged with glazed rim, spout unflanged with flared rim, hollowed and glazed base.

DESIGN: Cherubs with trumpets

INSCRIPTION: S:DE MECON:-

MEANING OF INSCRIPTION: *Syrupus de meconio*, syrup of poppies (*Papaverum somniferum*)

CONTEMPORARY ACCOUNT: "'Take Garden white Poppy-Heads with their Seeds ℔ ss. Heads of black Poppies ℥ vi. Steep them well bruised in ℔ viii. of Water 24 hours, and then boil it to ℔ iii. Press the Liquor out hard, and boil it up to a Syrup with ℔ iss. of white Sugar.'

"This, considering the Importance of its Intention, and the Certainty with which it answers it, is a better Medicine, and does more good than all under this Division besides put together. This ought by no means to be clarify'd, because it robs it of its chief Properties... This is used to procure Sleep, in which it acts as any other *Opiate*... It also, better than many other Forms of this kind, stops *Defluxions* and *Catarrhs*, with all Coughs from thin Rheum. It may be given from ℈ i. to ℈ iii. to Children, and from ℥ iii. to ℈ i. to grown Persons. In making this, more Sugar is generally used than what is order'd in the *Recipe*."
(J. Quincy, *A Compleat English Dispensatory*, 1718, pp. 377–378)

DATE OF MANUFACTURE: 1700–1740

PLACE OF MANUFACTURE: London, or possibly Bristol.

DIMENSIONS: Height 180 mm, maximum width 160 mm

PROVENANCE: Bought in 1957, Howard Collection.

CONDITION: Good; large chip off base, chip off glaze by spout, glaze damaged on rim, spout, handle and foot.

REFERENCE: Howard, Delftware Drug Jars, No. 54.

Cherub and shell

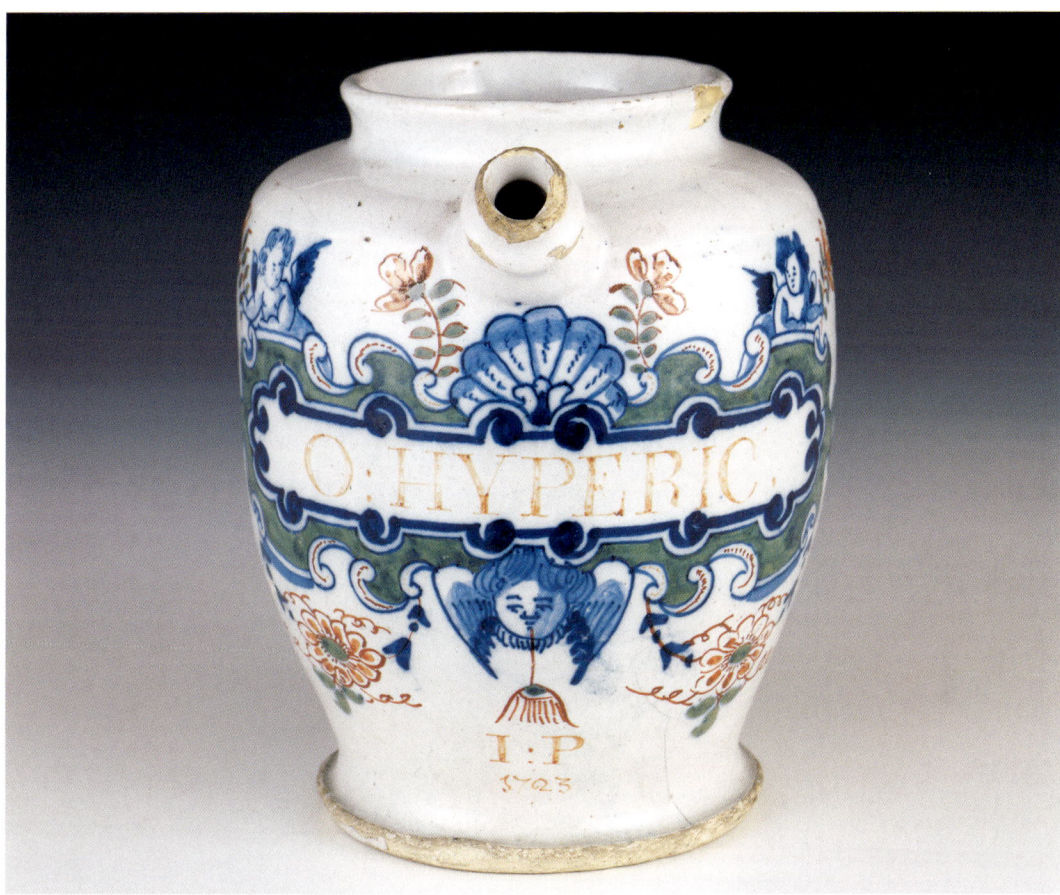

Wet drug jar (Cat.164)

ACCESSION NUMBER: KBN/P1

DESCRIPTION: Ovoid jar, tapering slightly towards splayed base, with spout and (broken) strap handle. White glaze with pinkish tinge and design in blue, green and rusty red. Label panel straight with navy strap-work frame. Neck ridged with glazed rim, flanged spout, slightly concave glazed base, with wide unglazed rim.

DESIGN: Cherub and shell

INSCRIPTION: O:HYPERIC; I:P 1723

MEANING OF INSCRIPTION: *Oleum hypericum* (*Hypericum perforatum*), hypericum or St John's Wort oil. 'I:P' are the initials of the apothecary who commissioned the jar, possibly James Pitson, or John Pocklington (Grigsby D408).

CONTEMPORARY ACCOUNT: "This plant flowers in *July*. It gives place to none as a *Vulnerary*. It is found in the Compositions of some *Alexipharmicks*, but 'tis never prescrib'd in that Intention in common Practice. It is likewise accounted *Aberstersive*, and good against the *Stone*, and Obstructions in the *Urinary Passages*. It has the Credit also of destroying *Worms*. It is much us'd in *Discutient Fomentations*; and the Oil made of its Flowers is in great esteem amongst our Surgeons, both for an excellent *Discutient* and *Deterger*. Some Authors, as *Sala*, have much commended the use of this Herb in *Melancholy* and Distraction, which seems to have given Occasions to some *Enthusiasts* to call it, *Fuga Daemonium*." (J. Quincy, *A Compleat English Dispensatory*, 1718, p. 123)

DATE OF MANUFACTURE: 1723

PLACE OF MANUFACTURE: London

DIMENSIONS: Height 175 mm, maximum width 143 mm

PROVENANCE: Bought in 1957, Howard Collection. Previously Gautier Collection.

CONDITION: Fair; some crazing of glaze, chip off glaze at neck rim, spout rim chipped, fragments of broken handle remaining.

COMMENT: It seems most likely that this jar belonged to James Pitson who became Upper Warden of the Society of Apothecaries in 1722, and Master in 1723: a good reason to commission jars dated in this year.

There are eight jars surviving from this set, four dry jars (three in the Wilkinson Collection, and one in the Longridge Collection), this oil jar and three pill pots (KAN/P1) (Cat. 165), one in the Victoria and Albert Museum, and one in the Greenfield Village and Henry Ford Museum, Dearborn, USA. KCNP/6 (Cat. 166) is in the same basic style, but undated, and obviously from a different batch.

REFERENCE: Grigsby, The Longridge Collection of English Slipware and Delftware. catalogue number D408.

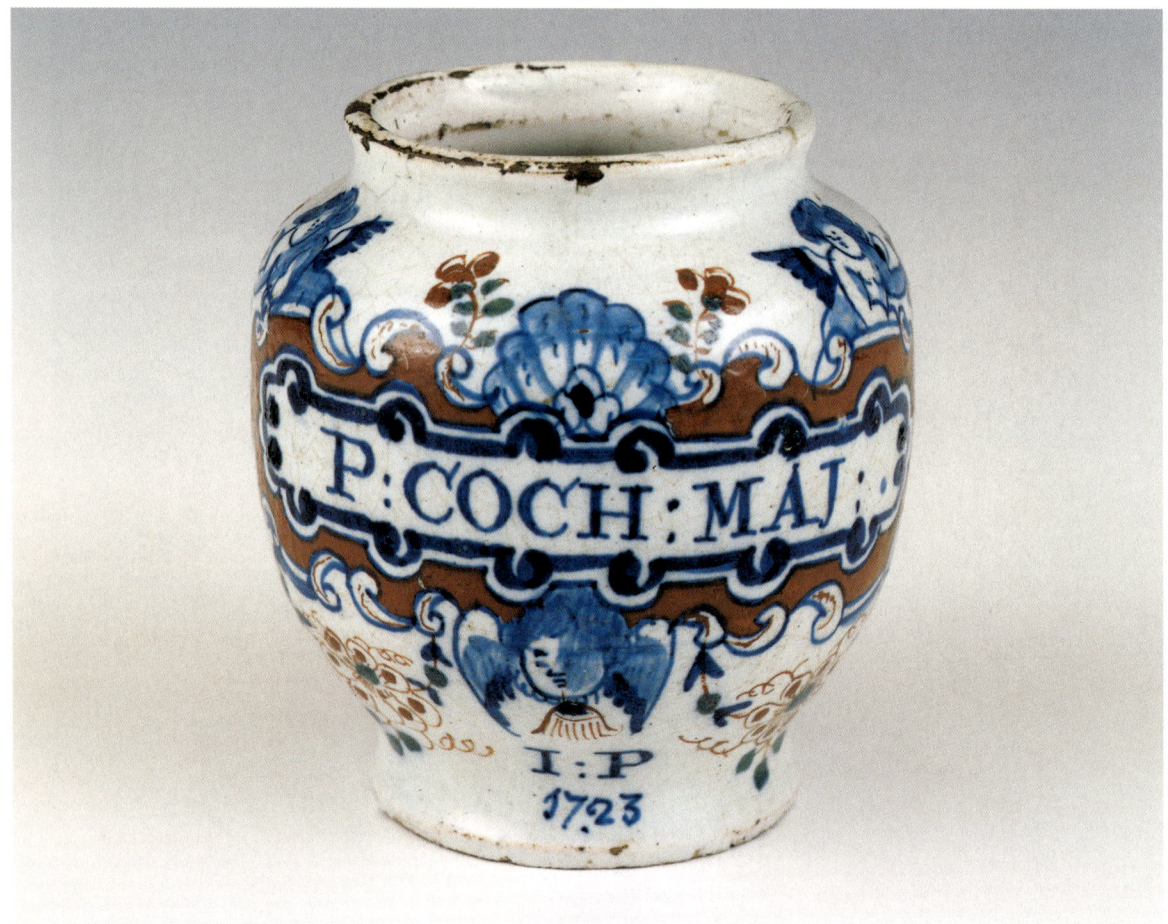

Dry drug jar (Cat.165)

ACCESSION NUMBER: KAN/P1
DESCRIPTION: Ovoid jar, tapering slightly towards splayed base. White glaze with pinkish tinge and design in blue, rusty red, and green. Label panel straight with wavy strap-work frame. Neck ridged with glazed rim, slightly concave unglazed base.
DESIGN: Cherub and shell
INSCRIPTION: P:COCH:MAJ: I:P 1723
MEANING OF INSCRIPTION: *Pilulae cochiae majores*, cochia major pills, used as a strong laxative. 'I:P' are the initials of the apothecary who commissioned the jar.
CONTEMPORARY ACCOUNT: "'Take of Hiera Picra ʒ x. of the Troches of Alhandal ʒ iiiss. of Diagrydium ʒ iiss. of the most resinous Turpeth ʒ v. and make them into a Constistence fit for Pills, with a sufficient quantity of Syrup of Buckthorn, S.A. ... it is hardly ever used in the present Practice." (J. Quincy, *A Compleat English Dispensatory*, 1718, p. 458)
DATE OF MANUFACTURE: 1723
PLACE OF MANUFACTURE: London

DIMENSIONS: Height 85 mm, maximum width 85 mm
PROVENANCE: Bought in 1957, Howard Collection.
CONDITION: Good; fine cracks descending from neck, glaze crazed.
COMMENT: It has been suggested that the apothecary who commissioned the jar was possibly James Pitson, or John Pocklington (Grigsby D408). It seems most likely that this jar belonged to James Pitson who became Upper Warden of the Society of Apothecaries in 1722, and Master in 1723: a good reason to commission jars dated in this year.

    There are eight jars surviving from this set, four dry jars (three in the Wilkinson Collection, Thackray Museum, Leeds, and one in the Longridge Collection), an oil jar KBN/P1 (Cat. 164) and three pill pots (this jar, one in the Victoria and Albert Museum, and one in the Greenfield Village and Henry Ford Museum, Dearborn, USA). KCNP/6 (Cat. 166) is in the same basic style, but undated, and obviously from a different batch.
REFERENCE: Grigsby, The Longridge Collection of English Slipware and Delftware. Catalogue number D408.

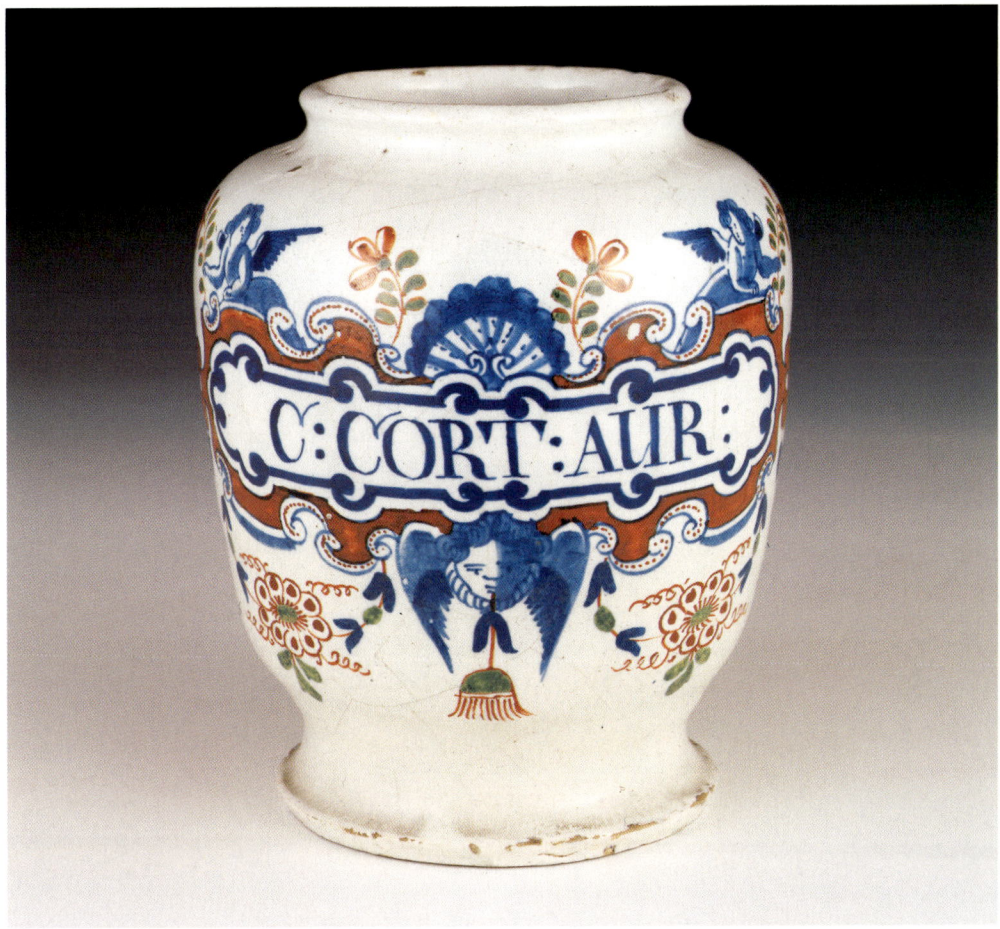

Dry drug jar (Cat.166)

ACCESSION NUMBER: KCN/P6

DESCRIPTION: Ovoid jar, tapering slightly towards splayed base. White glaze with greyish tinge and design in blue, rusty red and green. Label panel straight with wavy strap-work frame. Neck ridged, with glazed rim, concave glazed base.

DESIGN: Cherub and shell

INSCRIPTION: C:CORT:AUR

MEANING OF INSCRIPTION: *Conserva cortex aurantiorum*, conserve of orange peel

CONTEMPORARY ACCOUNT: "*Conserves* of the Peels of *Oranges*, *Citrons*, *Lemons*, and the like, are made with double the quantity of Sugar only, because their Warmth helps to keep them. The first of these is only in use, and requires great Labour to make it very fine: if therefore the Orange-Chips, as they are shave thin off the Orange, are put in an earthen Pan some weeks, with the sufficient quantity of Sugar, they will mellow, or as it were rot so together, that it will require much less trouble to reduce it into a good *Conserve*." (J. Quincy, *A Compleat English Dispensatory*, 1718, p. 401)

DATE OF MANUFACTURE: 1720–1740

PLACE OF MANUFACTURE: Probably Lambeth, London

DIMENSIONS: Height 175 mm, maximum width 150 mm

PROVENANCE: Bought in 1957, Howard Collection.

CONDITION: Good; glaze crazed and chipped on rim of neck and base, some pitting.

COMMENT: Howard described this as "a perfect example of the cherub decoration, but in magnificent polychrome" (p. 23).

This jar is similar to the dated I.P. 1723 jars (Cat. 164 and 165), but does not appear to be part of the same group, as it has a 'softer' look. In addition, the cherub's wings and the tendrils on the floral swags are both nearly horizontal, and the inner strapwork border to the cartouche is more spaced than the 1723 examples.

REFERENCES: Drey, Apothecary Jars. Plate G and p. 136.

Howard, English Delftware Drug Jars, No. 58.

Cherub and shell

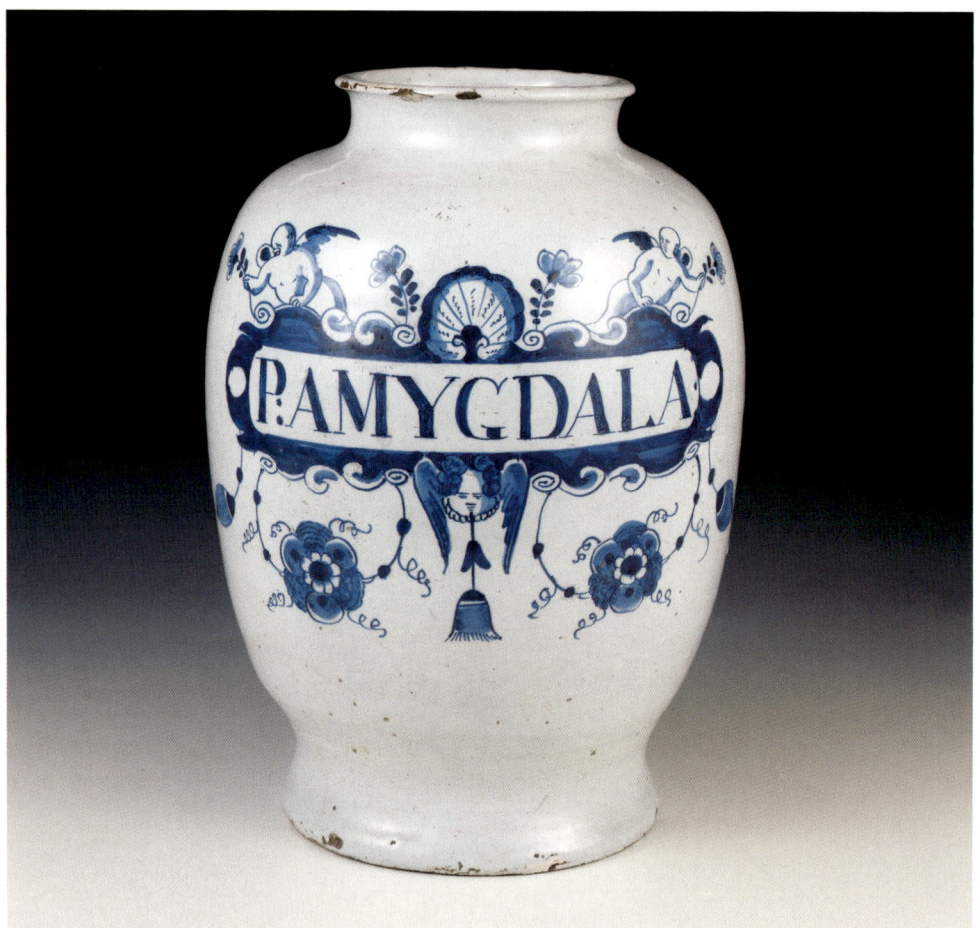

Dry drug jar (Cat.169)

ACCESSION NUMBER: KCN3

DESCRIPTION: Ovoid jar, tapering slightly towards splayed base. White glaze with bluish tinge and design in blue. Label panel straight with even outline. Neck everted with glazed rim, flat and partly glazed base.

DESIGN: Cherub (bald) and shell

INSCRIPTION: P:AMYGDALA

MEANING OF INSCRIPTION: *Pulvis amygdala dulcium*, powdered almonds (*Amygdala dulcium*)

CONTEMPORARY ACCOUNT: "These are of a soft, sweet, grateful Taste, and nutritive. They are much prescribed in Emulsions, in the common Practice, and are good in all Disorders from the cholerick and acrimonious Humours. They cool and cleanse the Kidneys and Urinary Passages, and give ease in cholick Pains, and all Irritations of the Bowels." (J. Quincy, *A Compleat English Dispensatory*, 1718, p. 114)

DATE OF MANUFACTURE: c. 1740

PLACE OF MANUFACTURE: London

DIMENSIONS: Height 320 mm, maximum width 245 mm

PROVENANCE: Bought in 1957.

CONDITION: Good; rim chipped, some pitting, glaze chipped on rim and base.

COMMENT: This jar is part of a group of over 40 jars which are closely related to, and probably by the same painter as, the set dated 1738 with the initials W.I., including KAN2 (Cat. 168), KCN9 (Cat. 171), KCN28 (Cat. 170) and KDN6 (Cat. 172).

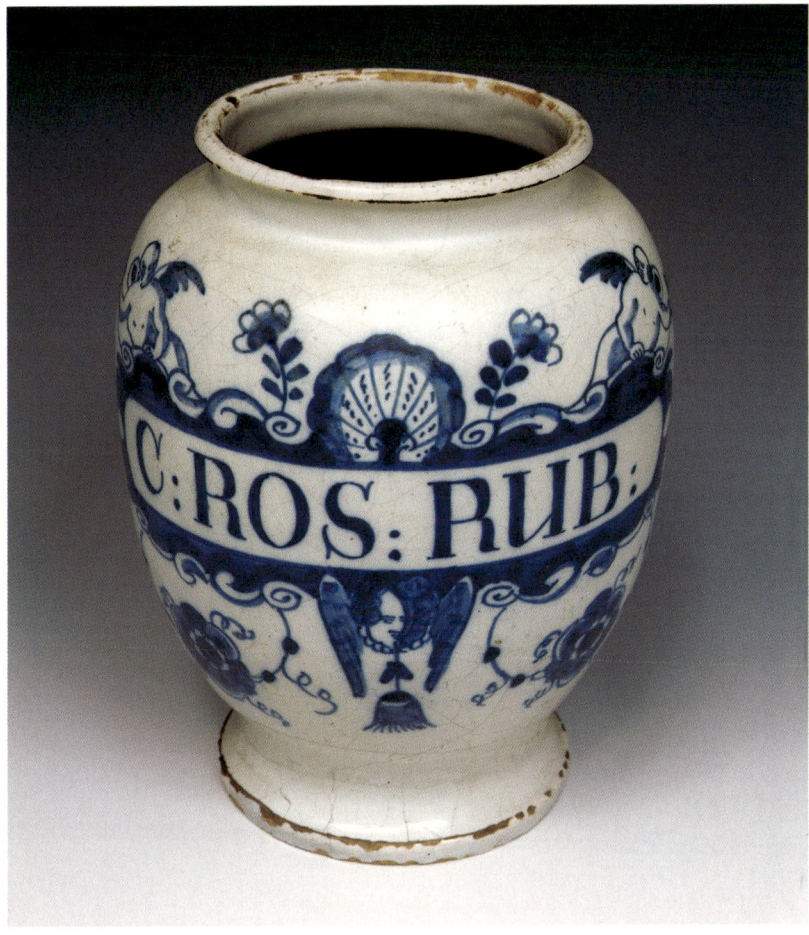

Dry drug jar (Cat.170)

ACCESSION NUMBER: KCN28

DESCRIPTION: Ovoid jar, tapering slightly towards splayed base. White glaze with bluish tinge and design in blue. Label panel straight with even outline. Neck everted.

DESIGN: Cherub and shell

INSCRIPTION: C:ROS:RUB

MEANING OF INSCRIPTION: *Conserva rosarum rubrum*, conserve of red roses

CONTEMPORARY ACCOUNT: "These blow in *May* and *June*. They are sufficiently known to all Persons. What are used in the Shops, unless for the distill'd Water, are the Buds before they quite blow; because then they are much rougher and more astringent. The Conserve made of them is deservedly in great esteem, but the common Notion of its being the better for Age, is an Error: for their Astringency, which arises from the Solidity and Asperity of their component Parts, by long lying in the Sugar, which mellows and softens them, very much decays. They are good in almost all Distempers of the Lungs, and particularly in Defluxions of *Rheum*." (J. Quincy, *A Compleat English*

Dispensatory, 1718, p. 99)

DATE OF MANUFACTURE: c. 1740

PLACE OF MANUFACTURE: London

DIMENSIONS: Height 170 mm maximum width 127 mm

PROVENANCE: Unknown.

CONDITION: Good; small losses of glaze and chips to rim and base. Some pitting and cracked glaze.

COMMENT: This jar seems to be part of a group of over 40 jars which are closely related to, and probably by the same painter as, the set dated 1738 with the initials W.I., including KAN2 (Cat. 168), KCN9 (Cat. 171), KCN3 (Cat. 169) and KDN6 (Cat. 172).

Cherub and shell

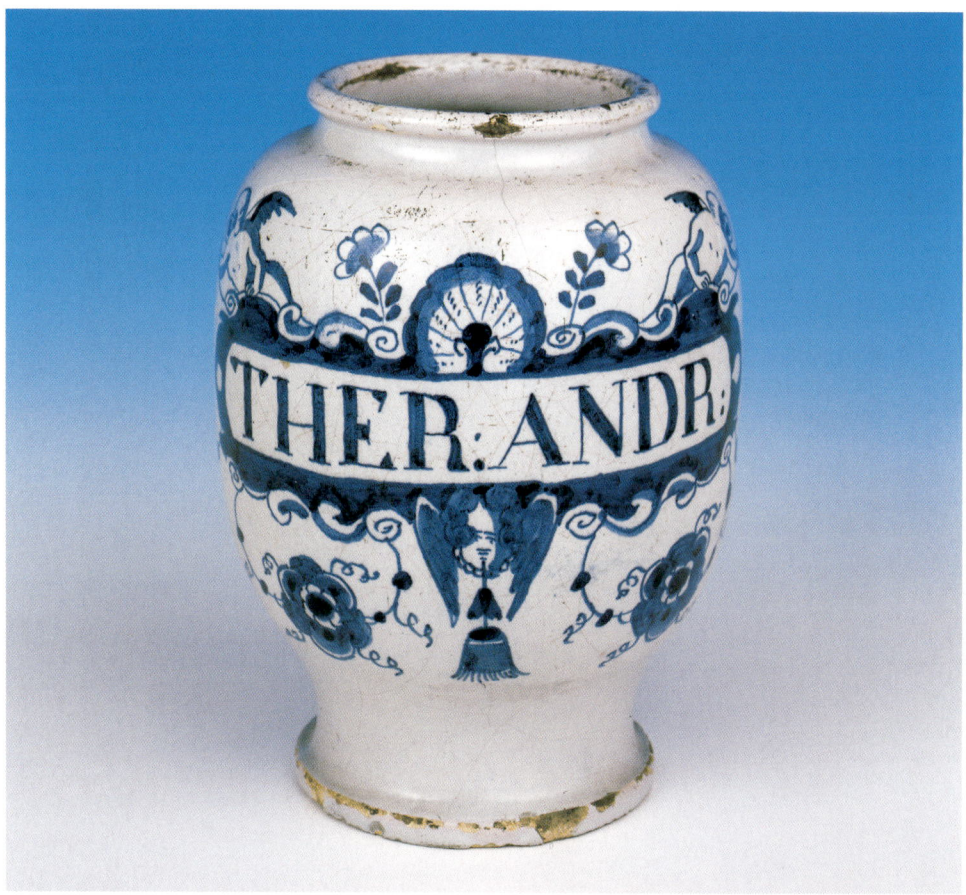

Dry drug jar (Cat.171)

ACCESSION NUMBER: KCN9

DESCRIPTION: Ovoid jar, tapering slightly towards splayed base. White glaze with pinkish tinge and design in blue. Label panel straight with even outline. Neck ridged with glazed rim, slightly concave glazed base with unglazed edge.

DESIGN: Cherub (bald) and shell

INSCRIPTION: THER:ANDR:

MEANING OF INSCRIPTION: *Theriaca Andromachi*, the treacle or theriaca of Andromachus, a preparation traced back to Andromachus, physician to the Emperor Nero (AD 37). This extraordinary preparation was supposed to be an antidote to all poisons. It was also used in the 1600s to prevent the plague.

CONTEMPORARY ACCOUNT: "Take *Troches of Squills* ℥ vi. Troches of Vipers, long Pepper, *Opium*, and Troches of Hedycroi, ana ℥ iii. *Red Rose Buds dry'd, Orrice, Juice of Liquorice, Seeds of Sweet Navew*, Tops of Scordium, Opobalsam, *Troches of Agarick*, Cinnamon, ana ℥ iss. Myrrh, Zedoary, Saffron, *Cassia-Bark*, Spikenard, Schoenanth, white and black Pepper, *Frankincense, Dittany of Crete, Rhapontick*, Staecha's, *Hore-Hound, Parsley-Seeds*, Calaminth, *Cyprus* Turpentine, *Roots of Cinque-foil*, and Ginger, ana ℥ vi. *Tops of Polymountain*, Ground-Pine, *Celtick* Spikenard, *Amomus*, Styrax, Meum-Root, Tops of Germander, *Phu-Root, Earth of* Lemnos, Indian Leaf, *Calcanthum, Gentian Root, Gum-Arabick, Juice of Hypocistis*, Cubebs, Seeds of Anise, Cardomoms, Fennel, of *Hartwort, German Acacia*, Seeds of Treacle-Mustard, Tops of St John's-wort, *Seeds of Bishop's-weed*, Sagapenum, ana ℥ iv. Castor, *long Birthwort, Amber*, or *Bitumen Judaicum, Seeds of Daucus*, Opoponax, *Centaury the lesser*, and Galbanum, ana ℥ ii. Canary ℥ xl. Honey, three times the weight of the whole Species when powder'd; and mix all into an Electuary." (J. Quincy, *A Compleat English Dispensatory*, 1718, p. 409)

DATE OF MANUFACTURE: c. 1740

PLACE OF MANUFACTURE: London

DIMENSIONS: Height 180 mm, maximum width 143 mm

PROVENANCE: Donation, 1953, Austen Collection.

CONDITION: Fair; large crack ascending from base, two holes and chips in base, glaze crazed and flaked on neck and base rims.

COMMENT: This jar seems to be part of a group of over 40 jars which are closely related to, and probably by the same painter as, the set dated 1738 with the initials W.I., including KAN2 (Cat. 168), KCN28 (Cat. 170) and KDN6 (Cat. 172).

REFERENCE: Lothian, 'The John Austen Collection' Figure 12 and p. 98.

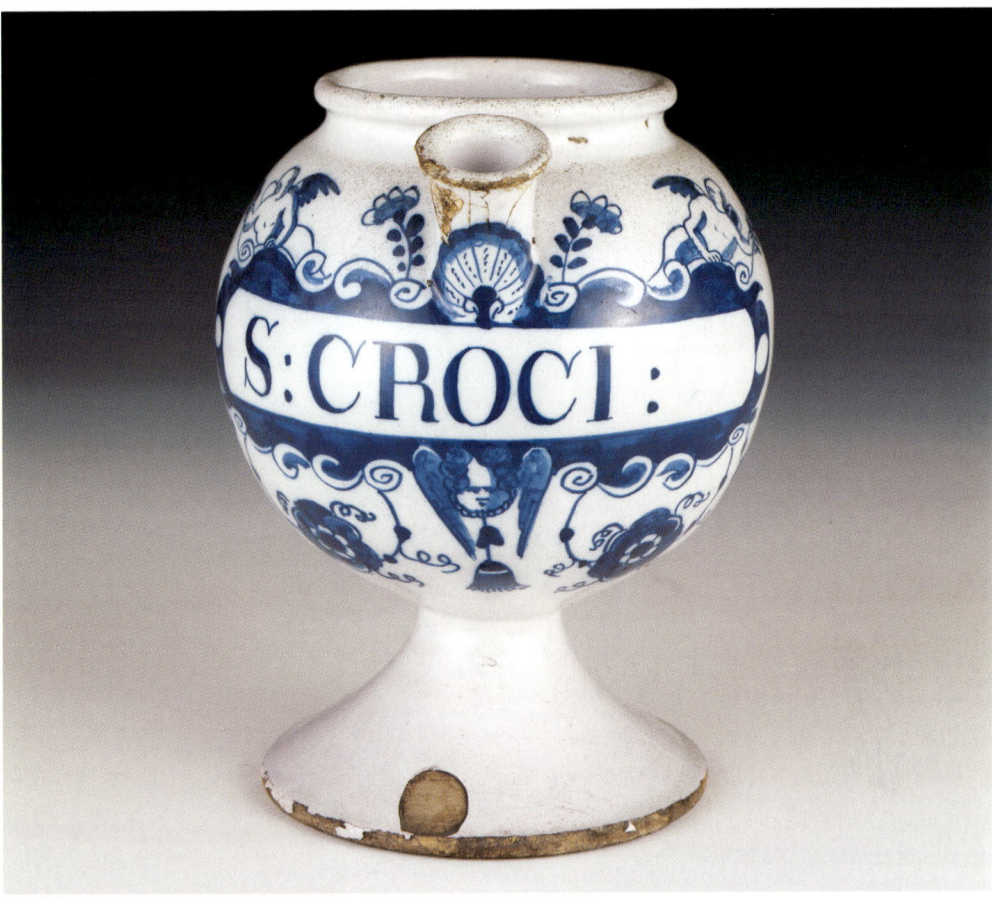

Wet drug jar (Cat.172)

ACCESSION NUMBER: KDN6

DESCRIPTION: Bulbous jar on spreading foot, with spout and fluted strap-like looped handle. White glaze with pinkish tinge and design in blue. Label panel straight with even outline. Neck ridged with glazed rim, spout slightly flared, hollowed and glazed base with unglazed edge.

DESIGN: Cherub (bald) and shell

INSCRIPTION: S:CROCI:

MEANING OF INSCRIPTION: *Syrupus croci*, syrup of saffron (*Crocus sativus*)

CONTEMPORARY ACCOUNT: "'Infuse of the best *English* Saffron ʒ i. in ℔ i. of Canary. Let it stand close stop'd in a gentle warmth two or three Days; then press out the Wine, and melt it in Sugar that is very fine ʒ xx., which will give it a proper Consistence.'

"This is much us'd, and is expected to have all the Virtues of the *Simple* from whence it is made: it may be given almost at pleasure, and is much prescrib'd for Childrens Juleps." (J. Quincy, *A Compleat English Dispensatory*, 1718, pp. 386–387)

DATE OF MANUFACTURE: c. 1740

PLACE OF MANUFACTURE: London

DIMENSIONS: Height 180 mm, maximum width 145 mm

PROVENANCE: Bought in 1957, Howard Collection.

CONDITION: Good; base chipped, glaze flaked on base (2 cm diameter) and on handle and spout.

COMMENT: This jar seems to be part of a group of over 40 jars which are closely related to, and probably by the same painter as, the set dated 1738 with the initials W.I., including KAN2 (Cat. 168), KCN9 (Cat. 171), KCN28 (Cat. 170) and KCN3 (Cat. 169).

REFERENCE: Howard, G. E. English Delftware Drug Jars, No. 48.

Cherub and shell

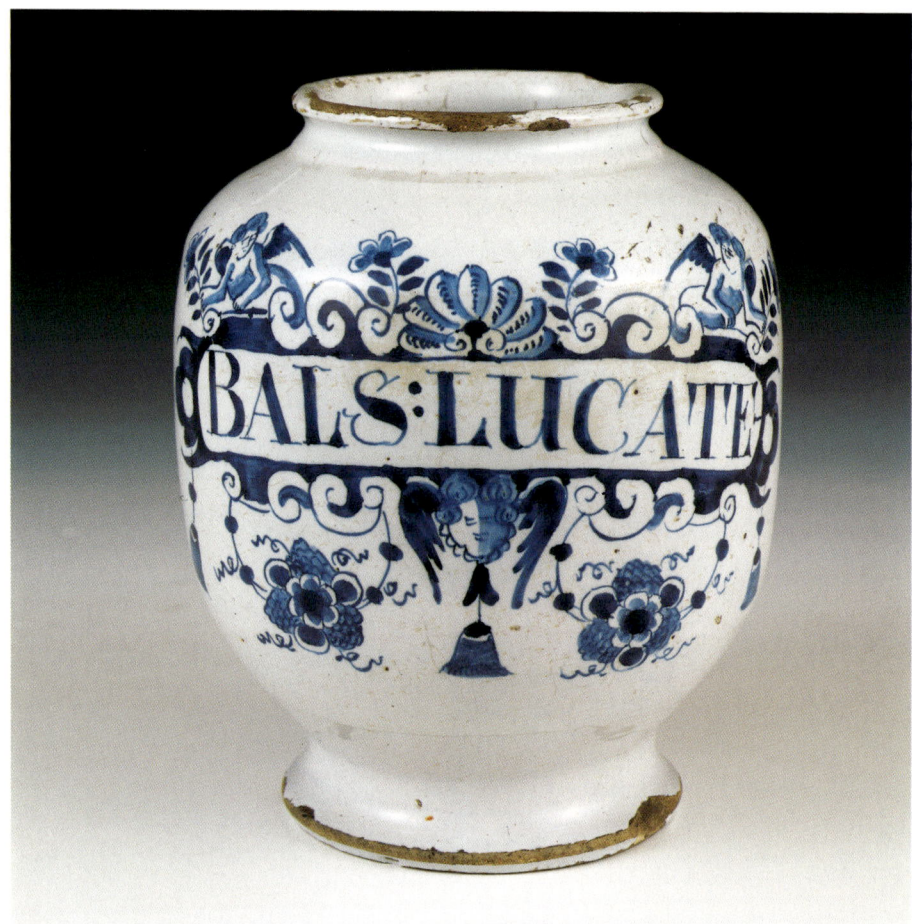

Dry drug jar (Cat.173)

ACCESSION NUMBER: KCN18
DESCRIPTION: Ovoid jar, tapering slightly towards splayed base. White glaze with pinkish tinge and design in blue. Label panel slightly curved upwards with even outline. Neck everted with glazed rim, slightly concave unglazed base.
DESIGN: Cherub and shell
INSCRIPTION: BALS:LUCATE-
MEANING OF INSCRIPTION: *Balsamum Locatelli*, Lucatellus balsam
CONTEMPORARY ACCOUNT: "'From the College. Take yellow Wax melted in a little Canary-Wine ℔ i. Oil of Olives, *Venice* – Turpentine wash'd in Rose-water, ana (pound) iss. Boil them till the Wine is evaporated, and when almost cold, stir in of red Sanders, finely powder'd ℥ ii. and preserve it for use... This Composition stands recommended for an internal *Vulnerary*, and is prescribed in such Coughs as give suspicion of *Tubercules* and *Ulcerations* in the Lungs; and also in all internal Decays from the like Causes, whether the Seat be in the Breast, or any other part. It is given likewise upon accidental Bruises and inward Bleeding.

Externally it is used to deterge and incarnate green Wounds and Ulcers that are not of too long standing." (J. Quincy, *A Compleat English Dispensatory*, 1718, p. 445)
DATE OF MANUFACTURE: 1740–1760
PLACE OF MANUFACTURE: London
DIMENSIONS: Height 180 mm, maximum width 160 mm
PROVENANCE: Bequest, Saville Peck, 1955.
CONDITION: Good; neck and base chipped, glaze crazed and flaked on neck and base rims.
REFERENCE: Illustrated in Medical Bulletin, July 1953, Plate 4C.

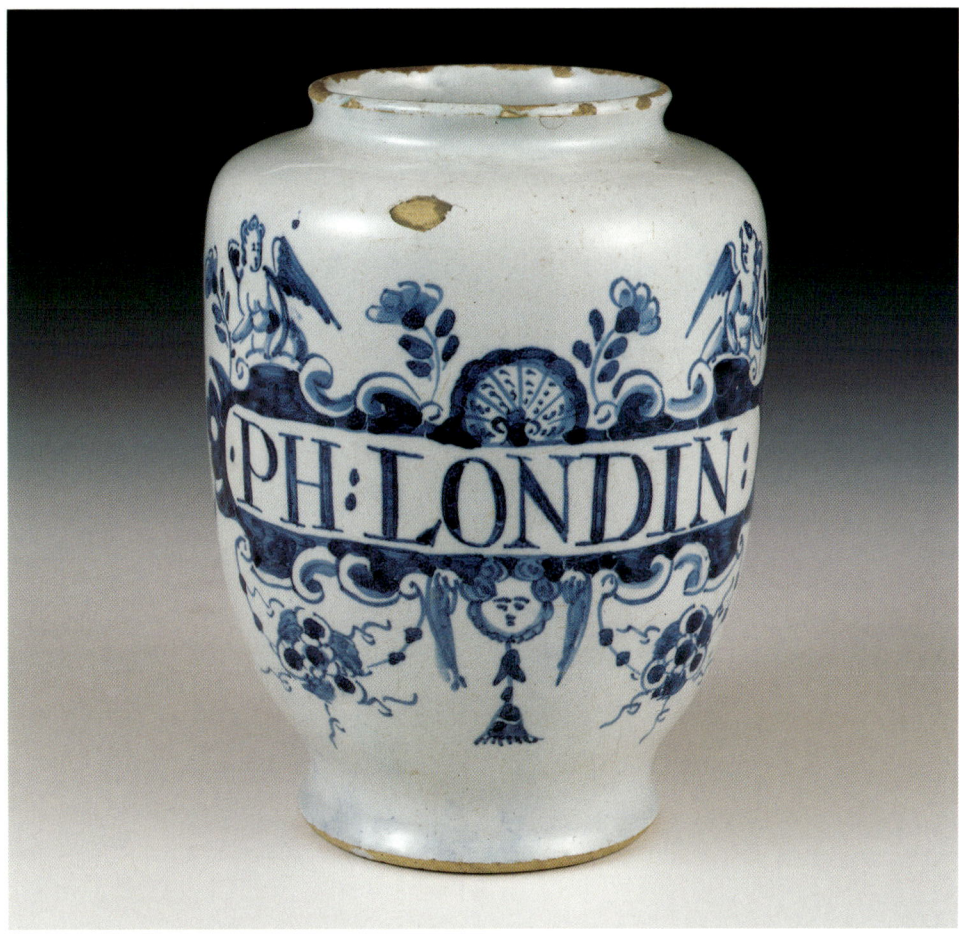

Dry drug jar (Cat.174)

ACCESSION NUMBER: KCN12

DESCRIPTION: Ovoid jar, tapering slightly towards splayed base. White glaze with pinkish tinge and design in blue. Label panel straight with even outline. Neck ridged with glazed rim, slightly concave glazed base with unglazed edge. Cross mark on base.

DESIGN: Cherub and shell

INSCRIPTION: PH:LONDIN:

MEANING OF INSCRIPTION: *Philonium Londinense.* Originally called Roman Philonium (or medicine), this substance became known as London Philonium in the 1746 London Pharmacopoeia. A preparation with many ingredients, including opium, and used in pain relief and to induce sleep. It was named after a first century physician, Philon of Tarsus.

CONTEMPORARY ACCOUNT: "'Take white Pepper, Seeds of white Henbane, ana ℥ v. *Opium* ℥ iiss. Cassia – Bark ℥ iss. Smallage – Seed ℥ i. Seeds of Parsly, Fennel and Daucus, ana gr. xlv. Saffron ℥ ss. Spikenard, Pellitory of *Spain*, and Zedoary, ana gr. xv. Cinnamon ℥ iss. Myrrh and Castor, ana ℥ i. Honey, three times the quantity of the whole. Mix them, S.A.'

"This is somewhat more us'd than the former [Philonum Persicum], but their Difference is not great. The proportion of *Opium* and *Henbane* is the same in both, and therefore their Doses also alike." (J. Quincy, *A Compleat English Dispensatory*, 1718, p. 408)

DATE OF MANUFACTURE: 1720–1750

PLACE OF MANUFACTURE: London

DIMENSIONS: Height 170 mm, maximum width 135 mm

PROVENANCE: Bequest, Saville Peck, 1955 (previously Prior Collection).

CONDITION: Good; glaze flaked on bowl, neck and base rims.

Cherub and shell

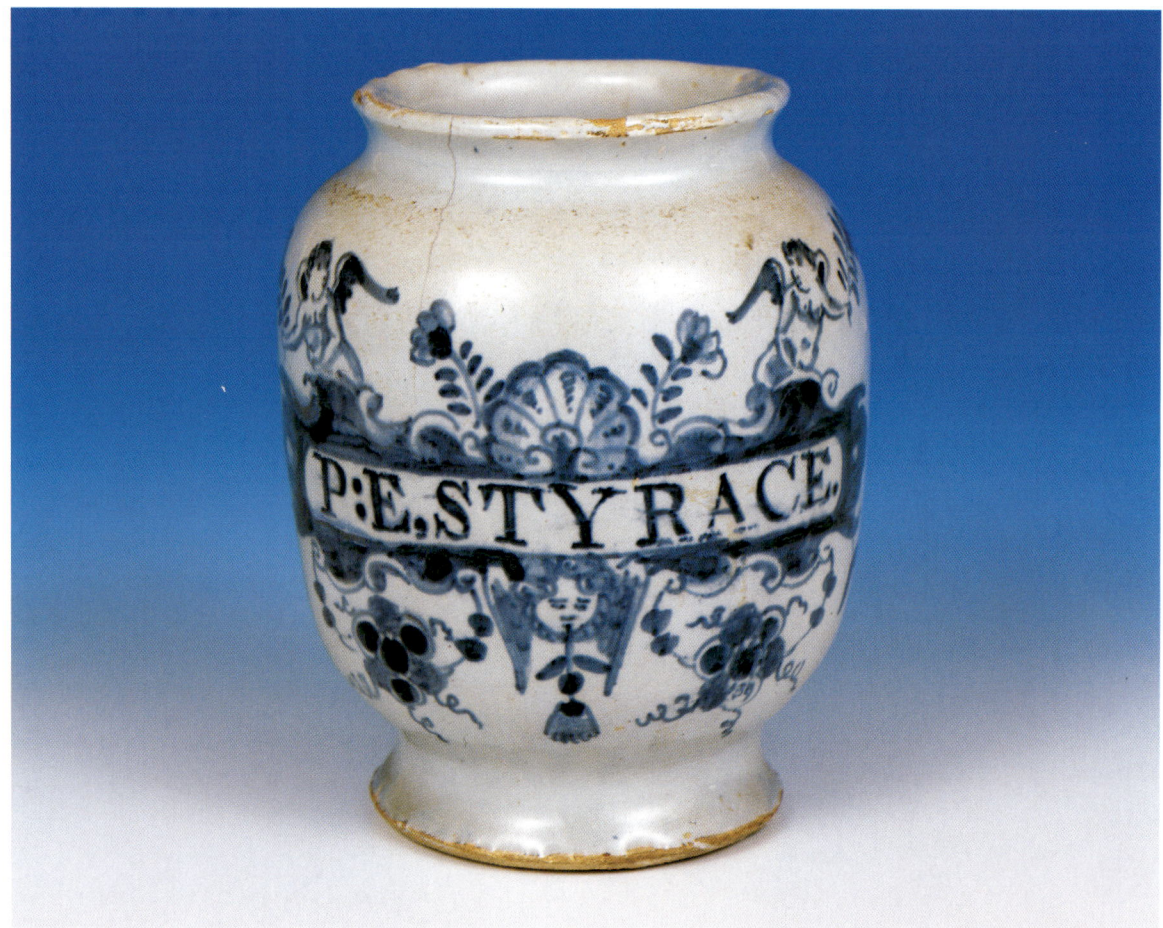

Dry drug jar (Cat.175)

ACCESSION NUMBER: KCN32
DESCRIPTION: Ovoid jar, tapering slightly towards splayed base. Bluish glaze and design in blue. Label panel straight with even outline. Neck ridged, glazed base.
INSCRIPTION: P:E. STYRACE
MEANING OF INSCRIPTION: *Pilulae e styrace*, pills made with styrax (*Styrax officinalis*)
CONTEMPORARY ACCOUNT: "'Take Styrax, Olibanum, Myrrh, Extract of Liquorice, Opium, ana ʒ ss. Saffron ʒ i. Syrup of white Poppies a sufficient quantity, to beat them into a Mass.

"In this Composition the *Styrax* must be strain'd, and the *Opium*, tho some dry and powder it, and beat together with the Extract of Liquorice into a Paste: and then receive the rest of the Ingredients in Powder. There is gr.i. of *Opium* in every gr.vi. of this Mass; and therefore it ought in the extreme Dose not to exceed xii. or xv. Gr... It is much more us'd than any other of this Intention; but it ought to be with caution." (J. Quincy, *A Compleat English Dispensatory*, 1718, p. 423)
DATE OF MANUFACTURE: 1740–1760

PLACE OF MANUFACTURE: London
DIMENSIONS: Height 100 mm, maximum width 60 mm
PROVENANCE: Bequest, Avis Fox, 1983.
CONDITION: Good; slight crack from neck downwards, slight chips round neck.

Cherub and shell

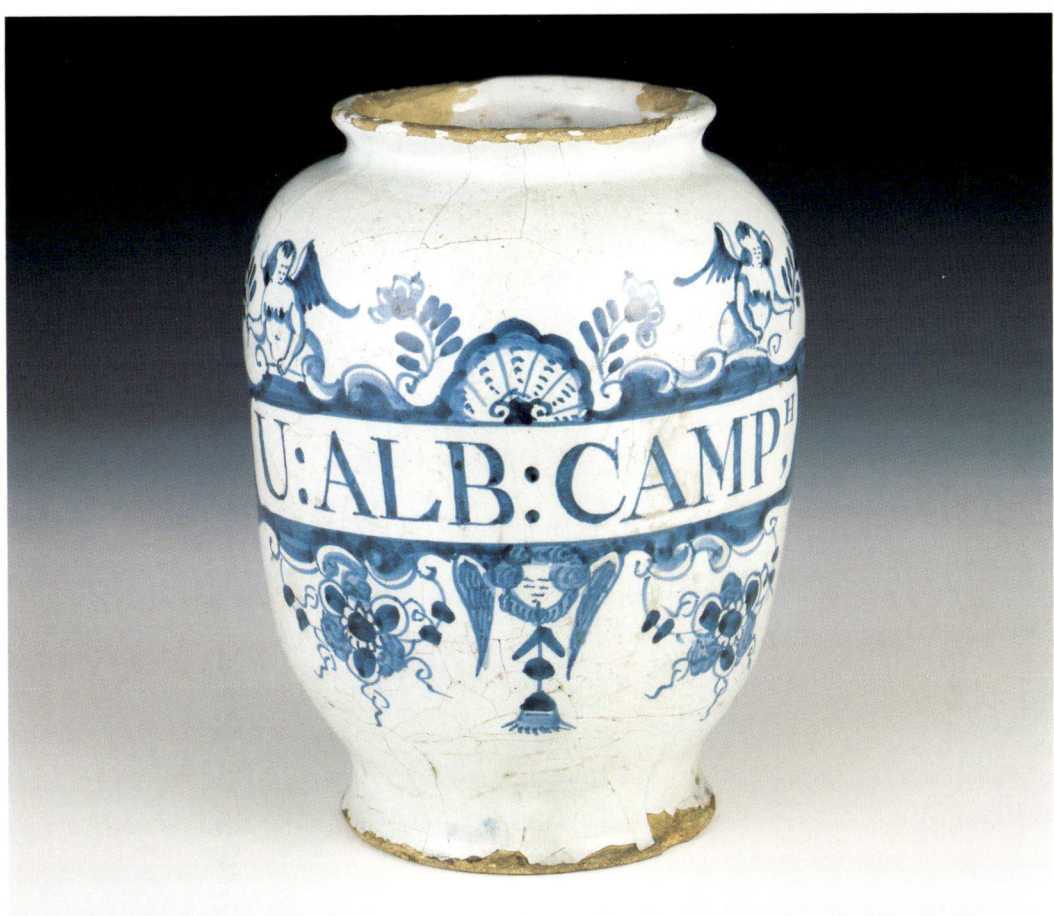

Dry drug jar (Cat.176)

ACCESSION NUMBER: KCN19

DESCRIPTION: Ovoid jar, tapering slightly towards splayed base. Bluish-white glaze with pinkish tinge and design in blue. Label panel straight with even outline. Neck everted with partly glazed rim, concave glazed base with unglazed edge. In blue on base: X.

DESIGN: Cherub and shell

INSCRIPTION: U:ALB:CAMPH;

MEANING OF INSCRIPTION: *Unguentum album camphorum*, camphorated white ointment

CONTEMPORARY ACCOUNT: "This is made by adding the former [white ointment – Unguentum Album] a dram and a half of camphire first beat with a few drops of oil of almonds... Remark...this unguent being often used to the frettings of the skin in young children." (H. Pemberton, *The Dispensatory*, 1746, p. 364)

DATE OF MANUFACTURE: 1740–1760

PLACE OF MANUFACTURE: London

DIMENSIONS: Height 180 mm, maximum width 145 mm

PROVENANCE: Bought in 1957, Howard Collection.

CONDITION: Fair; base chipped, glaze crazed and flaked from body, neck and base rims.

Cherub and shell

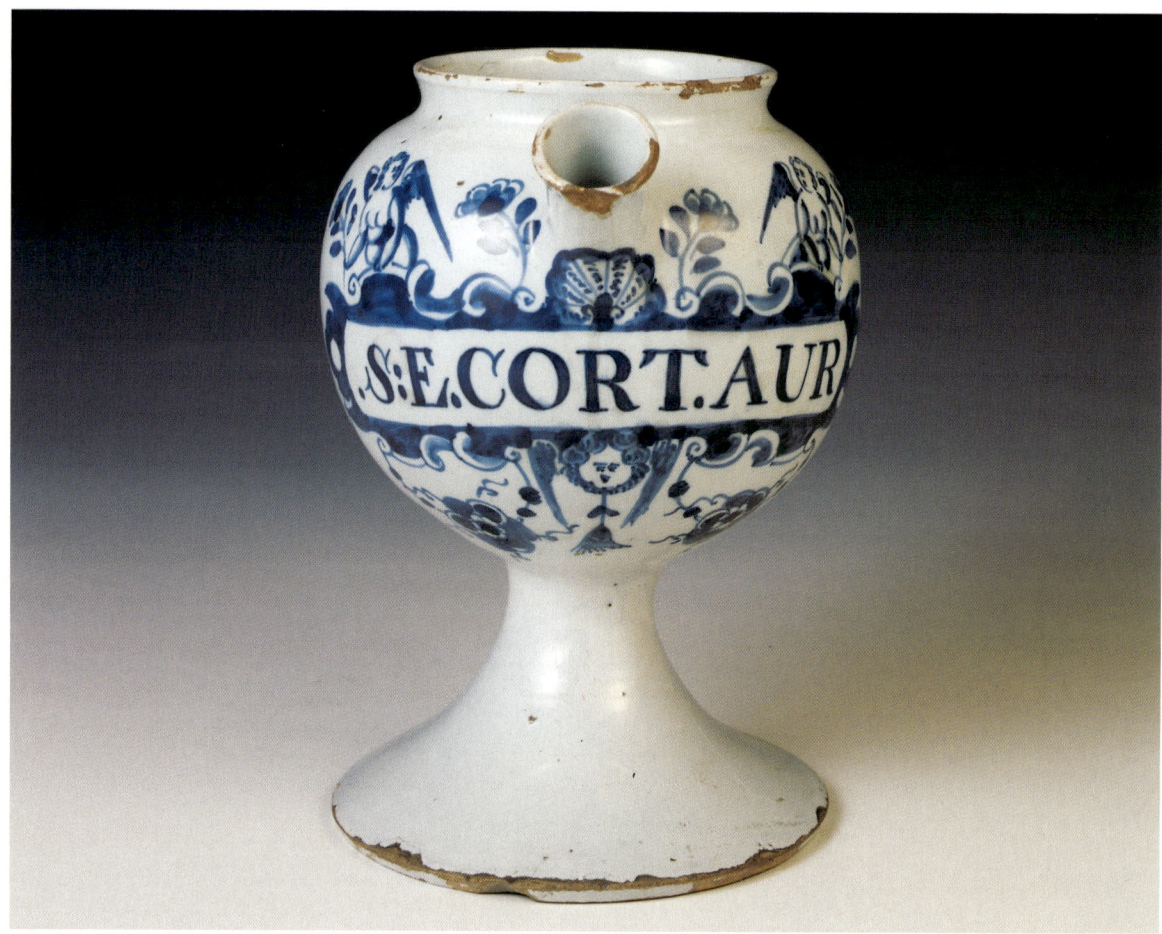

Wet drug jar (Cat.177)

ACCESSION NUMBER: KDN5

DESCRIPTION: Bulbous jar on spreading foot, with spout and fluted strap-like looped handle. White glaze with pinkish tinge and design in blue. Label panel curved slightly upwards with even outline. Neck everted with glazed rim, flared spout, hollowed and glazed base with unglazed edge. In blue on base: I.

DESIGN: Cherub and shell

INSCRIPTION: S:E.CORT.AUR

MEANING OF INSCRIPTION: *Syrupus e cortex aurantiorum*, syrup of orange peel

CONTEMPORARY ACCOUNT: "Take of the outer yellow rind of fresh Seville orange-peel eight ounces, of boiling water five pints. Steep the peel in the water for a night in a close vessel, and in the morning dissolve in the liquors strained of double refined sugar beaten to a powder as much, as is sufficient to make a syrup. Remark. Here powdering the sugar is particularly requisite, that it may the sooner dissolve, and the syrup not lose more than is necessary of the volatile flavour of the peel by the liquor's long continuing hot." (H. Pemberton, *The Dispensatory*, 1746, pp. 292–293)

DATE OF MANUFACTURE: 1740–1760

PLACE OF MANUFACTURE: London

DIMENSIONS: Height 185 mm, maximum width 143 mm

PROVENANCE: Bequest, Saville Peck, 1955 (previously Prior Collection).

CONDITION: Good; glaze flaked on handle, spout, neck and base rims.

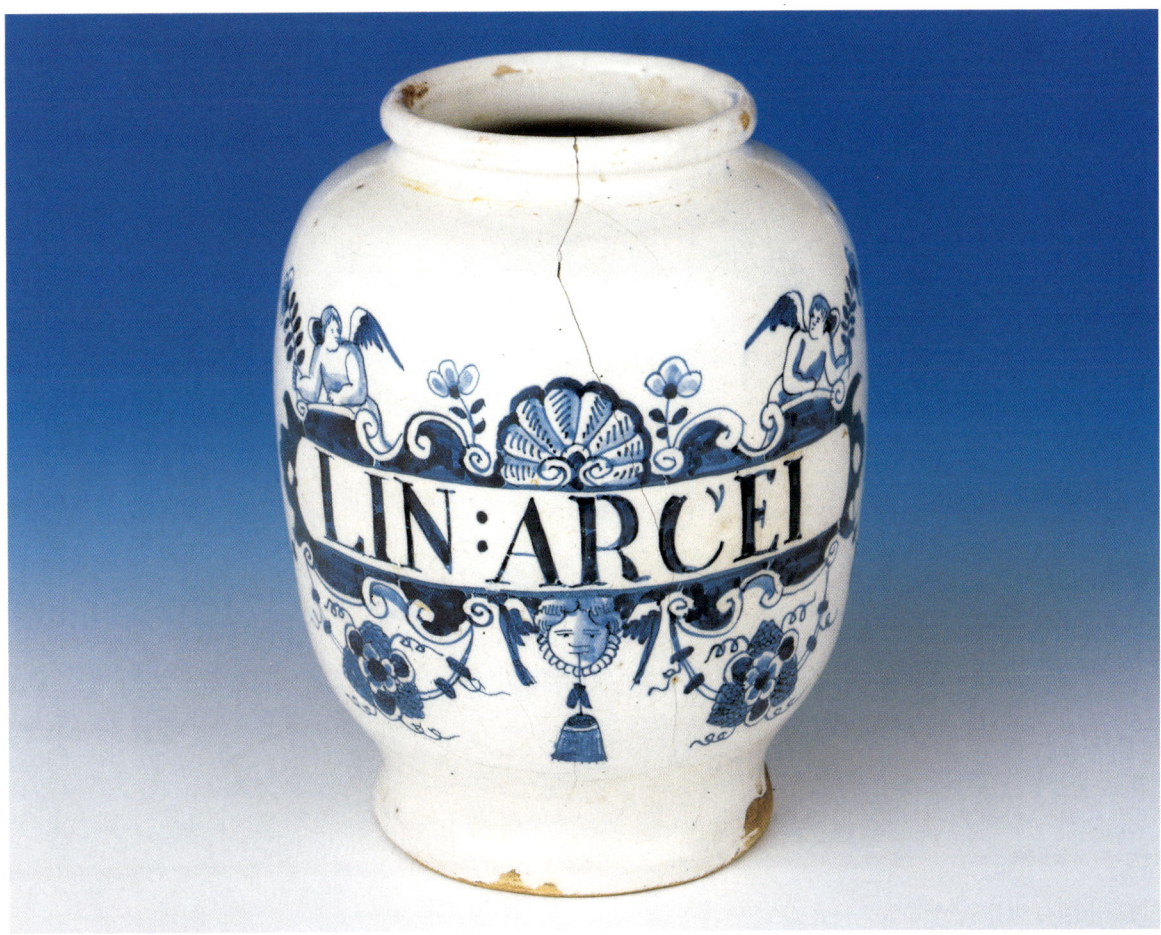

Dry drug jar (Cat. 178)

ACCESSION NUMBER: KCN21
DESCRIPTION: Ovoid jar, tapering slightly towards ridged base. White glaze with greyish tinge and design in blue. Label panel straight with even outline. Neck ridged with glazed rim, concave unglazed base.
DESIGN: Cherub and shell
INSCRIPTION: LIN:ARCEI
MEANING OF INSCRIPTION: *Linimentum Arcei*, Arceus Liniment. Astringent liniment for cleaning and 'digesting' wounds.
CONTEMPORARY ACCOUNT: "'Take Gum Elemi and Turpentine, ana ℥ iss, old Sheep's Suet ℥ ii. Lard ℥ i. Mix and make them into an Ointment S.A.'

   "This is troublesome to make, because there can be procured none of the *Gum Elemi*, but with so much Dross as to make it necessary to strain it. This is reckon'd a better Dressing in fresh Wounds than *Basilicon*; because it does not incarn too fast, and is so warm and detersive, as to make it useful even in Ulcers of some standing. This is now much us'd in Surgery; but it generally goes under the Appellation of *Linimentum Arcei*." (J. Quincy, *A Compleat English Dispensatory*, 1718, p. 455)
DATE OF MANUFACTURE: 1740–1760
PLACE OF MANUFACTURE: London
DIMENSIONS: Height 180 mm, maximum width 145 mm
PROVENANCE: Bequest, Saville Peck, 1955.
CONDITION: Fair; crack descending from neck, glaze crazed and flaked from neck and base rims.
REFERENCE: Walker, Ancient pharmacy jars pp. 251–252, No. II, 2.

Cherub and shell

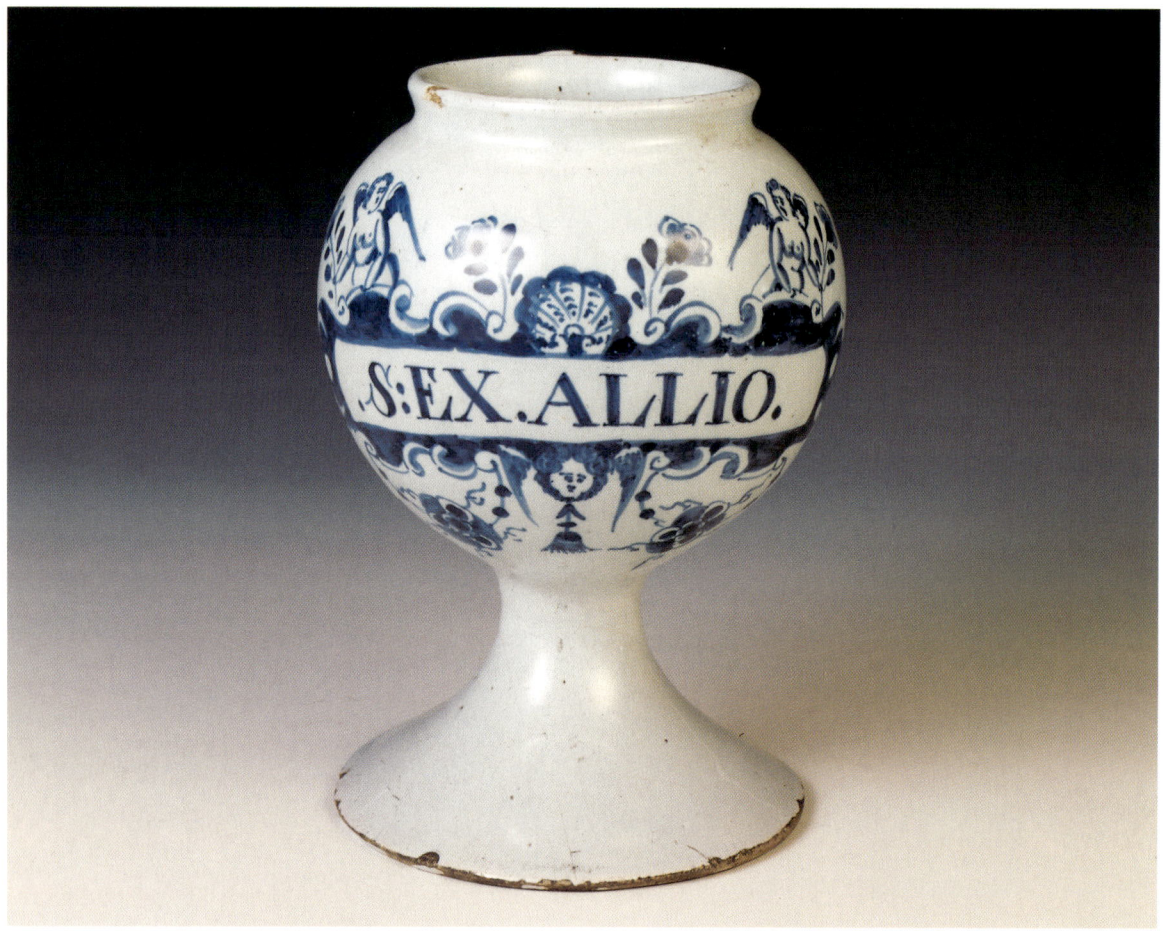

Wet drug jar (Cat.181)

ACCESSION NUMBER: KDN3
DESCRIPTION: Bulbous jar on spreading foot with spout only, on opposite side to label. White glaze with pinkish tinge and design in blue. Label panel straight with even outline. Neck ridged with glazed rim, unflanged spout with flared rim, hollowed and glazed base with unglazed edge. In blue on base: I.
DESIGN: Cherub and shell
INSCRIPTION: S:EX.ALLIO.
MEANING OF INSCRIPTION: *Syrupus ex allio*, syrup of garlic (*Allium sativum*). Used in the treatment of bronchitis, pneumonia and nervous afflictions.
CONTEMPORARY ACCOUNT: "Take of the root of garlick sliced one pound, of boiling water a quart. Steep the garlick in the water twelve hours in a close vessel, and in the liquor strained dissolve a sufficient quantity of sugar, so as to make the syrup." (H. Pemberton, *The Dispensatory*, 1746, p. 291)
DATE OF MANUFACTURE: 1740–1760
PLACE OF MANUFACTURE: London
DIMENSIONS: Height 185 mm, maximum width 140 mm

PROVENANCE: Bought in 1957, Howard Collection.
CONDITION: Good; base chipped, glaze crazed and flaked on spout, neck and base rims.
REFERENCE: Howard, English Delftware Drug Jars, p. 22 and No. 49.

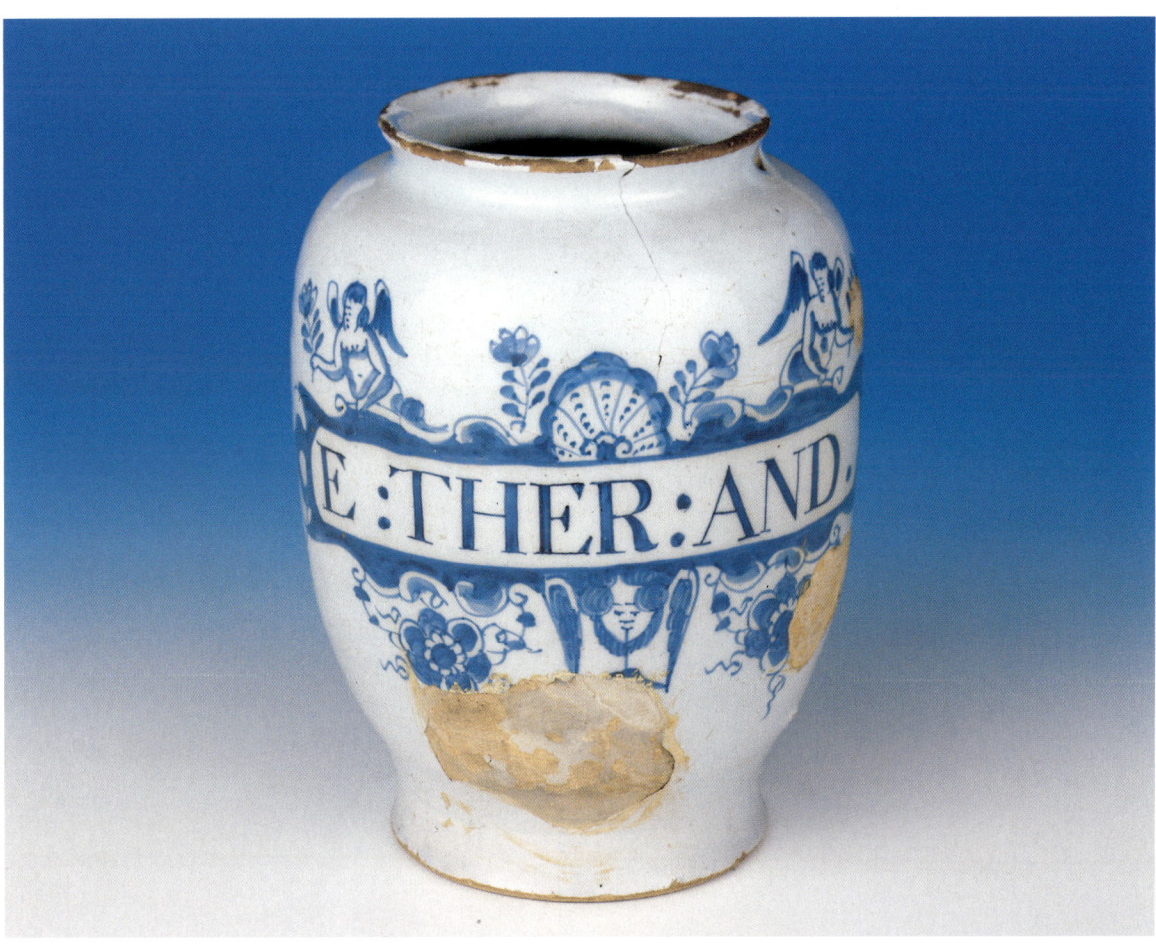

Dry drug jar (Cat.182)

ACCESSION NUMBER: KCN22
DESCRIPTION: Ovoid jar, tapering slightly towards slightly splayed base. White glaze with bluish tinge and design in blue. Label panel straight with even outline. Neck everted with glazed rim, concave glazed base with unglazed edge.
DESIGN: Cherub and shell
INSCRIPTION: E:THER:AND
MEANING OF INSCRIPTION: *Theriaca Andromachi*, the treacle or theriaca of Andromachus, a preparation traced back to Andromachus, physician to the Emperor Nero (AD 37). This extraordinary preparation was supposed to be an antidote to all poisons. It was also used in the 1600s to prevent the plague.
CONTEMPORARY ACCOUNT: "Take *Troches of Squills* ℥ vi. Troches of Vipers, long Pepper, *Opium*, and Troches of Hedycroi, ana ℥ iii. *Red Rose Buds dry'd, Orrice, Juice of Liquorice, Seeds of Sweet Navew*, Tops of Scordium, Opobalsam, *Troches of Agarick*, Cinnamon, ana ℥ iss. Myrrh, Zedoary, Saffron, *Cassia-Bark*, Spikenard, Schoenanth, white and black Pepper, *Frankincense, Dittany of Crete, Rhapontick*, Staecha's, *Hore-*

Hound, Parsley-Seeds, Calaminth, *Cyprus* Turpentine, *Roots of Cinque-foil*, and Ginger, ana ℥ vi. *Tops of Polymountain*, Ground-Pine, *Celtick* Spikenard, *Amomus*, Styrax, Meum-Root, Tops of Germander, *Phu-Root, Earth* of Lemnos, Indian Leaf, *Calcanthum, Gentian Root, Gum-Arabick, Juice of Hypocistis*, Cubebs, Seeds of Anise, Cardomoms, Fennel, of *Hartwort, German Acacia*, Seeds of Treacle-Mustard, Tops of St John's-wort, *Seeds of Bishop's-weed*, Sagapenum, ana ℥ iv. Castor, *long Birthwort, Amber*, or *Bitumen Judaicum*, Seeds of *Daucus*, Opoponax, *Centaury the lesser*, and Galbanum, ana ℥ ii. Canary ℥ xl. Honey, three times the weight of the whole Species when powder'd; and mix all into an Electuary.

"This is not only the Capital Alexipharmick of our Shops, but of all *Europe*; and has a great deal more wrote about it, than could be contain'd in the largest Volume" (J. Quincy, *A Compleat English Dispensatory*, 1718, p. 409)
DATE OF MANUFACTURE: 1740–1760
PLACE OF MANUFACTURE: London
DIMENSIONS: Height 185 mm, maximum width 150 mm
PROVENANCE: Bequest, Saville Peck, 1955.
CONDITION: Poor; crack descending from neck, four pieces of glaze flaked from bowl, glaze crazed and flaked from neck and base rims.

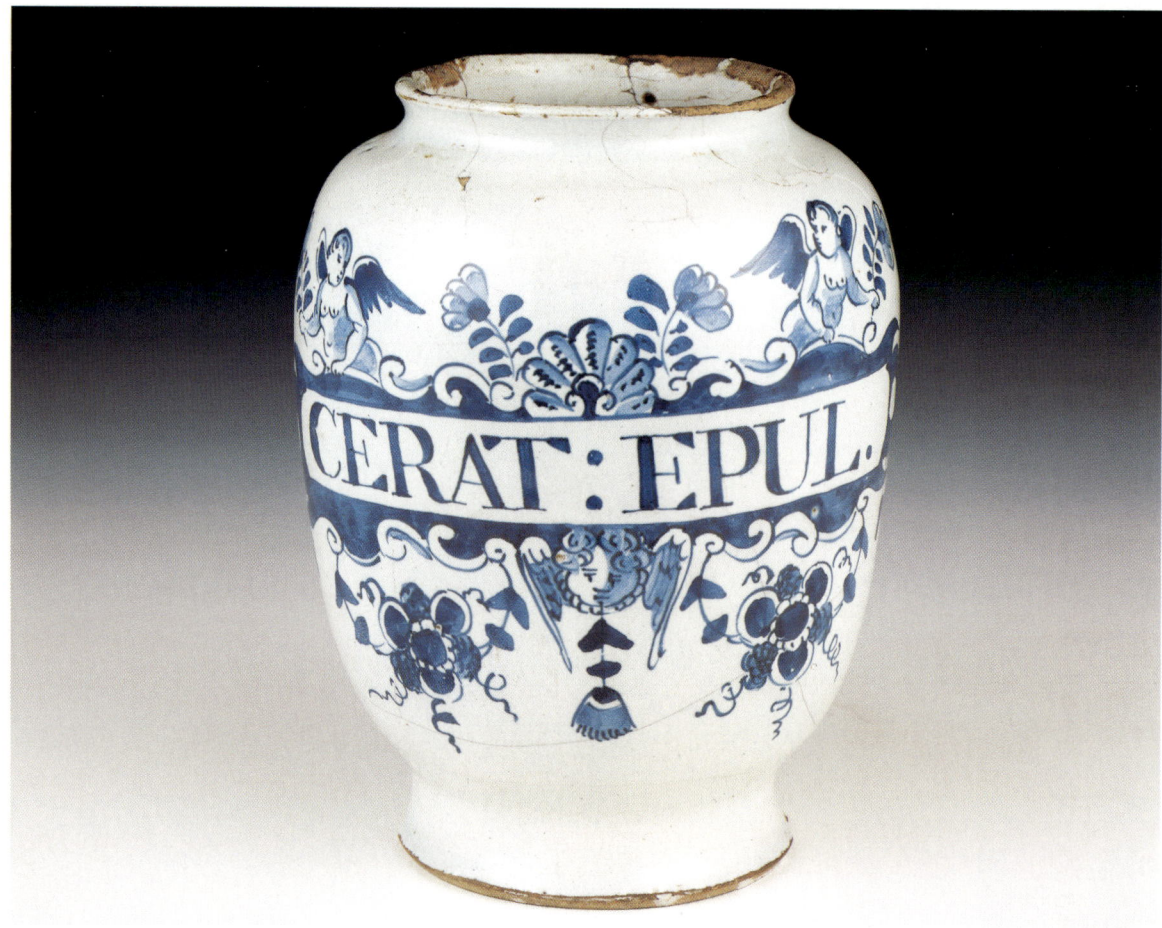

Dry drug jar (Cat.183)

ACCESSION NUMBER: KCN15

DESCRIPTION: Ovoid jar, tapering slightly towards splayed base. White glaze with pinkish tinge and design in blue. Label panel straight with even outline. Neck everted with glazed rim, slightly concave glazed base with unglazed edge. Cross mark on base.

DESIGN: Cherub and shell

INSCRIPTION: CERAT:EPUL.

MEANING OF INSCRIPTION: *Ceratum epuloticum*, cicatrizing cerate, to heal wounds

CONTEMPORARY ACCOUNT: "Take of oil olive a pound; yellow wax, prepared calamy, of each half a pound. Melt the wax with the oil, and as soon as the mixture begins to congeal, sprinkle in the calamy, and stir all well, till the cerate is quite cold." (H. Pemberton, *The Dispensatory*, 1746, p. 376)

DATE OF MANUFACTURE: 1740–1760

PLACE OF MANUFACTURE: London

DIMENSIONS: Height 185 mm, maximum width 150 mm

PROVENANCE: Bequest, Saville Peck, 1955 (previously Prior Collection).

CONDITION: Poor; large crack descending from neck almost to base and partly encircling bowl, base chipped, large pieces of glaze missing from bowl (2 cm) and below neck (1.5 cm), glaze flaked from neck and base rims.

REFERENCE: Walker, Ancient pharmacy jars p. 252, No. II, 6.

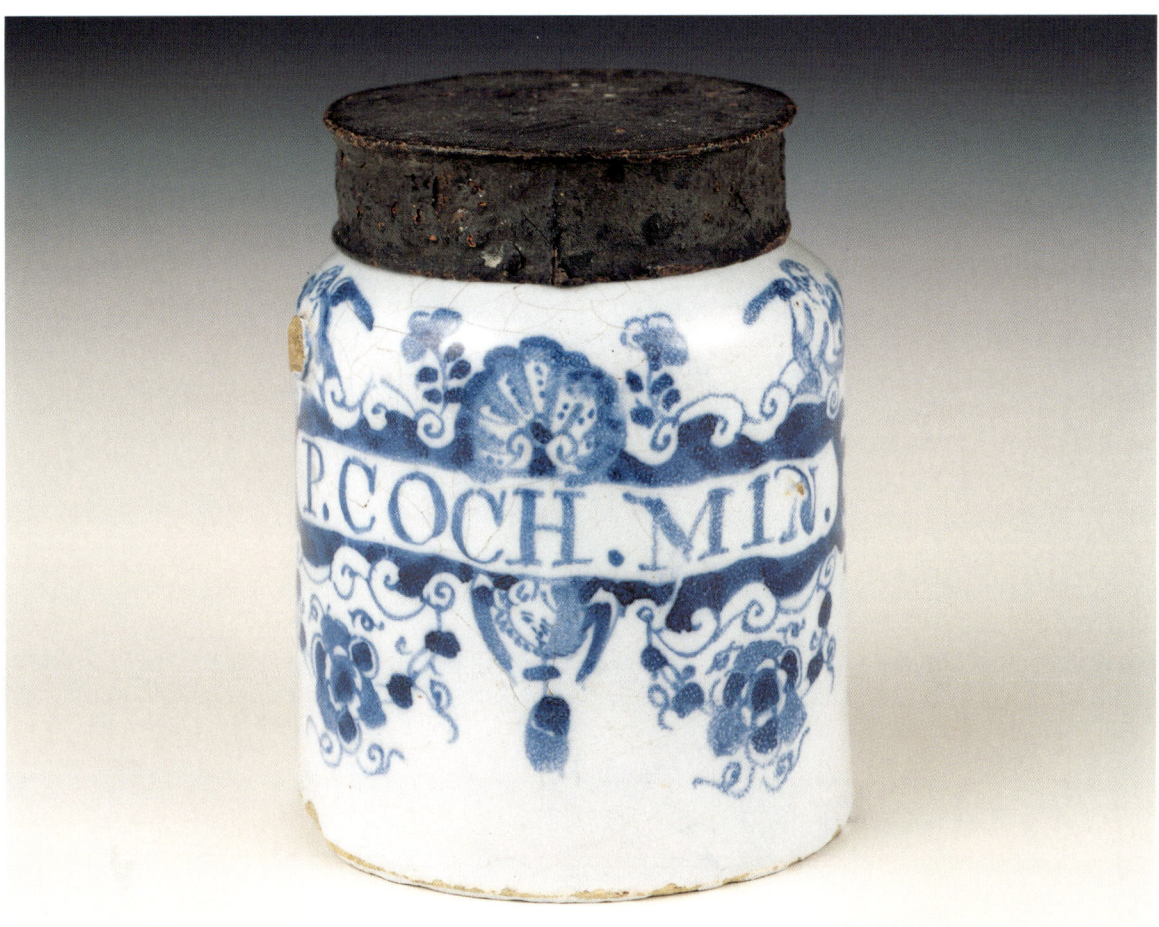

Dry drug jar (Cat.184)

ACCESSION NUMBER: KCN4

DESCRIPTION: Cylindrical jar. White glaze with bluish tinge and design in blue. Label panel straight. Neck everted with glazed rim, concave glazed base. Metal lid.

DESIGN: Cherub and shell

INSCRIPTION: P.COCH.MIN.

MEANING OF INSCRIPTION: *Pilulae cochiae minores*, cochia minor pills

CONTEMPORARY ACCOUNT: "'Tale Aloes *Succotrina*, Scammony, Colcynth, ana ʒ i. Oil of Cloves ℈ ii. Syr. of Buckthorn, a sufficient quantity to make them into a Mass.'

"This is the most common Purges in our Shops, and is indeed a very good one: it is sure in Operation, and not only cleanses the first Passages, but fetches Humours from remote Parts, and does good service in many obstinate chronick Cases, where the Constitution can bear with brisk purging." (J. Quincy, *A Compleat English Dispensatory*, 1718, p. 420)

DATE OF MANUFACTURE: 1750–1770

PLACE OF MANUFACTURE: London

DIMENSIONS: Height 90 mm, maximum width 75 mm

PROVENANCE: Bought in 1957, Howard Collection.

CONDITION: Good; rim and base chipped, glaze crazed.

Cherub and shell

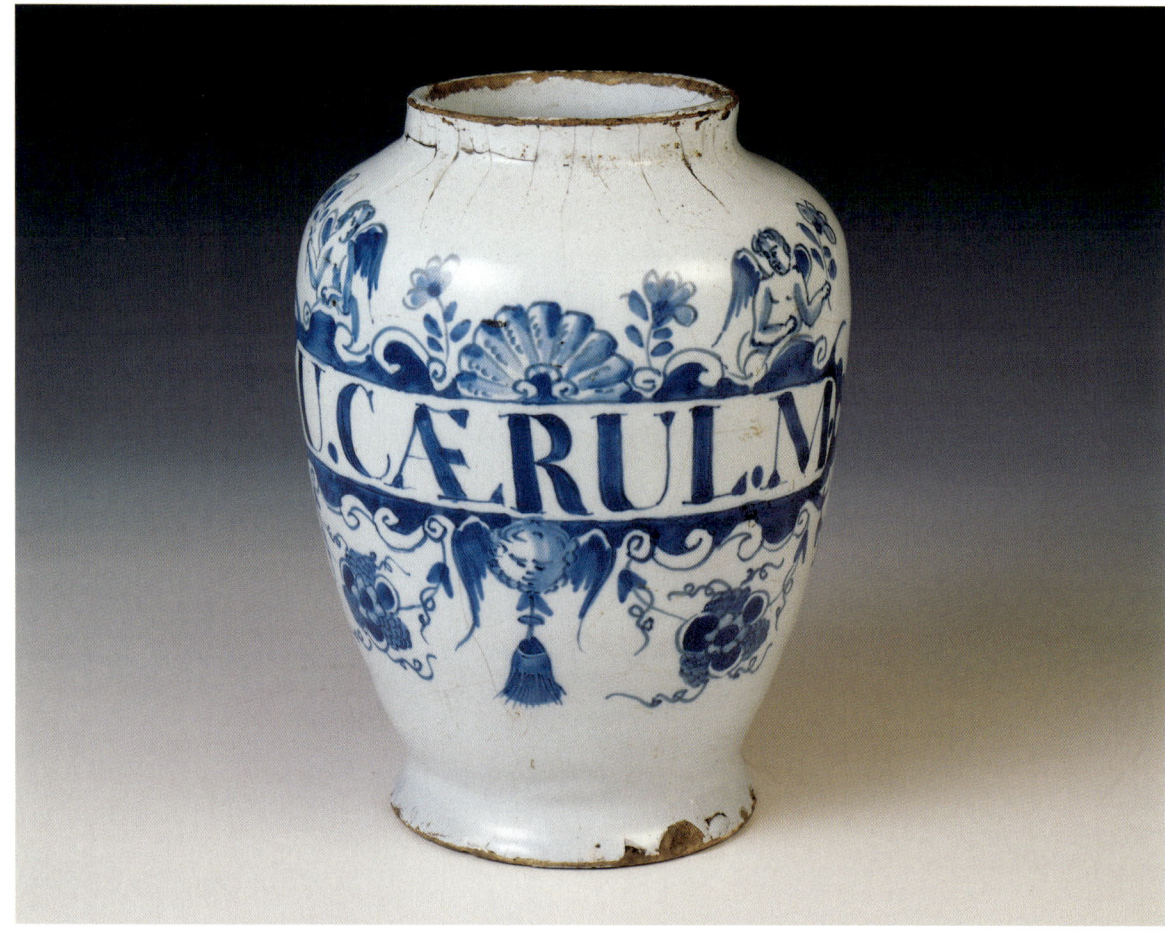

Dry drug jar (Cat.185)

ACCESSION NUMBER: KCN26

DESCRIPTION: Ovoid jar, tapering slightly towards splayed base. White glaze with bluish tinge and design in blue. Label panel straight with even outline. Neck straight with partly glazed edge, slightly concave glazed base with unglazed edge.

DESIGN: Cherub and shell

INSCRIPTION: U.CAERUL.M.

MEANING OF INSCRIPTION: *Unguentum caeruleum mitis*, weaker/milder blue ointment.

CONTEMPORARY ACCOUNT: "Take of tried hog's lard four pounds, of quicksilver one pound, of common turpentine an ounce. Rub the quicksilver in a mortar with the turpentine, till the quicksilver appears no longer; then add by degrees the lard warmed, and mix them diligently." (H. Pemberton, *The Dispensatory*, 1746, p. 367)

DATE OF MANUFACTURE: 1750–1770

PLACE OF MANUFACTURE: London

DIMENSIONS: Height 180 mm, maximum width 95 mm

PROVENANCE: Donation from Mr Hampton, date unknown.

CONDITION: Good; base chipped, glaze crazed and flaked from neck and base rims.

COMMENT: The inscriptions and designs seem to have been painted by the same hand as KCN27 (Cat. 186), KCN2 (Cat. 187), KCN16 (Cat. 188), KCN1 (Cat. 189) and KCN5 (Cat. 190).

Cherub and shell

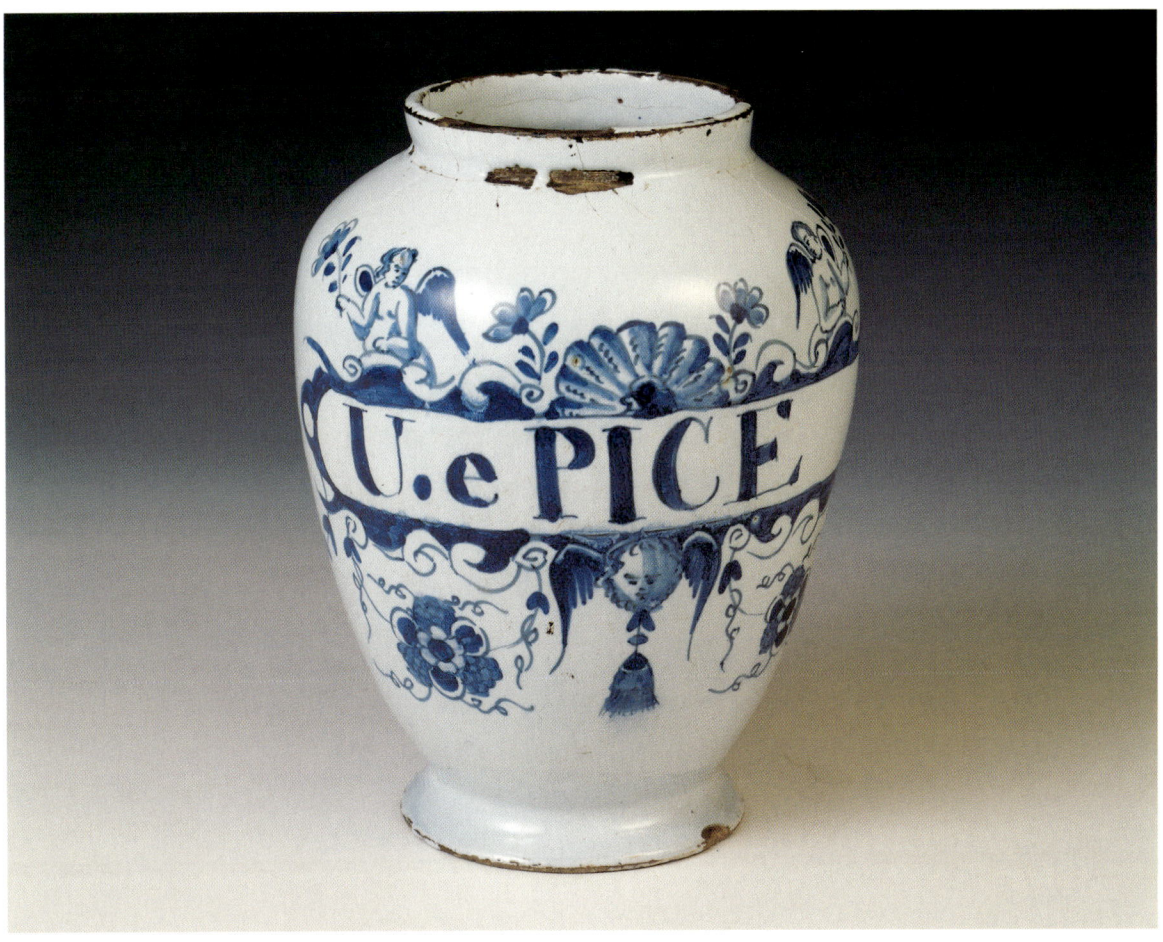

Dry drug jar (Cat.186)

ACCESSION NUMBER: KCN27

DESCRIPTION: Ovoid jar, tapering slightly towards splayed base. White glaze with bluish tinge and design in blue. Label panel straight with even outline. Neck straight with partly glazed edge, slightly concave glazed base with unglazed edge.

DESIGN: Cherub and shell

INSCRIPTION: U.e PICE

MEANING OF INSCRIPTION: *Unguentum e pice*, ointment of tar. Used in treatment of skin disorders.

CONTEMPORARY ACCOUNT: "Take of Tar, and of tried [dried?] Mutton sewet equal weights. Melt them together, and strain, while hot." (H. Pemberton, *The Dispensatory*, 1746, p. 368)

DATE OF MANUFACTURE: 1750–1770

PLACE OF MANUFACTURE: London

DIMENSIONS: Height 180 mm, maximum width 90 mm

PROVENANCE: Donated by Mr Hampton, date unknown.

CONDITION: Good; base chipped, glaze crazed and flaked from neck and base rims.

COMMENT: The inscriptions and designs seem to have been painted by the same hand as KCN26 (Cat. 185), KCN2 (Cat. 187), KCN16 (Cat. 188), KCN1 (Cat. 189) and KCN5 (Cat. 190).

Cherub and shell

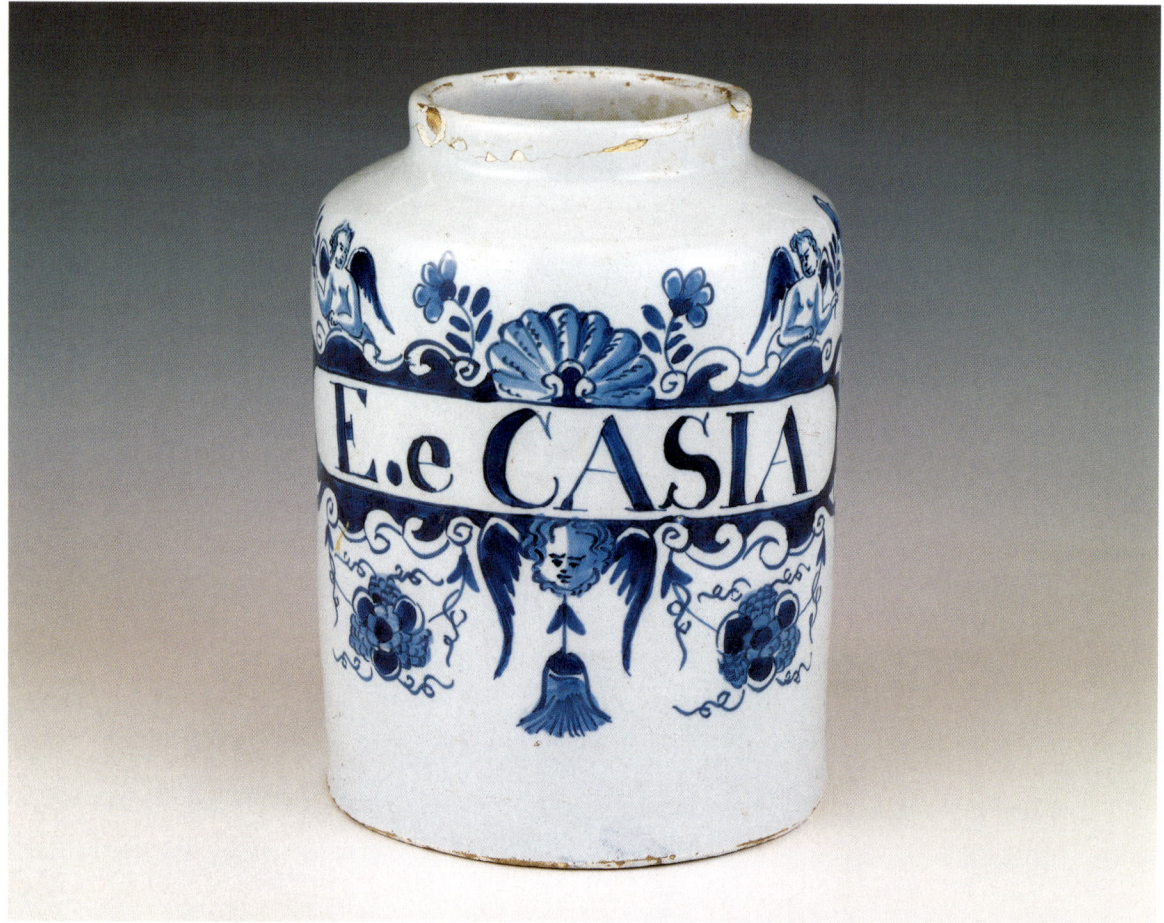

Dry drug jar (Cat.189)

ACCESSION NUMBER: KCN1
DESCRIPTION: Cylindrical jar. White glaze with bluish tinge and design in blue. Label panel straight with even outline. Neck straight with glazed rim, concave glazed base with unglazed outer rim. Metal lid.
DESIGN: Cherub and shell
INSCRIPTION: E. e CASIA
MEANING OF INSCRIPTION: *Electuarium e cassia*, electuary of cassia (*Cassia fistula*)
CONTEMPORARY ACCOUNT: "Take the solutive syrup of roses, the pulp of cassia fresh extracted, of each half a pound; of manna two ounces; of the pulp of tamarinds one ounce. Rub the manna in a mortar, and with a small heat dissolve it in the syrup, then add the pulps, and the heat being continued reduce the whole to a proper consistence." (H. Pemberton, *The Dispensatory*, 1746, p. 334)
DATE OF MANUFACTURE: 1750–1770
PLACE OF MANUFACTURE: London
DIMENSIONS: Height 180 mm, maximum width 140 mm

PROVENANCE: Donated by Mr Hammond, date unknown.
CONDITION: Good; crack at base of neck.
COMMENT: The inscriptions and designs seem to have been painted by the same hand as KCN26 (Cat. 185), KCN27 (Cat. 186), KCN2 (Cat. 187), KCN16 (Cat. 188) and KCN5 (Cat. 190).

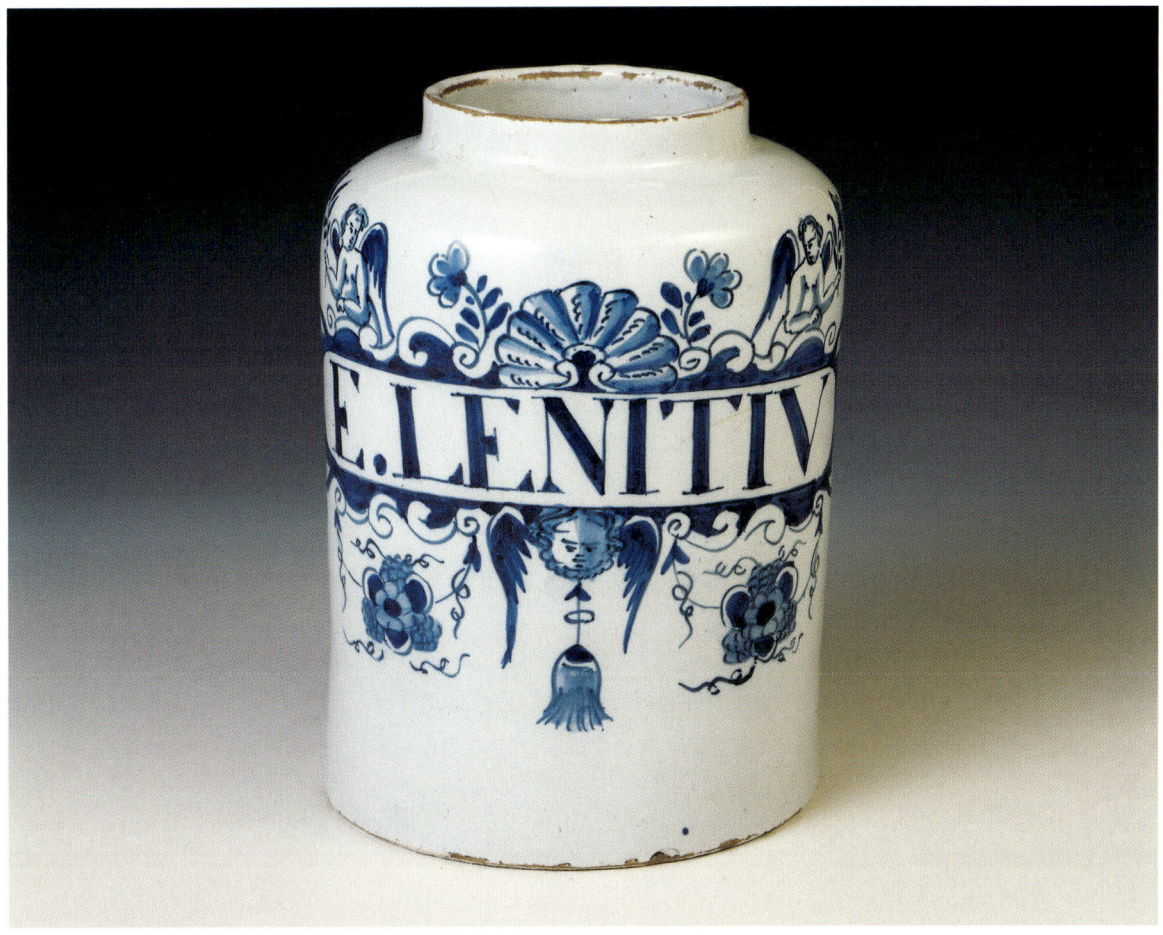

Dry drug jar (Cat.190)

ACCESSION NUMBER: KCN5
DESCRIPTION: Cylindrical jar. White glaze with bluish tinge. Label panel straight with even outline. Neck straight, with glazed rim, slightly concave partly glazed base.
DESIGN: Cherub and shell
INSCRIPTION: E.LENITIV
MEANING OF INSCRIPTION: *Electuarium lenitivum*, lenitive (laxative) electuary
CONTEMPORARY ACCOUNT: "'Take Raisins, Polypody of the Oak, Sena ana ℥ ii. Mercury m.iss. Jujebs, Sebestians, ana no xx. Maiden-hair, Violet-Leaves, Barley, ana m.i. Prunes, Tamarings, ana ℥ vi. Liquorice ℥ ss. Boil all in a sufficient quantity of Water, and add to the strain'd Liquor, Sugar of Violets ℥ vi. Common Sugar ℔ ii, which boil into a thick Syrup, to which add the Pulps of Tamarinds, Cassia, and Prunes, ana ℥ vi. Powder of Sena ℥ vi. Aniseeds ℥ i., and mix all into an Electuary.'

"This is the only officinal Lenitive Purge in use, and well enough answers that End, but it is a very un-artful Composition..." (J. Quincy, *A Compleat English Dispensatory*, 1718, p. 405)

DATE OF MANUFACTURE: 1750–1770
PLACE OF MANUFACTURE: London
DIMENSIONS: Height 180 mm, maximum width 140 mm
PROVENANCE: Bought in 1956.
CONDITION: Good; glaze chipped on base and rim.
COMMENT: The inscriptions and designs seem to have been painted by the same hand as KCN26 (Cat. 185), KCN27 (Cat. 186), KCN2 (Cat. 187), KCN16 (Cat. 188) and KCN1 (Cat. 189).

Cherub and shell

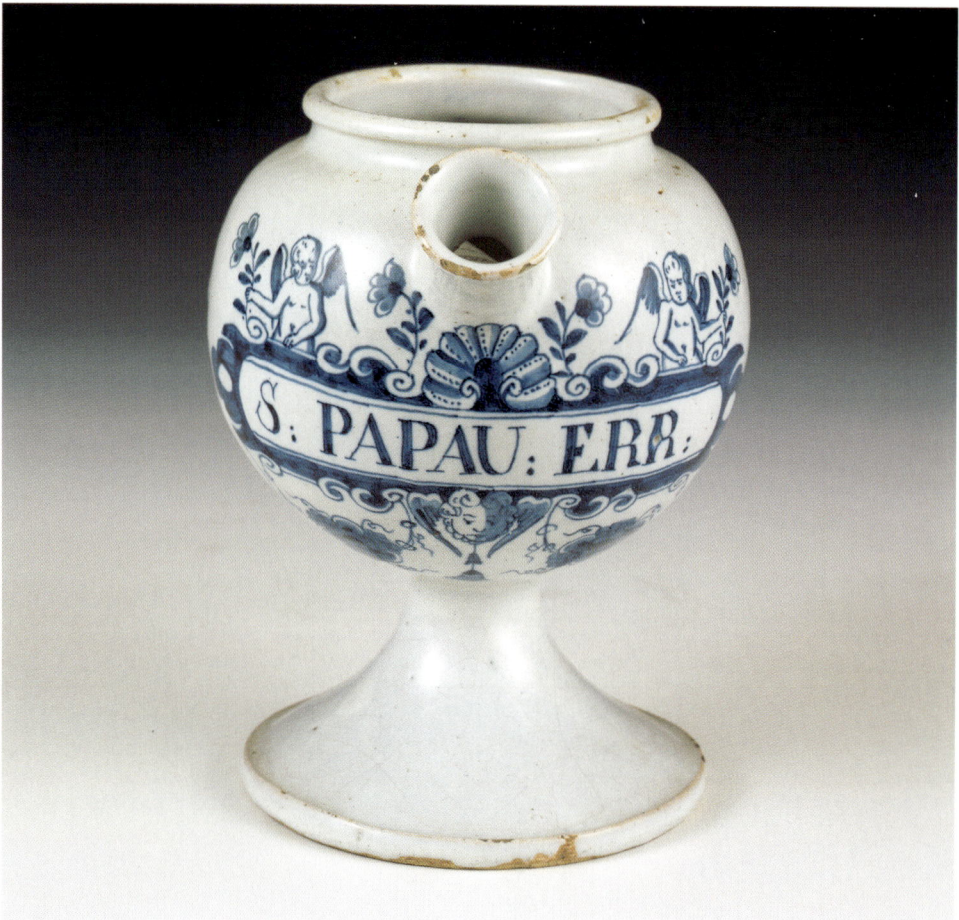

Wet drug jar (Cat.191)

ACCESSION NUMBER: KDN2

DESCRIPTION: Bulbous jar on spreading foot, with spout and fluted strap-like looped handle. White glaze with pinkish tinge and design in blue. Label panel straight with even outline and parallel lines inside top and bottom edges. Neck ridged with glazed rim, unflanged spout with flared rim, hollowed and glazed base with unglazed edge.

DESIGN: Cherub and shell

INSCRIPTION: S:PAPAU:ERR:

MEANING OF INSCRIPTION: *Syrupus de papavere erratico*, syrup of wild poppy (*Papaver rhoeas*)

CONTEMPORARY ACCOUNT: "'Take Flowers of the Wild or Corn-Poppy ℔ ii. Pour upon them boiling Water ℔ iv. and make into a Syrup, after another Infusion with fresh Flowers, with the same quantity of fine Sugar as there is Liquor press'd out.'

"This is better done by one Infusion, pouring no more upon the Flowers than will just scald them, and then putting to each Pound, of Sugar ℔ ii. which will melt into a due Consistence without boiling: for so much boiling prejudices the Colour, which is beautiful enough in Juleps or any liquid Forms; whereas the medicinal Virtues are not much worth regarding: for altho these Flowers are accounted both *Anodyne* and *Alexipharmic*, yet in such a small quantity as we have of them in half an Ounce of Syrup, (the usual Dose) it is so very little, as not to be regarded." (J. Quincy, *A Compleat English Dispensatory*, 1718, pp. 378–379)

DATE OF MANUFACTURE: 1720–1740

PLACE OF MANUFACTURE: London

DIMENSIONS: Height 160 mm, maximum width 123 mm

PROVENANCE: Bought in 1957, Howard Collection.

CONDITION: Good; glaze crazed and flaked on handle, spout, neck and base rims.

COMMENT: Howard commented that this jar was "remarkably small for a Syrup jar" (p. 22). This is part of a small group of eleven jars including one in the Wellcome Collection, and two at Colonial Williamsburg with added parallel lines at top and bottom inside the cartouche.

REFERENCE: Howard, English Delftware Drug Jars, p. 22 and No. 46.

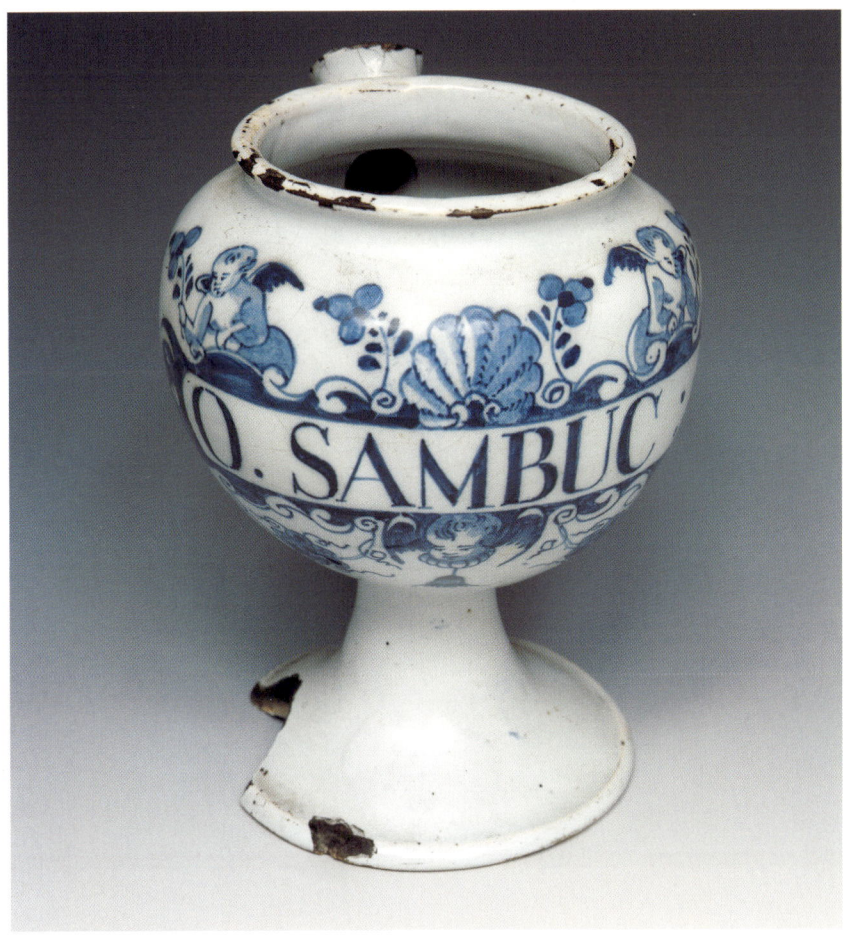

Wet drug jar (Cat.192)

ACCESSION NUMBER: KDN10

DESCRIPTION: Bulbous jar on spreading foot, with spout only (on opposite side to label). White glaze with bluish tinge and design in blue. Label panel straight with even outline. Neck everted with glazed rim, flared spout, hollowed base.

DESIGN: Cherub and shell

INSCRIPTION: O.SAMBUC

MEANING OF INSCRIPTION: *Oleum sambucinum*, oil of elder (*Sambucus nigra*)

CONTEMPORARY ACCOUNT: "This Tree has not one part free from the Tortures of Pharmacy...we shall just take notice here, that the green Leaves are only us'd in the Shops to make an *Oil* with for some external Intentions, and that they are sometimes, by way of *Cataplasms*, applied hot to *Erysipela's* and *Inflammatory Tumours*." (J. Quincy, *A Compleat English Dispensatory*, 1718, pp. 131–132)

DATE OF MANUFACTURE: 1730–1750

PLACE OF MANUFACTURE: London

DIMENSIONS: Height 178 mm, maximum width 147 mm

PROVENANCE: Donation from Mr Appleton, 1938.

CONDITION: Fair; glaze flaked from spout, neck and base rims, chip from foot.

COMMENT: This jar is part of a group of 20 jars with a very characteristic style of clover-shaped flower with a pellet on the tip of the middle petal (see also KDN4 – Cat. 194, KDN9 – Cat. 193, and KDN11 – Cat. 195). This same style of flower also appears on two of the plates with the Apothecaries' arms in the Ashmolean Museum, Oxford and Saffron Walden Museum and a pill tile (Lot 12 Christies 2/6/1986, present whereabouts unknown).

Cherub and shell

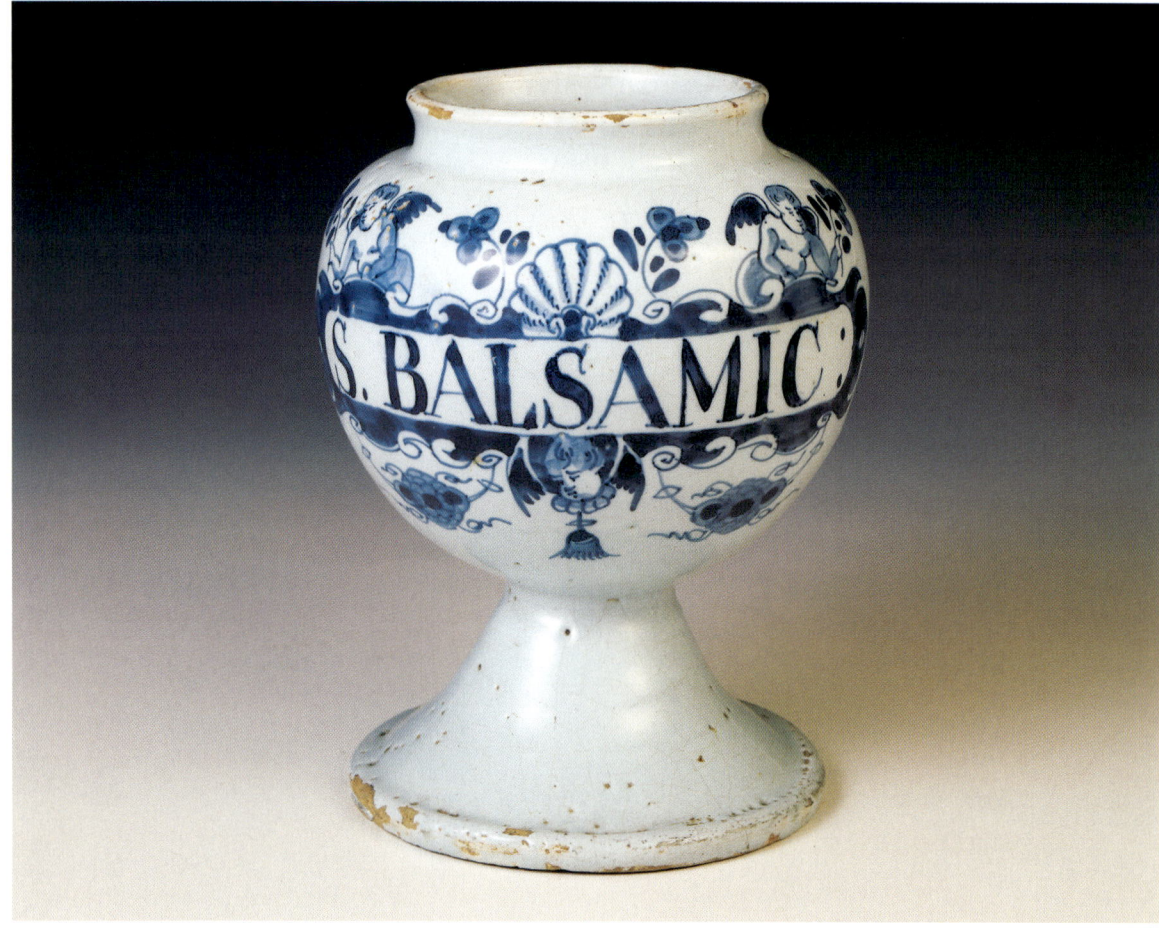

Wet drug jar (Cat.193)

ACCESSION NUMBER: KDN9

DESCRIPTION: Bulbous jar on spreading foot, with spout only (on opposite side to label). White glaze with bluish tinge and design in blue. Label panel straight with even outline. Neck slightly everted with glazed rim, flared spout, hollowed, ridged, glazed base with unglazed edge.

DESIGN: Cherub and shell (cherubs look outwards)

INSCRIPTION: S.BALSAMIC:

MEANING OF INSCRIPTION: *Syrupus balsamicus*, balsamic syrup, later known as syrup of tolu.

CONTEMPORARY ACCOUNT: "'Take Balsam of *Tolu* ℥ ii. Colts-Foot-Water ℥ xii. Boil them in a circulatory Vessel with the Juncture well luted, in a Sand-Heat three hours. When it is cold, in the strain'd Water by degrees dissolve ℥ xx. of Sugar without any heat.'

"This is very judiciously contriv'd yet many neglect the Care here enjoin'd, and boil in an open Vessel, by which they lose the finer parts of the Balsam. As for the Water here order'd, common Water will do as well. But if it be done with Rose or Orange-Water, it will be a most delightful Medicine, and much more of a Cordial..." (J. Quincy, *A Compleat English Dispensatory*, 1718, pp. 384–385)

DATE OF MANUFACTURE: 1730–1750

PLACE OF MANUFACTURE: London

DIMENSIONS: Height 170 mm, maximum width 145 mm

PROVENANCE: Bought in 1957, Howard Collection.

CONDITION: Good; base chipped, glaze pitted and flaked from spout, neck and base rims.

COMMENT: This jar is part of a group of 20 jars with a very characteristic style of clover-shaped flower with a pellet on the tip of the middle petal (see also KDN4 – Cat. 194, KDN10 – Cat. 192, and KDN11 – Cat. 195). This same style of flower also appears on two of the plates with the Apothecaries' arms in the Ashmolean Museum, Oxford and Saffron Walden Museum and a pill tile (Lot 12 Christies 2/6/1986, present whereabouts unknown).

REFERENCE: Howard, English Delftware Drug Jars, No. 51.

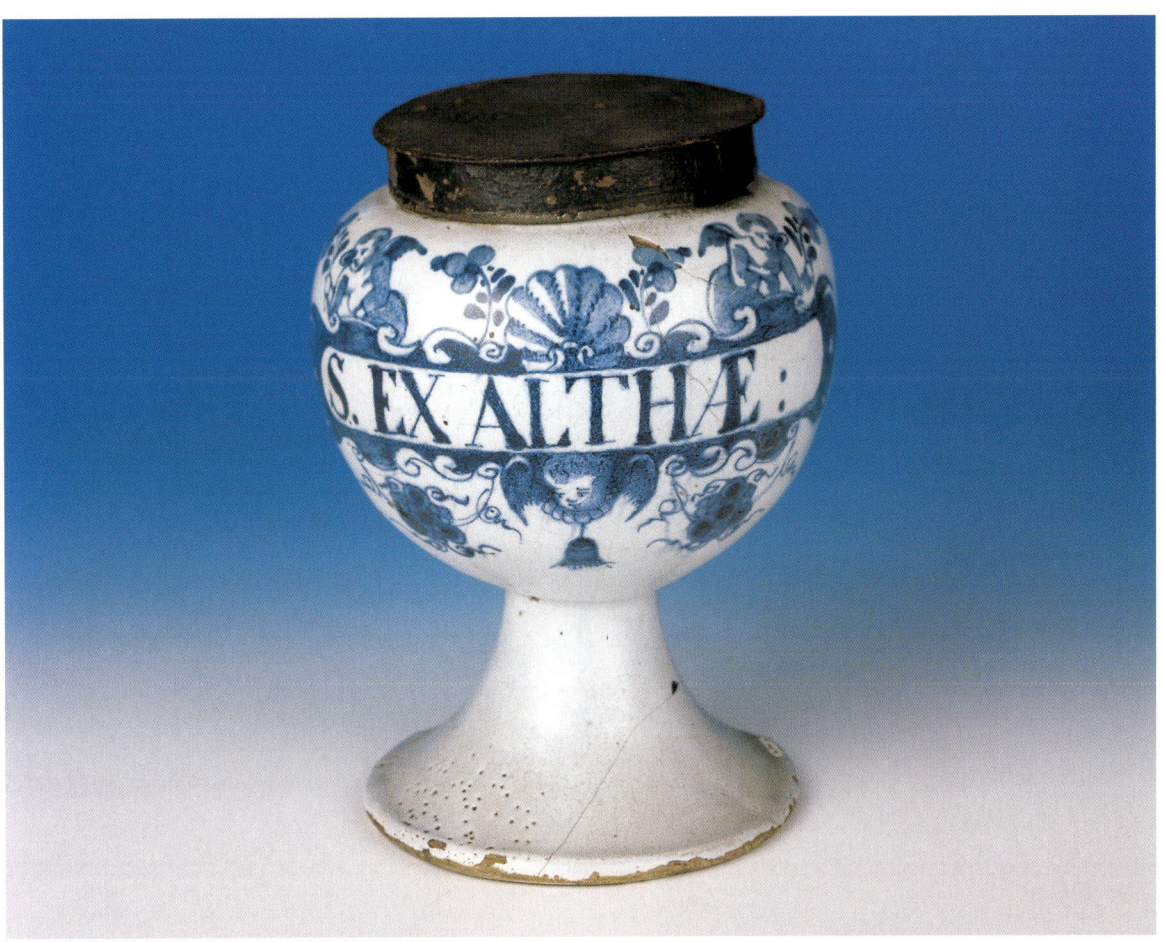

Wet drug jar (Cat.194)

ACCESSION NUMBER: KDN4

DESCRIPTION: Bulbous jar on spreading foot with spout only (on opposite side to label). White glaze with pinkish tinge and design in blue. Label panel straight with even outline. Metal cover glued to neck. Flared spout, hollowed and glazed base with unglazed edge.

DESIGN: Cherub and shell

INSCRIPTION: S.EX ALTHAE:

MEANING OF INSCRIPTION: *Syrupus ex althea*, syrup of marshmallow (*Althaea officinalis*)

CONTEMPORARY ACCOUNT: "Take Marsh-Mallow Roots ℥ ii. of Grass, Asparagus, Liquorise, Roots and Raisins ston'd, ana ℥ ss. Leaves of Marsh-Mallows, common Mallows, Pellitory of the Wall, Pimpernel, Saxifrage, Plantain, white and black Maidenhair, ana m.i. red Chiches ℥ i. The four greater and lesser cold Seeds, ana ℥ iii. Boil them in a Sufficient quantity of Water, strain the Liquor out hard and boil it up when clarify'd into a Syrup, with ℔ iiiss. of white Sugar."

"This Syrup is originally ascrib'd to *Fernelius*, and hath remain'd un-alter'd in all the *College Dispensatories*; but 'tis by many though a very indifferent Medicine, tho' greatly us'd, and much prescrib'd." (J. Quincy, *A Compleat English Dispensatory*, 1718, pp. 394–395)

DATE OF MANUFACTURE: 1730–1750

PLACE OF MANUFACTURE: London

DIMENSIONS: Height 185 mm, maximum width 145 mm

PROVENANCE: Donation, 1953, Austen Collection.

CONDITION: Very poor; large portion of base missing, part of spout missing, large cracks descending from neck and encircling bowl (has been repaired), glaze crazed and pitted.

COMMENT: This jar is part of a group of 20 jars with a very characteristic style of clover-shaped flower with a pellet on the tip of the middle petal (see also KDN9 – Cat. 193, KDN10 – Cat. 192, and KDN11 – Cat. 195). This same style of flower also appears on two of the plates with the Apothecaries' arms in the Ashmolean Museum, Oxford and Saffron Walden Museum and a pill tile (Lot 12 Christies 2/6/1986, present whereabouts unknown).

REFERENCE: Lothian, 'The John Austen Collection' Plate 12 and p. 97.

Cherub and shell

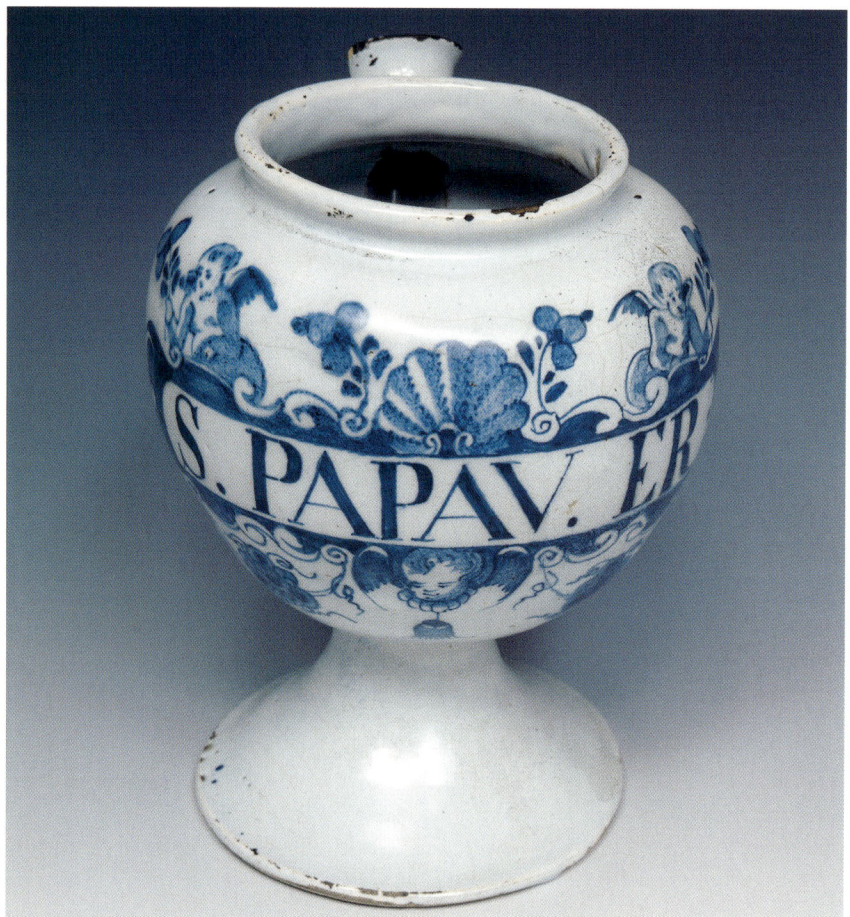

Wet drug jar (Cat.195)

ACCESSION NUMBER: KDN11
DESCRIPTION: Bulbous jar on spreading foot, with spout only (on opposite side to label). White glaze with bluish tinge and design in blue. Label panel straight with even outline. Neck ridged with glazed rim, flared spout, hollowed base.
DESIGN: Cherub and shell
INSCRIPTION: S.PAPAV. ER
MEANING OF INSCRIPTION: *Syrupus de papavere erratico*, syrup of wild poppy (*Papaver rhoeas*)
CONTEMPORARY ACCOUNT: "'Take Flowers of the Wild or Corn-Poppy ℔ ii. Pour upon them boiling Water ℔ iv. and make into a Syrup, after another Infusion with fresh Flowers, with the same quantity of fine Sugar as there is Liquor press'd out.'

"This is better done by one Infusion, pouring no more upon the Flowers than will just scald them, and then putting to each Pound, of Sugar ℔ ii. which will melt into a due Consistence without boiling: for so much boiling prejudices the Colour, which is beautiful enough in Juleps or any liquid Forms; whereas the medicinal Virtues are not much worth regarding: for altho these Flowers are accounted both *Anodyne* and *Alexipharmic*, yet in such a small quantity as we have of them in half an Ounce of Syrup, (the usual Dose) it is so very little, as not to be regarded." (J. Quincy, *A Compleat English Dispensatory*, 1718, pp. 378–379)

DATE OF MANUFACTURE: 1730–1750
PLACE OF MANUFACTURE: London
DIMENSIONS: Height 185 mm, maximum width
PROVENANCE: Donation from Mr Appleton, 1938.
CONDITION: Good; 1.5 cm chip from spout.
COMMENT: This jar is part of a group of 20 jars with a very characteristic style of clover-shaped flower with a pellet on the tip of the middle petal (see also KDN9 – Cat. 193, KDN10 – Cat. 192, and KDN4 – Cat. 194). This same style of flower also appears on two of the plates with the Apothecaries' arms in the Ashmolean Museum, Oxford and Saffron Walden Museum and a pill tile (Lot 12 Christies 2/6/1986, present whereabouts unknown).

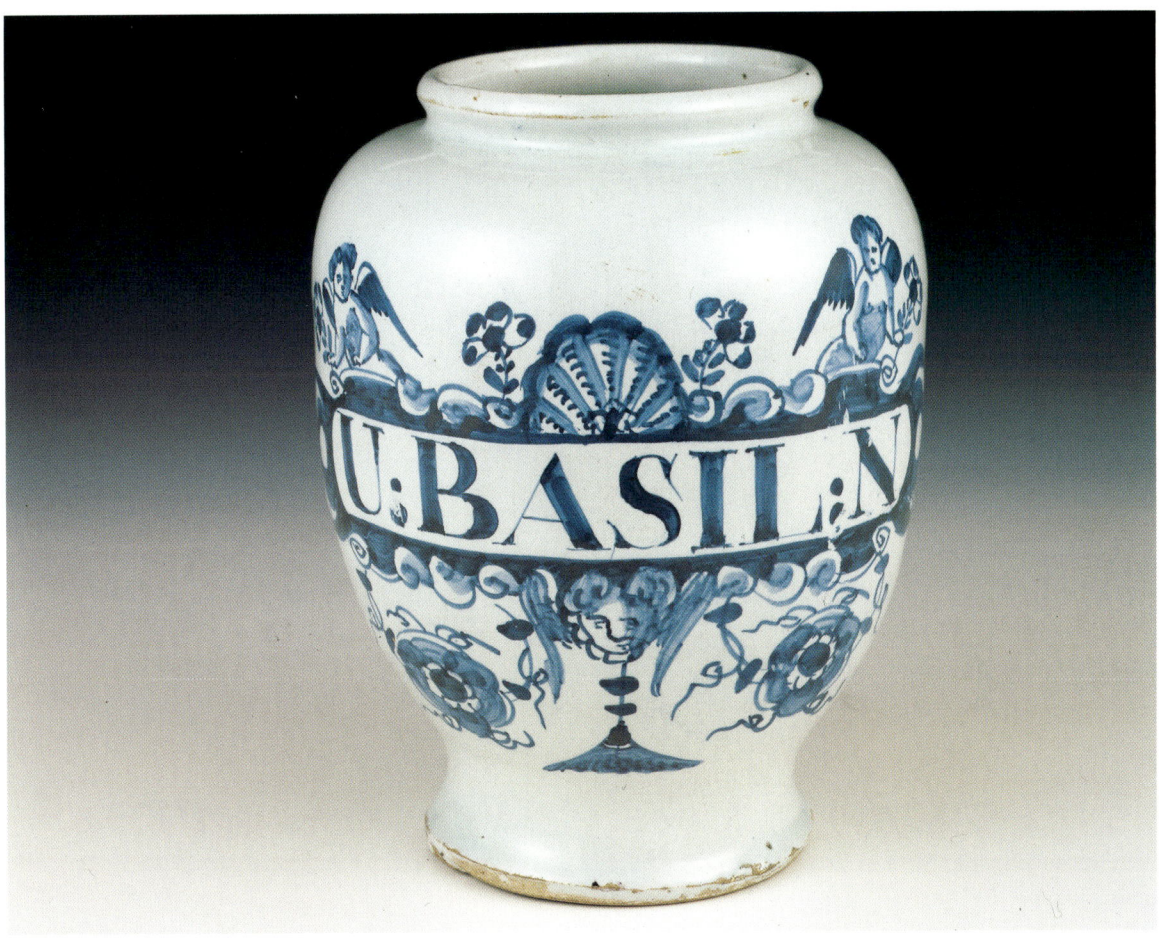

Dry drug jar (Cat.196)

ACCESSION NUMBER: KCN17

DESCRIPTION: Ovoid jar, tapering slightly towards splayed base. White glaze with bluish tinge and design in blue. Label panel straight with even outline. Neck ridged with glazed rim, concave glazed base with unglazed edge.

DESIGN: Cherub and shell

INSCRIPTION: U:BASIL:N

MEANING OF INSCRIPTION: *Unguentum basilicum nigrum*, black basilicum (basilicon) ointment

CONTEMPORARY ACCOUNT: "Take of oil olive a pint; yellow wax, yellow rosin, common pitch, of each nine ounces. Melt all together, and strain the mixture off, while hot." (H. Pemberton, *The Dispensatory*, 1746, p. 365)

DATE OF MANUFACTURE: 1750–1770

PLACE OF MANUFACTURE: Possibly Mortlake, London

COMMENT: Lothian suggested that this was a pair with KCN24 (Cat. 197).

DIMENSIONS: Height 180 mm, maximum width 150 mm

PROVENANCE: Bequest, Saville Peck, 1955 (previously Prior Collection).

CONDITION: Good; hair cracks encircling bowl, glaze flaked on rim of base and neck.

REFERENCE: Walker, Ancient pharmacy jars pp. 251–252, No. II, 3.

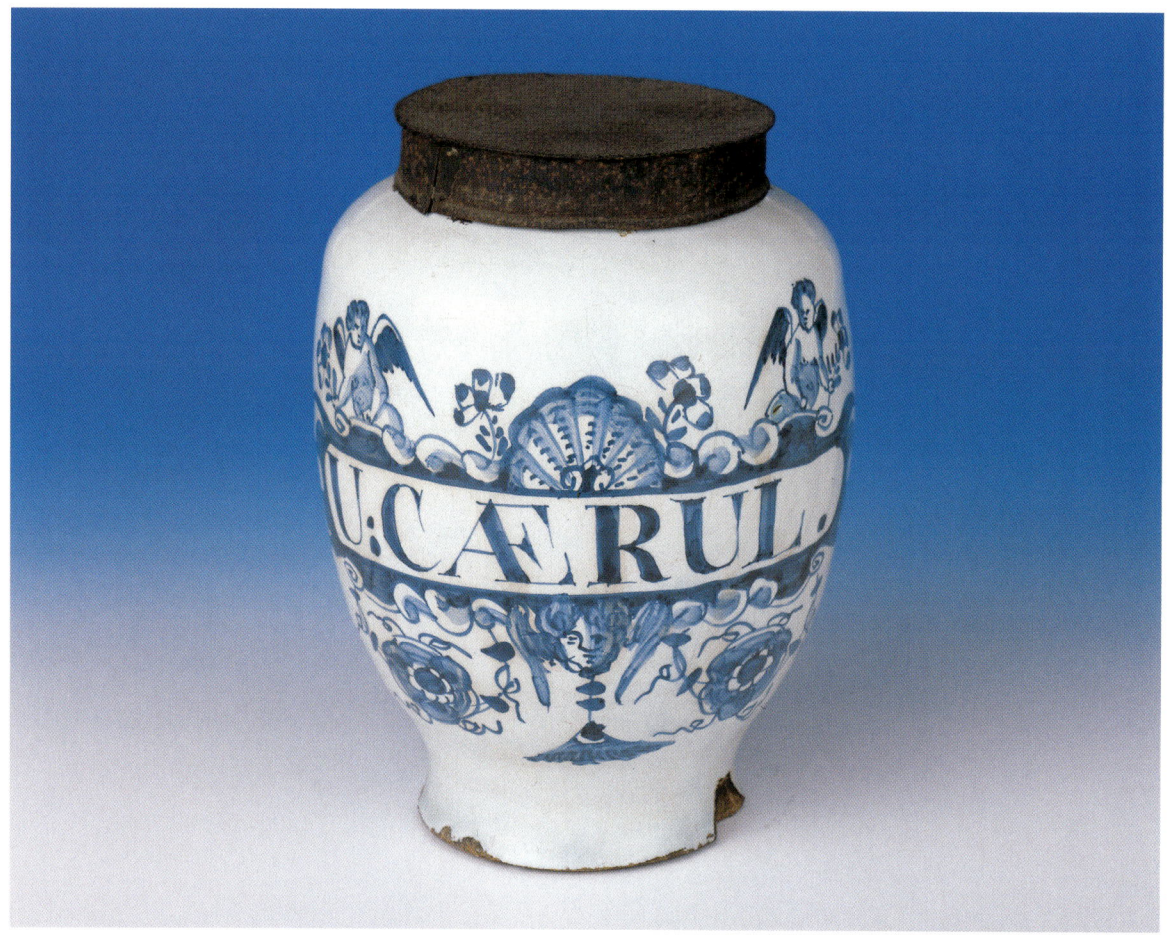

Dry drug jar (Cat.197)

ACCESSION NUMBER: KCN24
DESCRIPTION: Ovoid jar, tapering slightly towards splayed base. White glaze with bluish tinge and design in blue. Label panel straight with even outline. Neck ridged with glazed rim, slightly concave glazed base with unglazed edge. Metal lid.
DESIGN: Cherub and shell
INSCRIPTION: U:CAERUL
MEANING OF INSCRIPTION: *Unguentum caeruleum* (mitius), (weaker/milder) blue ointment
CONTEMPORARY ACCOUNT: "Take of tried hog's lard four pounds, of quicksilver one pound, of common turpentine an ounce. Rub the quicksilver in a mortar with the turpentine, till the quicksilver appears no longer; then add by degrees the lard warmed, and mix them diligently." (H. Pemberton, *The Dispensatory*, 1746, p. 367)
DATE OF MANUFACTURE: 1750–1770
PLACE OF MANUFACTURE: Possibly Mortlake, London
COMMENT: Lothian suggested that this was a pair with KCN17 (Cat. 196)

DIMENSIONS: Height 180 mm, maximum width 148 mm
PROVENANCE: Bequest, Saville Peck, 1955.
CONDITION: Good; 2.5 cm chip in base, glaze crazed.
REFERENCE: Walker, Ancient pharmacy jars pp. 251–252, No. II, 4.

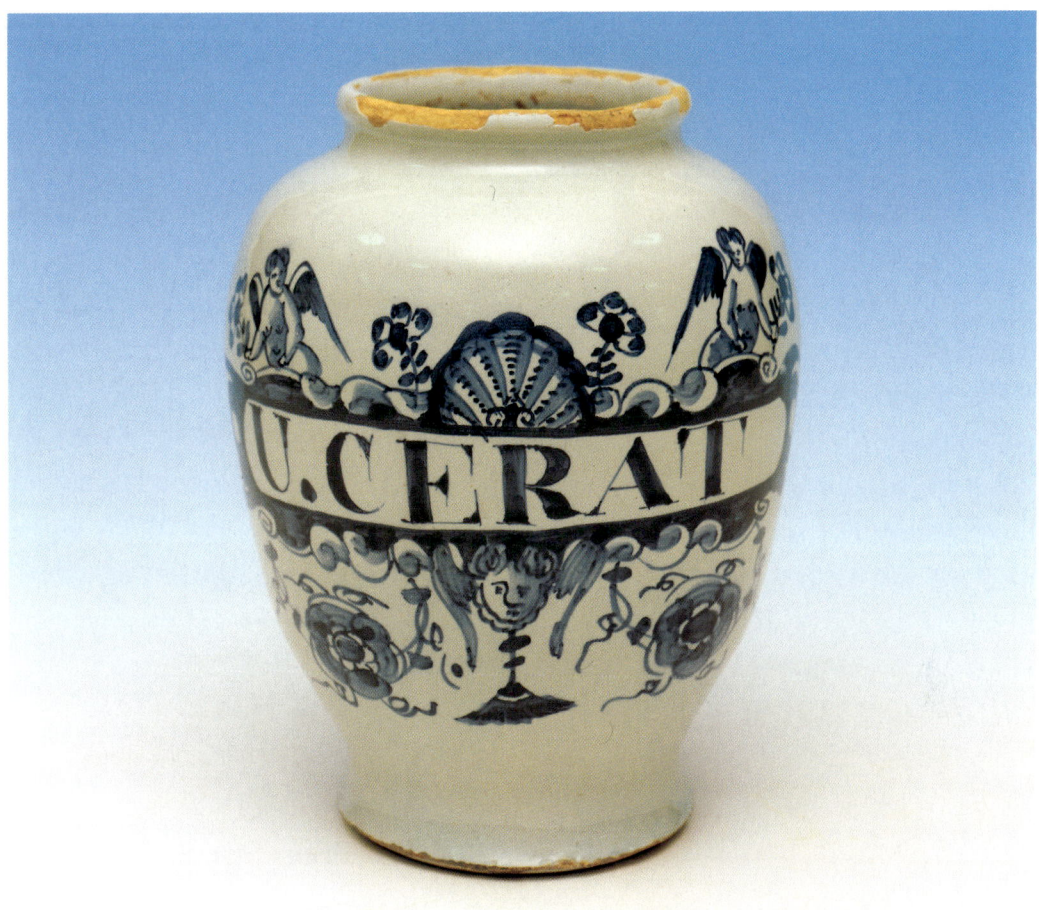

Dry drug jar (Cat.198)

ACCESSION NUMBER: KCN29

DESCRIPTION: Ovoid jar, tapering slightly towards splayed base. White glaze with bluish tinge and design in blue. Label panel straight with even outline. Neck ridged.

DESIGN: Cherub and shell

INSCRIPTION: U.CERAT

MEANING OF INSCRIPTION: *Unguentum cerae*, wax ointment. This name first becomes official in the 1788 pharmacopoeia, having been *Unguentum album* up until then.

CONTEMPORARY ACCOUNT: "Take of white wax, four ounces by weight. Spermaceti, three ounces by weight. Olive oil, one pint. Melt with a slow fire, and stir them constantly and briskly, until cold." (T. Healde, *The Pharmacopoeia of the Royal College of Physicians of London*, 1796, p. 305.)

DATE OF MANUFACTURE: 1750–1800

PLACE OF MANUFACTURE: Possibly Mortlake, London

DIMENSIONS: Height 183 mm, maximum width 137 mm.

PROVENANCE: Unknown

CONDITION: Good, some loss of glaze to rim.

Cherub and shell

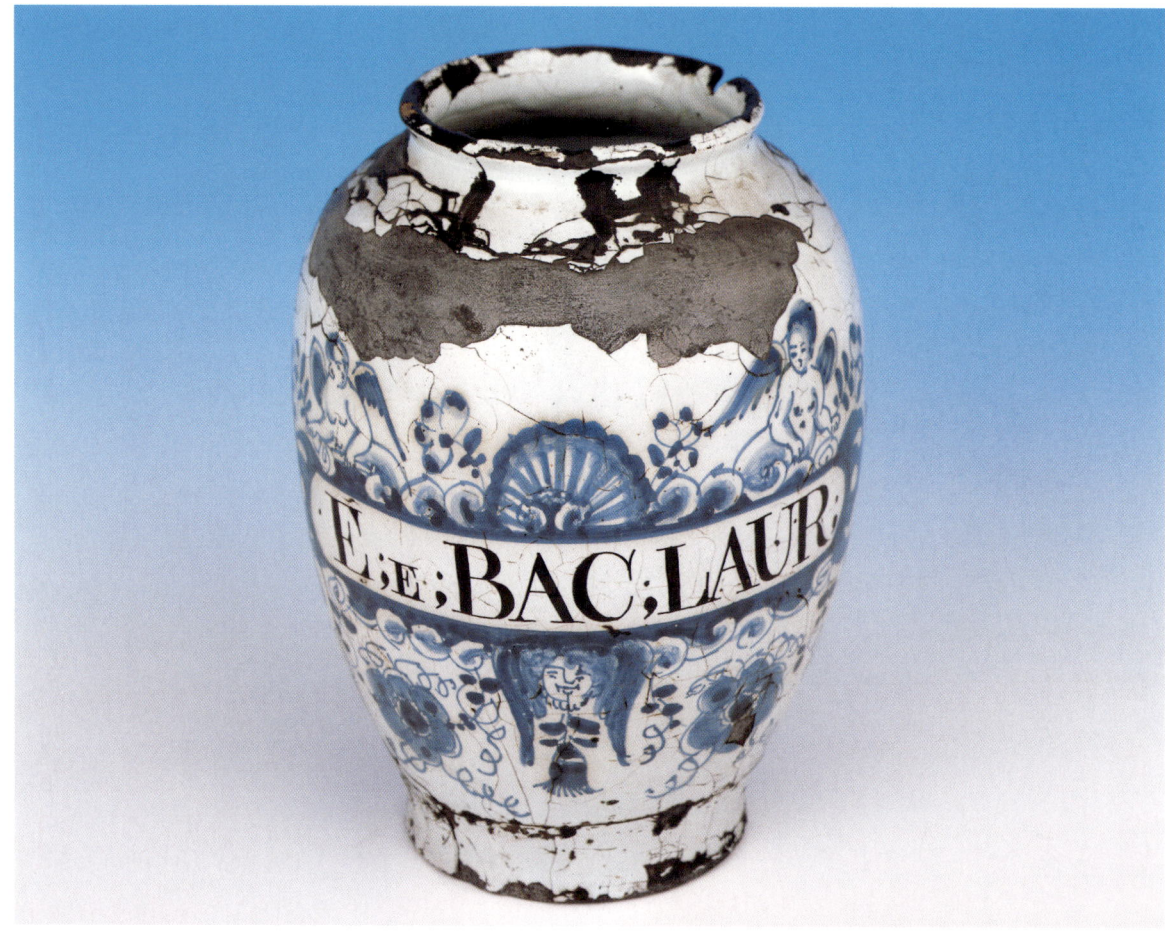

Dry drug jar (Cat.199)

ACCESSION NUMBER: KCN23

DESCRIPTION: Ovoid jar, tapering slightly towards base. White glaze with bluish tinge and design in blue and black. Label panel straight with even outline. Neck everted with partly glazed rim, slightly concave glazed base with unglazed edge.

DESIGN: Cherub and shell

INSCRIPTION: E;E;BAC;LAUR;

MEANING OF INSCRIPTION: *Emplastrum e baccis lauri*, plaster of bayberries (*Laurus nobilis*)

CONTEMPORARY ACCOUNT: "Colledg. Take of Bay-berries husked, Turpentine of each two ounces; Frankincense, Mastich, Mirrh, of each an ounce; Cyperus, Costus, of each half an ounce; Honey warmed and * not scummed [*and why not scummed? I had forgot, the Colledg is not bound to give a reason for what they do] four ounces; make it into a plaister according to Art."

Culpeper: "It is an excellent plaister to ease any pains coming of cold of wind, in any part of the body, whether Stomach, Liver, Belly, Reins or Bladder. It is an excellent remedy for the Cholick and Wind in the Bowels." (N. Culpeper, *The Physicians Library*, 1667, p. 237)

DATE OF MANUFACTURE: 1750–1770

PLACE OF MANUFACTURE: Possibly Mortlake, London

DIMENSIONS: Height 190 mm, maximum width 153 mm

PROVENANCE: Donation, 1953, Austen Collection.

CONDITION: Poor; chip in neck, crack encircling bowl, large portions of glaze flaked from body.

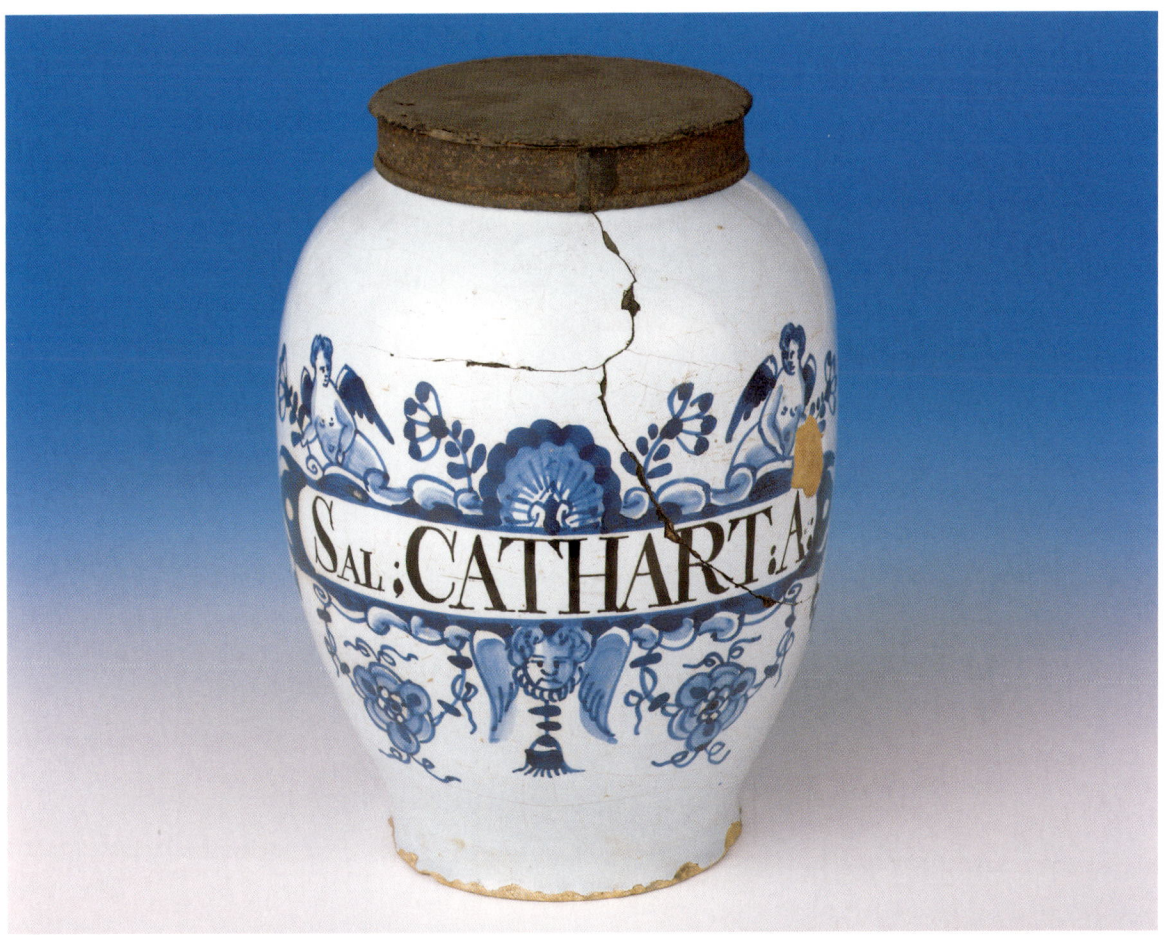

Dry drug jar (Cat.200)

ACCESSION NUMBER: KCN25

DESCRIPTION: Ovoid jar, tapering slightly towards slightly splayed base. White glaze with bluish tinge and design in blue and black. Label panel straight with even outline. Neck ridged with unglazed rim, slightly concave glazed base with unglazed edge. Metal lid.

DESIGN: Cherub and shell

INSCRIPTION: SAL;CATHART:A:

MEANING OF INSCRIPTION: *Sal catharticum amarus*, bitter purging salt

CONTEMPORARY ACCOUNT: "The bitter purging salt; extracted from the bitter liquor remaining after the crystalization of common salt from sea water. It was first prepared as a cheap substitute to the salt of the Epsom, and other purging mineral waters, from which it does not considerably differ, either in sensible qualities, or medical effects… The sal catharticus is a mild and gentle purgative, operating with sufficient efficacy, and in general with ease and safety, rarely occasioning any gripes, sickness, or the other inconveniencies which purgatives of the resinous kind are too often accompanied with. Six or eight drams may be dissolved for a dose in a proper quantity of common water; or four, five, or more in a pint, or quart of the purging waters. These liquors may likewise be so managed as to promote evacuation, by the other emunctories; if the patient is kept warm, they increase perspiration; by moderate exercise in a cool air, the urinary discharge." (W. Lewis, *The New Dispensatory*, 1770, pp. 214–215)

DATE OF MANUFACTURE: 1750–1770

PLACE OF MANUFACTURE: Possibly Mortlake, London

DIMENSIONS: Height 190 mm, maximum width 153 mm

PROVENANCE: Bequest, Saville Peck, 1955.

CONDITION: Poor; large crack descending from neck and encircling body, also several smaller cracks, glaze crazed and flaked from bowl and neck and base rims.

Cherub and shell

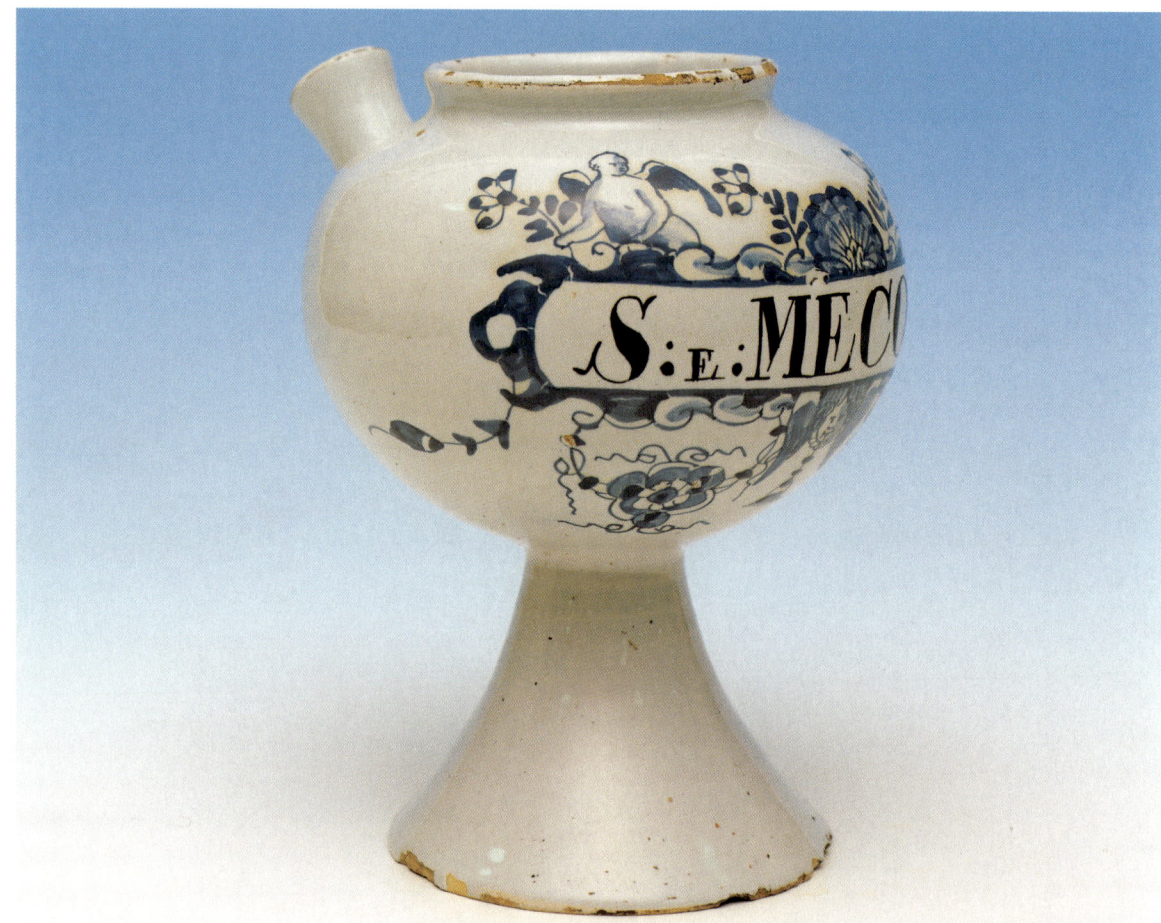

Wet drug jar (Cat.201)

ACCESSION NUMBER: KDN7

DESCRIPTION: Bulbous jar on elongated spreading foot, with spout only (on opposite side to label). White glaze with bluish tinge and design in blue and black. Label panel straight with even outline. Neck ridged, with glazed rim, flared spout, hollowed and glazed base with unglazed edge.

DESIGN: Cherub (bald) and shell.

INSCRIPTION: S:E:MECON.

MEANING OF INSCRIPTION: *Syrupus de meconio*, syrup of poppy juice (*Papaver somniferum*)

CONTEMPORARY ACCOUNT: "'Take Garden white Poppy-Heads with their Seeds ℔ ss. Heads of black Poppies ʒ vi. Steep them well bruised in ℔ viii. of Water 24 hours, and then boil it to ℔ iii. Press the Liquor out hard, and boil it up to a Syrup with ℔ iss. of white Sugar.'

"This, considering the Importance of its Intention, and the Certainty with which it answers it, is a better Medicine, and does more good than all under this Division besides put together. This ought by no means to be clarify'd, because it robs it of its chief Properties... This is used to procure Sleep, in which it acts as any other *Opiate*... It also, better than many other Forms of this kind, stops *Defluxions* and *Catarrhs*, with all Coughs from thin Rheum. It may be given from ʒ i. to ʒ iii. to Children, and from ʒ iii. to ℥ i. to grown Persons. In making this, more Sugar is generally used than what is order'd in the *Recipe*." (J. Quincy, *A Compleat English Dispensatory*, 1718, pp. 377–378)

DATE OF MANUFACTURE: 1700–1800

PLACE OF MANUFACTURE: Possibly Mortlake, London

DIMENSIONS: Height 190 mm, maximum width 150 mm

PROVENANCE: Donation from Mr Appleton, 1938.

CONDITION: Good; base chipped, glaze discoloured on and around blue design and flaked from spout, neck and base rims.

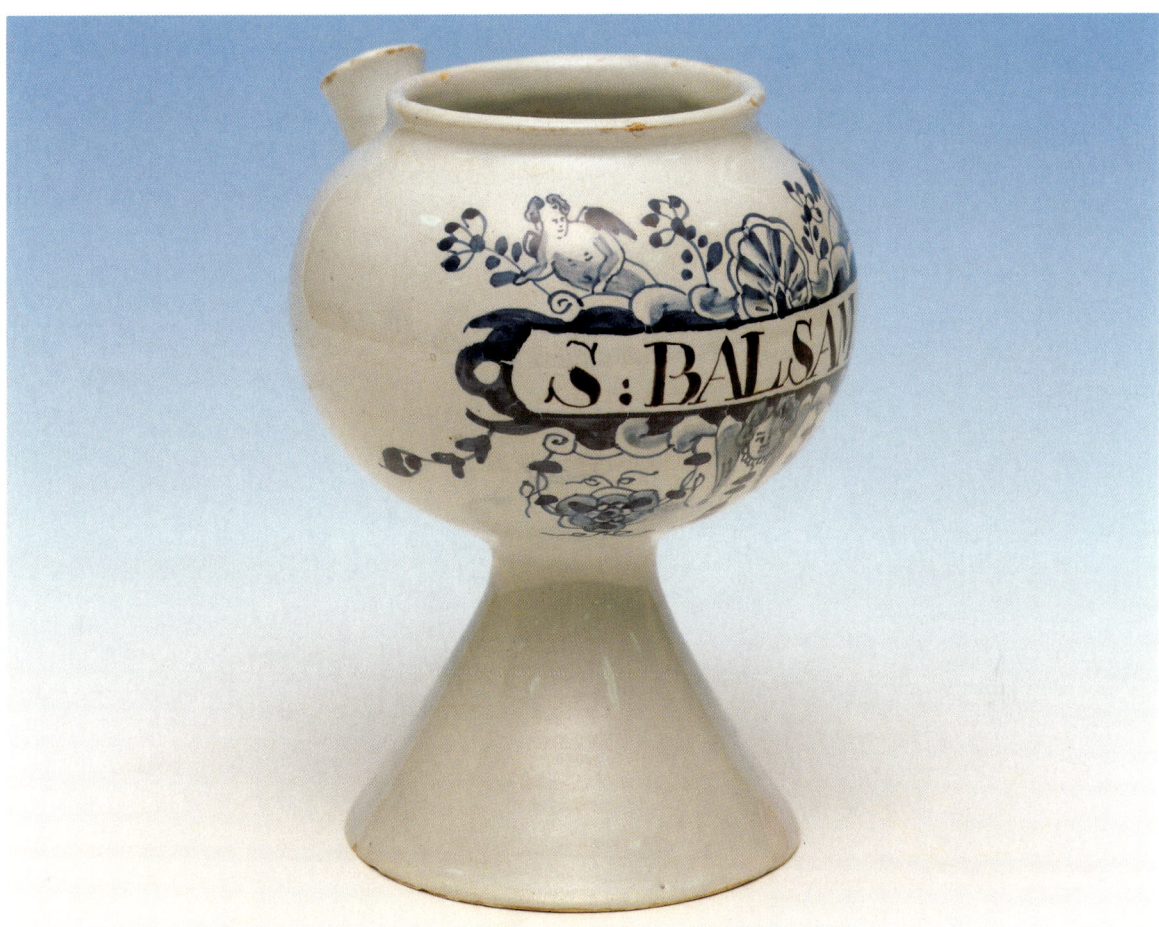

Wet drug jar (Cat. 202)

ACCESSION NUMBER: KDN8

DESCRIPTION: Bulbous jar on elongated spreading foot, with spout only (on opposite side to label). White glaze with bluish tinge and design in blue and black. Label panel straight with even outline. Neck ridged, with glazed rim and metal cover. Spout slightly flared, hollowed and glazed base with unglazed edge.

DESIGN: Cherub and shell

INSCRIPTION: S:BALSAM

MEANING OF INSCRIPTION: *Syrupus balsamicus*, balsamic syrup, later known as syrup of tolu

CONTEMPORARY ACCOUNT: "'Take Balsam of *Tolu* ℥ ii. Colts-Foot-Water ℥ xii. Boil them in a circulatory Vessel with the Juncture well luted, in a Sand-Heat three hours. When it is cold, in the strain'd Water by degrees dissolve ℥ xx. of Sugar without any heat.'

"This is very judiciously contriv'd yet many neglect the Care here enjoin'd, and boil in an open Vessel, by which they lose the finer parts of the Balsam. As for the Water here order'd, common Water will do as well. But if it be done with Rose or Orange-Water, it will be a most delightful Medicine, and much more of a Cordial..." (J. Quincy, *A Compleat English Dispensatory*, 1718, pp. 384–385)

DATE OF MANUFACTURE: 1730–1770

PLACE OF MANUFACTURE: Possibly Mortlake, London.

DIMENSIONS: Height 180 mm, maximum width 140 mm

PROVENANCE: Bequest, Saville Peck, 1955. Previously Prior Collection.

CONDITION: Good; 4 cm chip in base, glaze crazed and flaked from spout, neck and base rims.

COMMENT: Crellin notes that this jar has an unusual spherical body on a cone-shaped foot (p. 40).

REFERENCES: Crellin, Medical Ceramics p. 40.
 Walker, Ancient pharmacy jars p. 253, No. V, 2.

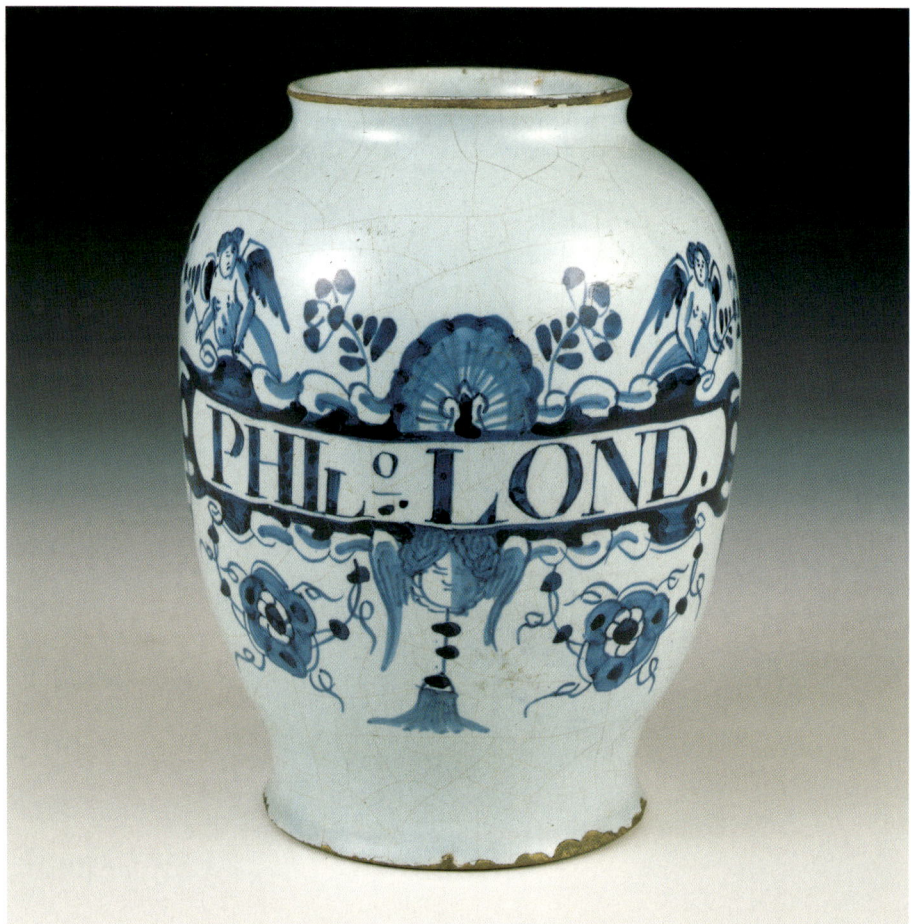

Dry drug jar (Cat.205)

ACCESSION NUMBER: KCN10

DESCRIPTION: Ovoid jar, tapering slightly towards splayed base. White glaze with greenish-blue tinge and design in blue. Label panel straight with even outline. Neck slightly everted with unglazed rim, slightly concave glazed base with unglazed edge.

DESIGN: Cherub and shell

INSCRIPTION: PHIL° LOND.

MEANING OF INSCRIPTION: *Philonium Londinense.* Originally called Roman Philonium (or medicine), this substance became known as London Philonium in the 1746 London Pharmacopoeia. A preparation with many ingredients, including opium, and used in pain relief and to induce sleep. It was named after a first century physician, Philon of Tarsus.

CONTEMPORARY ACCOUNT: "'Take white Pepper, Seeds of white Henbane, ana ʒ v. *Opium* ʒ iiss. Cassia – Bark ʒ iss. Smallage – Seed ʒ i. Seeds of Parsly, Fennel and Daucus, ana gr. xlv. Saffron ʒ ss. Spikenard, Pellitory of *Spain*, and Zedoary, ana gr. xv. Cinnamon ʒ iss. Myrrh and Castor, ana ʒ i. Honey, three times the quantity of the whole. Mix them, S.A.'

"This is somewhat more us'd than the former [Philonum Persicum], but their Difference is not great. The proportion of *Opium* and *Henbane* is the same in both, and therefore their Doses also alike." (J. Quincy, *A Compleat English Dispensatory*, 1718, p. 408)

DATE OF MANUFACTURE: 1720–1760

PLACE OF MANUFACTURE: Possibly Mortlake, London

DIMENSIONS: Height 185 mm, maximum width 145 mm

PROVENANCE: Bought in 1949.

CONDITION: Good; base chipped, glaze crazed and flaked on neck and base rims.

REFERENCES: Lothian, Cherub Designs pp. 610 and 612.

Lothian, English Delftware in the Pharmaceutical Society's Collection. p. 4 and Plate 6a.

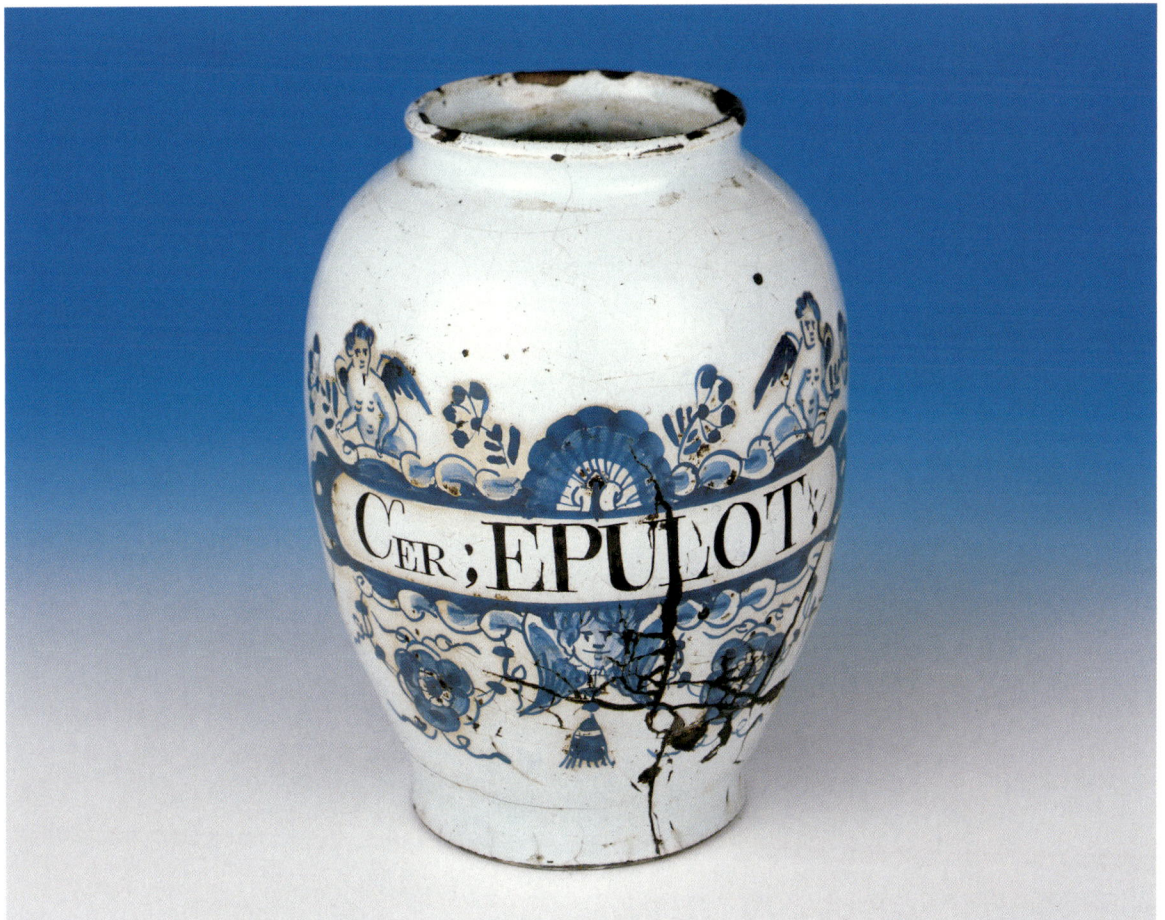

Dry drug jar (Cat.206)

CONDITION: Poor; large crack encircling bowl, glaze badly crazed and flaked on body, and on neck rim.

ACCESSION NUMBER: KCN14

DESCRIPTION: Ovoid jar, tapering slightly towards base. White glaze with pinkish tinge and design in blue and black. Label panel straight with even outline. Neck ridged with glazed rim, slightly concave glazed base with unglazed edge.

DESIGN: Cherub and shell

INSCRIPTION: CER;EPULOT;

MEANING OF INSCRIPTION: *Ceratum epuloticum*, cicatrising cerate, to heal wounds.

CONTEMPORARY ACCOUNT: "Take of oil olive a pound; yellow wax, prepared calamy, of each half a pound. Melt the wax with the oil, and as soon as the mixture begins to congeal, sprinkle in the calamy, and stir all well, till the cerate is quite cold." (H. Pemberton, *The Dispensatory*, 1746, p. 376)

DATE OF MANUFACTURE: 1745–1765

PLACE OF MANUFACTURE: Possibly Mortlake, London

DIMENSIONS: Height 185 mm, maximum width 150 mm

PROVENANCE: Donation, 1953, Austen Collection.

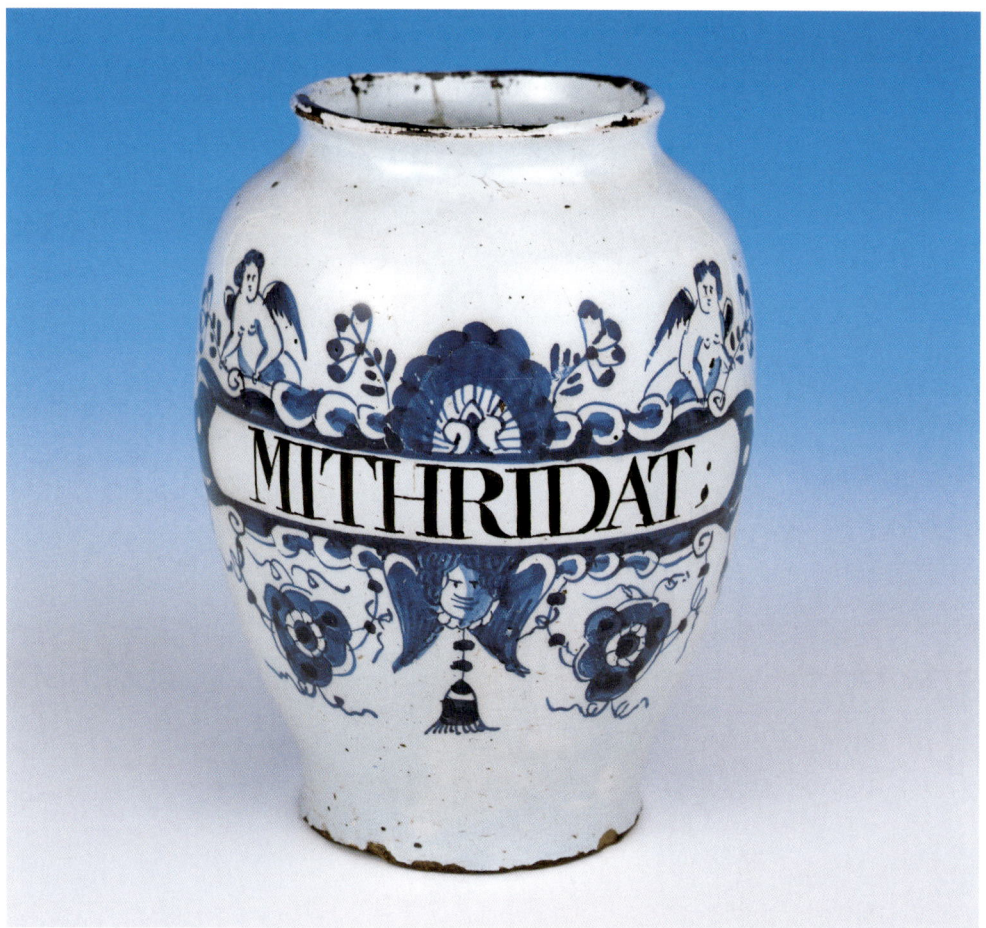

Dry drug jar (Cat.207)

ACCESSION NUMBER: KCN11

DESCRIPTION: Ovoid jar, tapering slightly towards base. White glaze with bluish tinge and design in blue and black. Label panel straight with even outline. Neck everted with glazed rim, slightly concave glazed base with unglazed edge.

DESIGN: Cherub and shell

INSCRIPTION: MITHRIDAT

MEANING OF INSCRIPTION: *Electuarium Mithridatum*, Mithridates' electuary. One of several forms of theriac (treacle) still popular in the 17th century as a universal antidote against poisons and infectious diseases. The name Mithridate is derived from Mithridates VI, king of Pontus (132–63 BC), who was believed to have rendered himself immune to poisoning by the constant use of antidotes.

CONTEMPORARY ACCOUNT: "Take of Arabian Myrrh, Saffron, Agaric, Ginger, Cinnamon, Spikenard, Frankincense, and Seeds of Treacle-Mustard, ana ʒ x. of the Seeds of Hartwort, Opobalsamum, or in its stead, expressed Oil of Nutmegs, Sweet-Rush, Arabian Stoechas, the true Costus, Galbanum, Cyprus Turpentine, Long Pepper, Castor, Juice of Hypocistis, Styrax, Opoanax, and Indian Leaf, or in its stead Mace, ana ʒ i. of Cassia Bark, Polymountain, white Pepper, Scordium, Seeds of wild Carrot, Carpobalsam, or Cubebs, Troches of Cypheos, and Bdellium, ana ʒ vii. of Spikenard cleansed, Gum Arabic, Macedonian Parsley Seed, Opium, the lesser Cardamoms, Fennel Seeds, Gentian Root, red Rose Flowers, and Dittany of Crete, ana ʒ v. of Aniseeds, Asarum, Acorus or Calamus Aromaticus, Orrice, the greater Valerian, and Sagapenum, ana ʒ iii. of Meum Root, Acacia, Stinks, and the tops of St. John's Wort, ana ʒ iiss. of the best Canary, enough to dissolve the Gums and Juices, which will take up about ʒ xxvi. of clarify'd Honey as much as the Weight of all the Ingredients, except the Wine; and make into an Electuary, S.A." (J. Quincy, *A Compleat English Dispensatory*, 1718, pp. 431–432)

DATE OF MANUFACTURE: 1740–1800

PLACE OF MANUFACTURE: Possibly Mortlake, London

DIMENSIONS: Height 190 mm, maximum width 150 mm

PROVENANCE: Donation, 1953, Austen Collection.

CONDITION: Fair; three cracks descending from neck, base and neck chipped, glaze flakes on neck and base rims, with some pitting.

REFERENCE: Lothian, 'The John Austen Collection' Plate 12 and pp. 97–98.

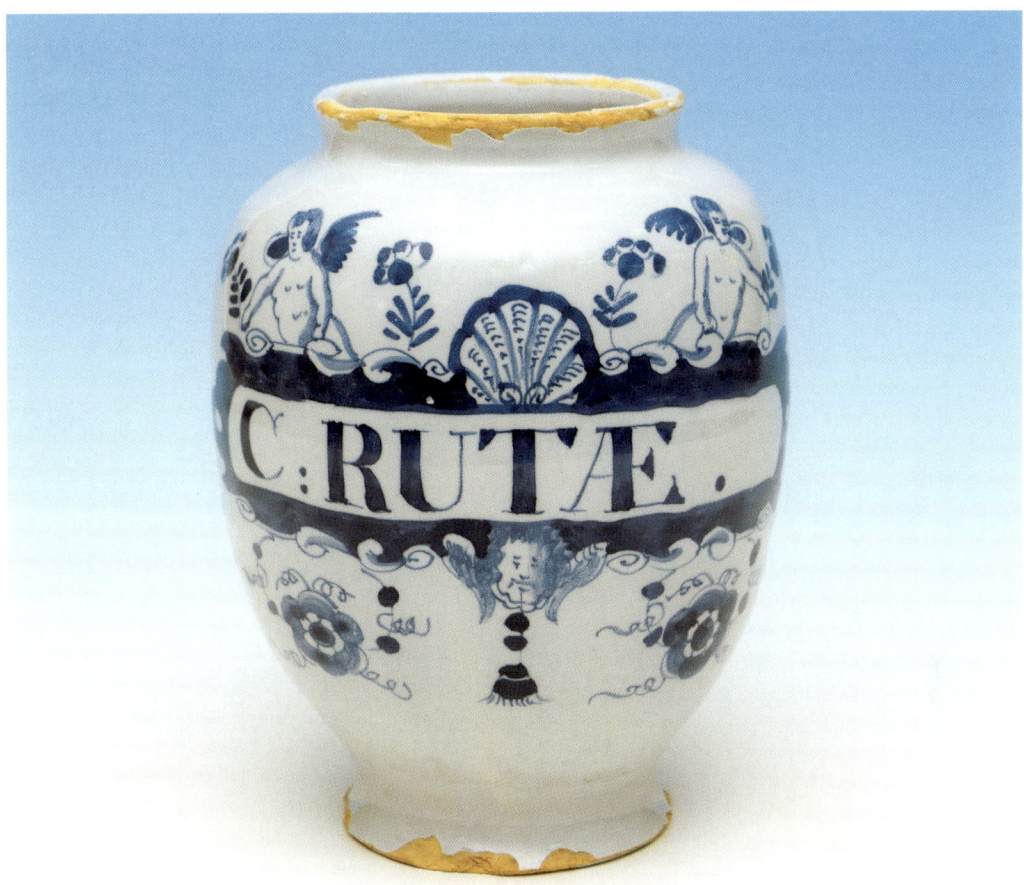

Dry drug jar (Cat.208)

ACCESSION NUMBER: KCN30

DESCRIPTION: Ovoid jar, tapering slightly towards splayed base. White glaze with bluish tinge and design in blue. Label panel straight with even outline. Neck everted.

DESIGN: Cherub and shell

INSCRIPTION: C.RUTAE

MEANING OF INSCRIPTION: *Conserva rutae*, conserve of rue (*Ruta graveolens*)

CONTEMPORARY ACCOUNT: "It flowers in *June*. This plant is very deservedly of great use in Medicine. Schroder [presumably Johann Schroder (1600-64), author of *The Compleat Chymical Dispensatory*, published in English in 1669] commends it as an *Alexipharmick* and a *Cephalick*; says it resists all kinds of Poisons and Malignities, and is therefore to be used in *Fevers*; and that it is good in all convulsive Cases. It is replete with a fat viscous Juice, and by that means yields little to any purpose in Distillation, unless where first digested in a spiritous *Menstruum*. Hence its simple Water in the shops is worth little, how much soever set by some. It ought to be raised with a spiritous Liquor, or used in *Conserve*, or, which is best of all, eat alone fresh gather'd, as many do with Bread and Butter. It is of excellent Service in all nervous Cases, and particularly in such as arise from the *Womb*, as it deterges the Glands, and by its Viscidity bridles those inordinate Motions, which frequently begin there, and affect the whole Constitution." (J. Quincy, *A Compleat English Dispensatory*, 1718, p. 91)

DATE OF MANUFACTURE: 1700–1800

PLACE OF MANUFACTURE: London

DIMENSIONS: Height 182 mm, maximum width 135 mm

PROVENANCE: Unknown.

CONDITION: Fair; significant chips to base, and large losses of glaze to rim.

Cherub and shell

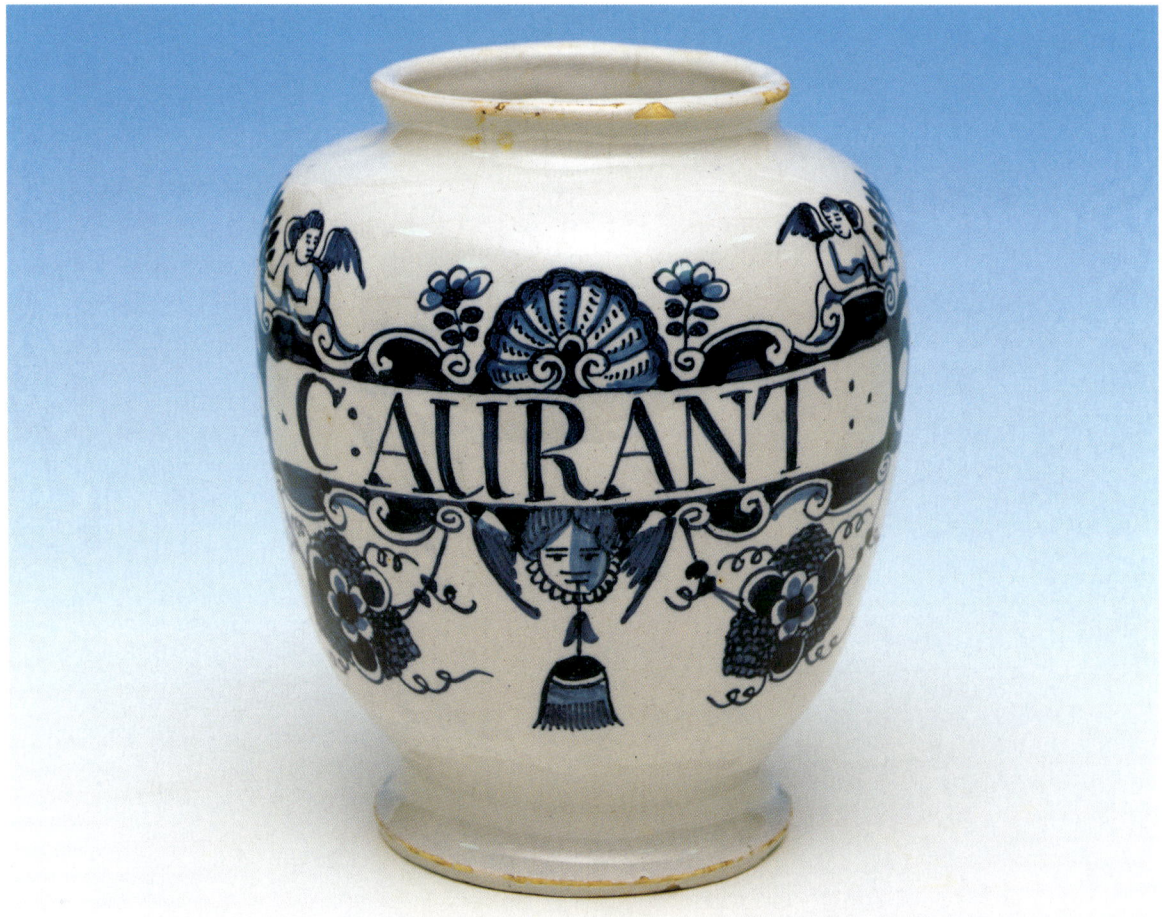

Dry drug jar (Cat.209)

ACCESSION NUMBER: KCN31

DESCRIPTION: Ovoid jar, tapering slightly towards splayed base. White glaze with bluish tinge and design in blue. Label panel straight with even outline. Neck everted.

DESIGN: Cherub and shell

INSCRIPTION: C.AURANT

MEANING OF INSCRIPTION: *Cortex aurantiorum*, rind of Spanish or Seville oranges. Used as an ingredient in other preparations, such as conserve or syrup of orange peel.

CONTEMPORARY ACCOUNT: "*Conserves* of the Peels of *Oranges*, *Citrons*, *Lemons*, and the like, are made with double the quantity of Sugar only, because their Warmth helps to keep them. The first of these is only in use, and requires great Labour to make it very fine: if therefore the Orange-Chips, as they are shave thin off the Orange, are put in an earthen Pan some weeks, with the sufficient quantity of Sugar, they will mellow, or as it were rot so together, that it will require much less trouble to reduce it into a good *Conserve*." (J. Quincy, *A Compleat English Dispensatory*, 1718, p. 401)

DATE OF MANUFACTURE: 1700–1800

PLACE OF MANUFACTURE: London

DIMENSIONS: Height 180 mm, maximum width 143 mm

PROVENANCE: Unknown.

CONDITION: Good; small chips to base and rim, crazed glaze.

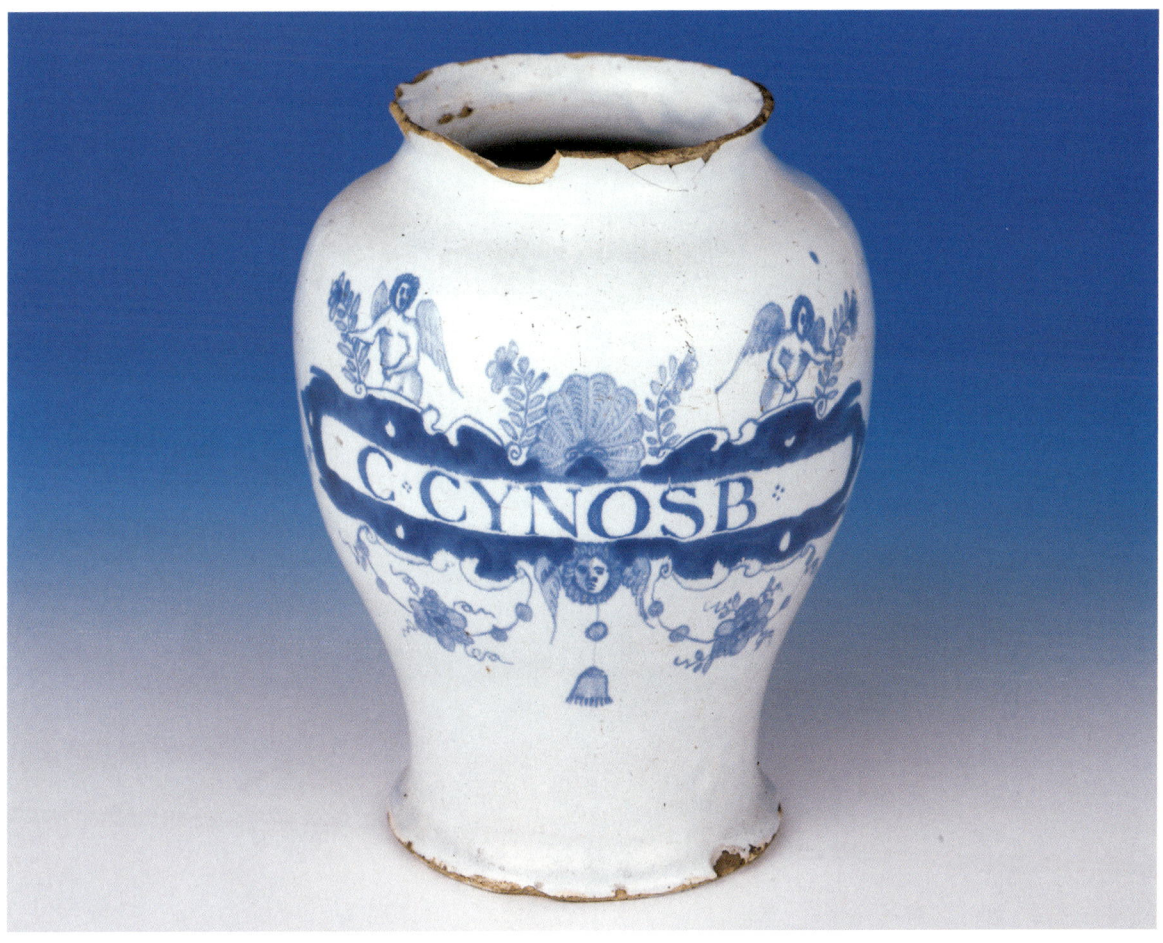

Dry drug jar (Cat.210)

ACCESSION NUMBER: KCN8

DESCRIPTION: Ovoid jar, tapering slightly towards splayed base. White glaze with bluish tinge and design in blue. Label panel straight with even outline. Neck everted with unglazed rim, slightly concave glazed base with unglazed rim.

DESIGN: Cherub and shell

INSCRIPTION: C CYNOSB

MEANING OF INSCRIPTION: *Conservus cynobastus*, conserve of rosehips from the dog rose (*Rosa caninus*). Used as a binding and flavouring agent.

CONTEMPORARY ACCOUNT: "Take of the pulp of ripe hips one pound, of double refined sugar twenty ounces; and mix them into a conserve." (H. Pemberton, *The Dispensatory*, 1746, p. 157)

DATE OF MANUFACTURE: 1750–1760

PLACE OF MANUFACTURE: London or possibly Liverpool

DIMENSIONS: Height 180 mm, maximum width 150 mm

PROVENANCE: Donation, 1953, Austen Collection.

CONDITION: Fair; neck rim badly chipped, base chipped, glaze flaked on neck and base.

Cherub and shell

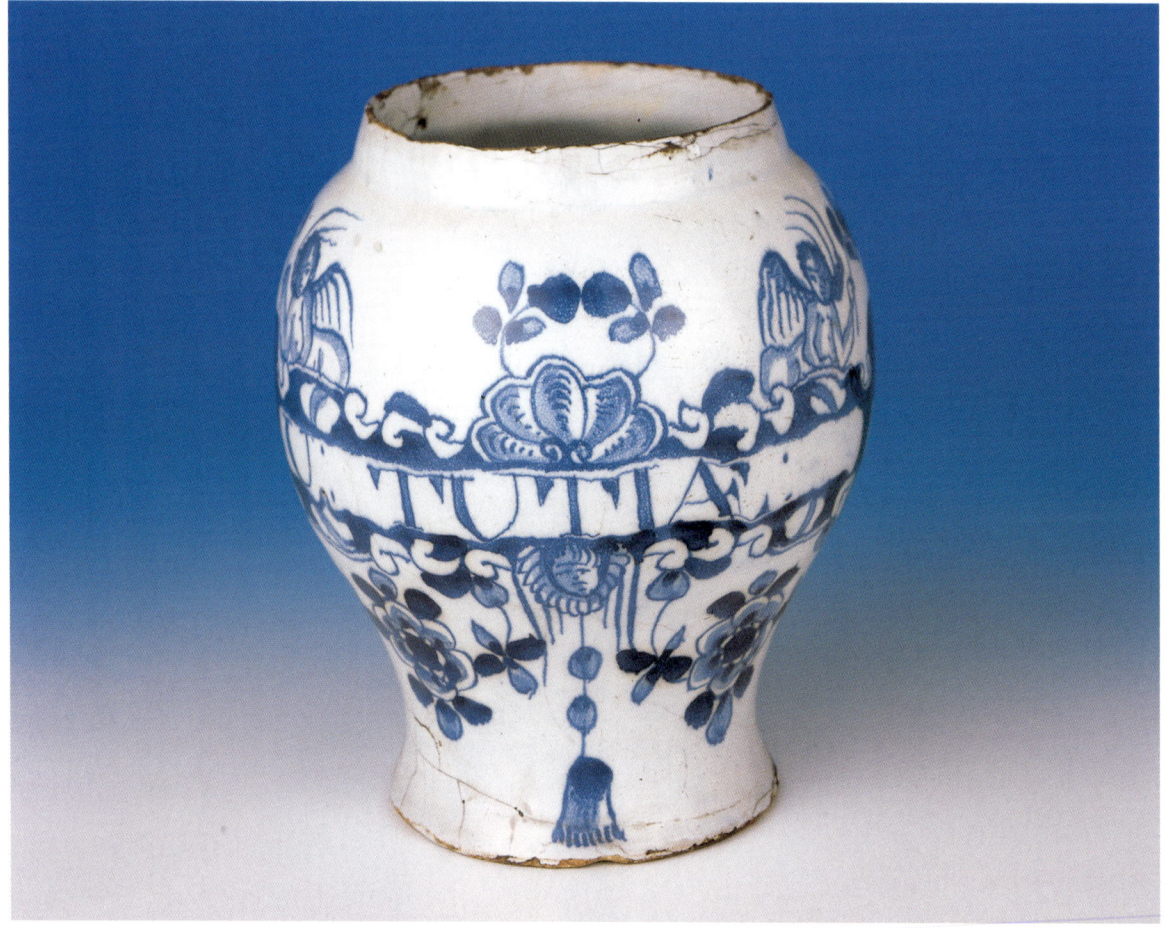

Dry drug jar (Cat.211)

ACCESSION NUMBER: KCN7

DESCRIPTION: Bulbous jar, tapering slightly towards slightly splayed base. White glaze with bluish tinge and design in blue. Label panel straight, with even outline. Neck straight with unglazed rim, slightly concave and partly glazed base.

DESIGN: Cherub and shell

INSCRIPTION: U:TUTIAE

MEANING OF INSCRIPTION: *Unguentum tutiae*, ointment of tutty. Tutiae, impure zinc oxide, is a Latinisation of an unknown word of Sanskrit origin.

CONTEMPORARY ACCOUNT: "Take Tutty finely levigated ℨ ii. Calamine ℨ i. Ointment of Roses ℔ iss. Mix S.A. This is chiefly used for sore Eyes, which proceed from hot Rheums: but most, if not all, use plain *Lard* in making it, instead of the *Rose-Ointments*; and do not seem to be chargeable with any blame for it, because that answers the Intention as well. This is much in esteem and use amongst the common People, but seldom met with in Prescription." (J. Quincy, *A Compleat English Dispensatory*, 1718, p. 460)

DATE OF MANUFACTURE: 1690–1750

PLACE OF MANUFACTURE: London or possibly Liverpool.

DIMENSIONS: Height 180 mm, maximum width 165 mm

PROVENANCE: Bought in 1957, Howard Collection.

CONDITION: Good; two cracks descending from neck and several ascending from base, glaze crazed and flaking on neck and above base.

COMMENT: Howard felt that this jar had "a distinctly early feeling", and that the decoration did not correspond with the "stereotyped perfection of design" that became common later in the 18th century (p. 20). However, the upright rim suggests a mid-18th century date.

REFERENCE: Howard, English Delftware Drug Jars, p. 20 and No. 39.

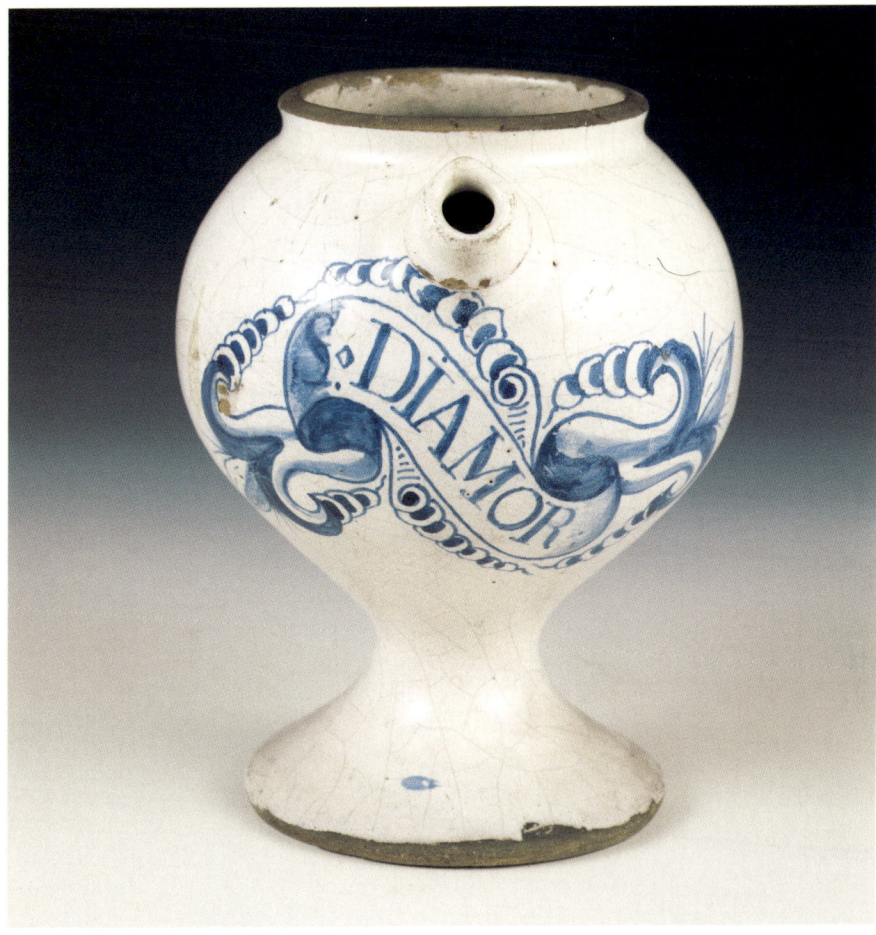

Dry drug jar (Cat.212)

ACCESSION NUMBER: KDE1

DESCRIPTION: Bulbous jar on spreading foot, with spout and fluted, strap-like looped handle. White glaze with pinkish tinge and design in blue. Label panel in the form of an S-shaped scroll, descending diagonally from left to right. Neck slightly everted with unglazed rim, flanged spout, hollowed and unglazed base.

DESIGN: A roughly 'S' shaped scroll, with ends in the form of fleur-de-lys

INSCRIPTION: S DIAMOR:

MEANING OF INSCRIPTION: *Syrupus diamoron*, syrup of mulberries (*Morus nigra*)

CONTEMPORARY ACCOUNT: "This is cooling and subastringent, and chiefly used for Gargarisms; and is sometimes acuated with Spirit of Vitriol." (J. Quincy, *A Compleat English Dispensatory*, 1718, p. 378)

DATE OF MANUFACTURE: c. 1680

PLACE OF MANUFACTURE: Possibly Brislington/Bristol

DIMENSIONS: Height 190 mm, maximum width 155 mm

PROVENANCE: Bought in 1957, Howard Collection.

CONDITION: Good; glaze badly crazed, flaked on spout, handle and base.

REFERENCE: Howard, English Delftware Drug Jars, p. 18 and No. 34.

Miscellaneous and transitional designs

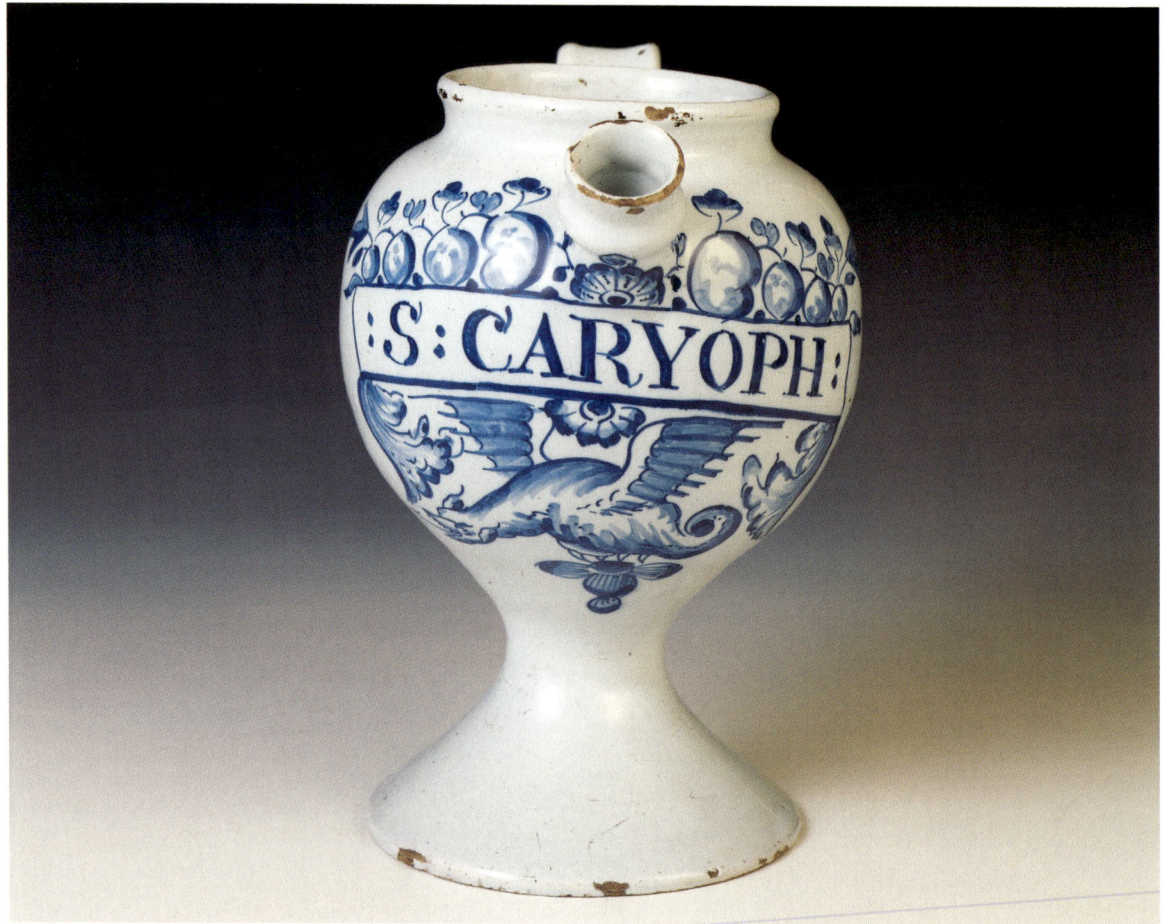

Wet drug jar (Cat.213)

ACCESSION NUMBER: KDY1

DESCRIPTION: Bulbous jar on spreading foot, with spout and fluted strap-like looped handle. White glaze with bluish tinge and design in blue. Label panel curved slightly upwards with even outline. Neck ridged with glazed rim, flanged spout, hollowed and glazed base.

DESIGN: Above label: shell (centre) with leaf and ovoid fruit motif; below label: shell (centre) with dragon or wyvern (volent) below

INSCRIPTION: S:CARYOPH:

MEANING OF INSCRIPTION: *Syrupus caryophylli*, syrup of clove gillyflowers or clove July flowers (*Dianthus caryophyllus*)

CONTEMPORARY ACCOUNT: "CARIOPHYLLI HORTENSES, Clove Gillyflowers; call'd also very commonly, Flores Tunica... They blow in June. They are a fine Aromatick, and very grateful to Smell and Taste. They have place in the Syrup made of them, and most Cephalic and Cordial Juleps. There is also a Conserve made of them, but it is hardly ever used." (J. Quincy, *A Compleat English Dispensatory*, 1718, p. 81)

DATE OF MANUFACTURE: c. 1700–1720

PLACE OF MANUFACTURE: Possibly Liverpool

DIMENSIONS: Height 195 mm, maximum width 145 mm

PROVENANCE: Bought in 1957, Howard Collection.

CONDITION: Good; base chipped, glaze crazed and flaked on handle, neck, spout and base.

COMMENT: Austin suggests that the dragon is more likely to be Python, the dragon being slain by Apollo on the arms of the Company of Apothecaries, than a Welsh dragon (p. 216). There are 24 jars of this type known, 14 dry drug jars, 9 wet drug jars and 1 pill pot.

REFERENCES: Austin, British Delft at Williamsburg, No. 466.
   Howard, G. E. English Delftware Drug Jars, p. 18 and No. 35.

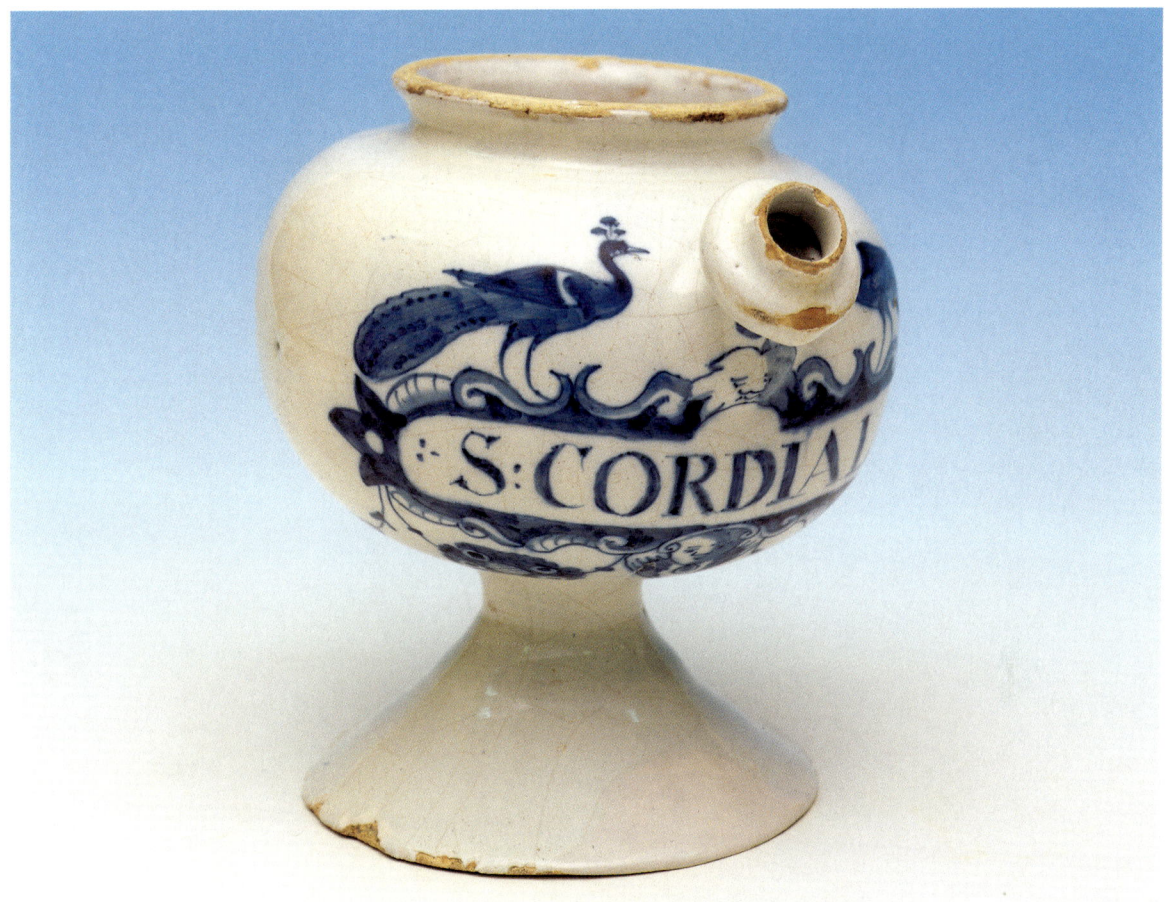

Dry drug jar (Cat.214)

ACCESSION NUMBER: KDY2

DESCRIPTION: Bulbous jar on spreading foot with spout only. White glaze with pinkish tinge and design in blue. Label panel straight with even outline. Neck ridged with unglazed rim, flanged spout, hollowed and glazed base, with unglazed rim.

DESIGN: Two peacocks

INSCRIPTION: S:CORDIAL

MEANING OF INSCRIPTION: *Syrupus cordialis*, cordial syrup

CONTEMPORARY ACCOUNT: Quincy includes two S.Cordials in his dispensatory. Here is one: "'Take Rhenish Wine ℔ ii. Rose Water ℥ iiss. Cloves, Ginger, ana ℈ ii. Cinnamon ℥ ss. Sugar ℥ iii. Ambergrease. Gr. iii. Musk gr. i. Rub the Sugar with the Sweets, and let them stand in Infusion in a slow warmth some hours; then pour off the liquor clear.'

"This is a pleasant Cordial enough, but not fit for an officinal Medicine; and is rarely order'd; when it is, it may be drank at discretion." (J. Quincy, *A Compleat English Dispensatory*, 1718, p. 375)

DATE OF MANUFACTURE: 1700–1730

PLACE OF MANUFACTURE: London

DIMENSIONS: Height 170 mm, maximum width 158 mm

PROVENANCE: Donation, 1953, Austen Collection.

CONDITION: Poor; several chips on base, glaze crazed and flaked on spout and neck rims.

COMMENT: This is one of a very small group of just seven jars which have fairly distinctly English body shapes, but which are painted with a typically Dutch design. There are two dry jars in the Wilkinson Collection at the Thackray Museum, Leeds, four pill pots in private collections in London and Scotland, and this syrup jar. The other six jars with a peacocks design are very uniform in style, with small, rather stiff, peacocks, whilst those on these jars are much more realistic. It has been suggested that these were painted by an immigrant Dutch painter.

REFERENCE: Lothian, 'The John Austen Collection', Figure 11 and pp. 97–98.

Miscellaneous and transitional designs

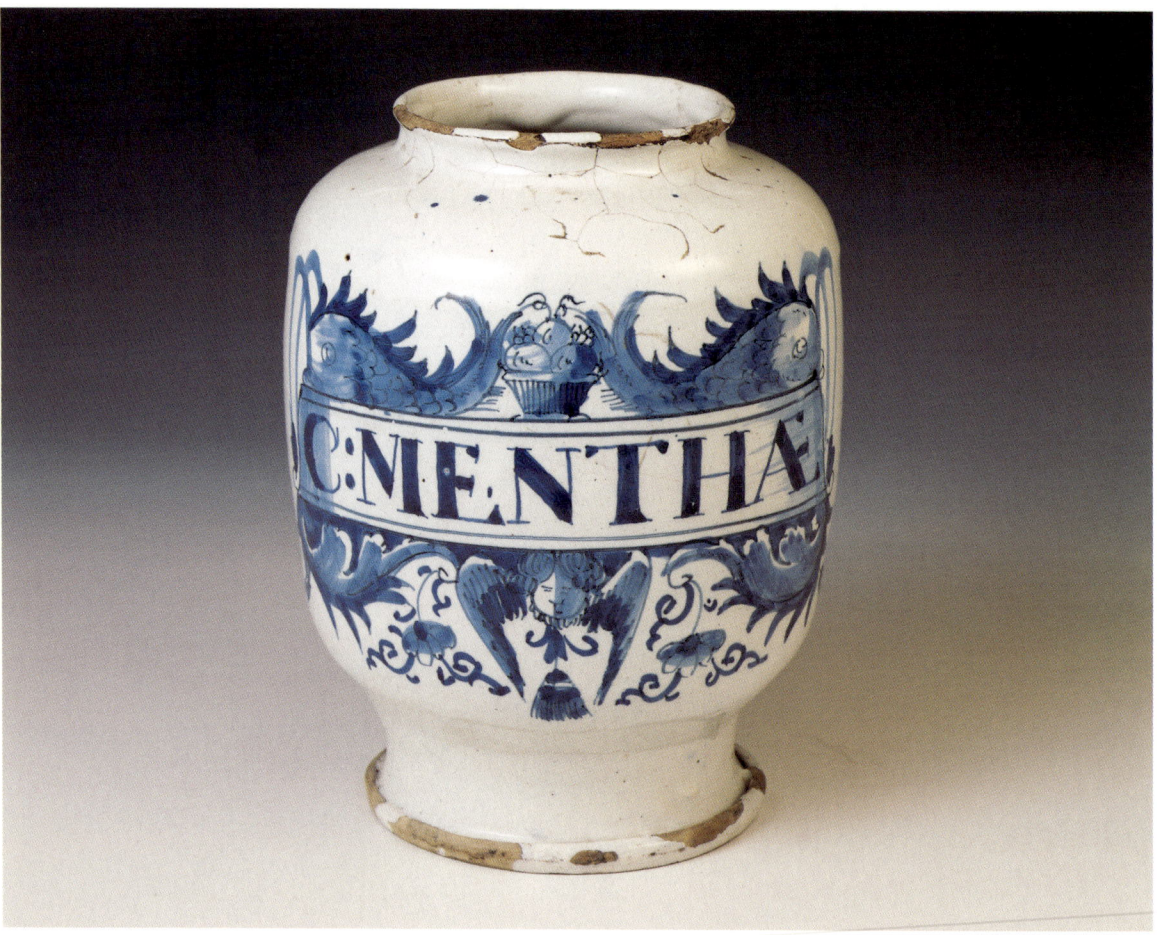

Wet drug jar (Cat.215)

ACCESSION NUMBER: KCY3

DESCRIPTION: Ovoid jar, tapering slightly towards splayed and ridged base with two faint narrow ridges encircling bowl, one below the neck and the other below the label. White glaze with pinkish tinge and design in blue. Label panel straight, framed with two thin even lines. Neck everted with glazed rim, slightly concave glazed base with unglazed edge.

DESIGN: Dolphins and basket of fruit

INSCRIPTION: C:MENTHAE

MEANING OF INSCRIPTION: Conserve of spearmint (*Mentha spicata*). Used as a tonic, a carminative and an antispasmodic.

CONTEMPORARY ACCOUNT: "The leaves are to be plucked from their stalks, and the flowers from their calix's...every one of them, when thus prepared, is to be pounded in a mortar with a wooden pestle, first by itself, and then with the addition of three times its weight of double refined sugar, till they are well incorporated together." (H. Pemberton, *The Dispensatory*, 1746, p. 156)

DATE OF MANUFACTURE: c. 1720–1730

PLACE OF MANUFACTURE: London, or possibly Liverpool

DIMENSIONS: Height 180 mm, maximum width 153 mm

PROVENANCE: Bought in 1966.

CONDITION: Good; neck and base chipped, glaze crazed and flaked on neck and base rims.

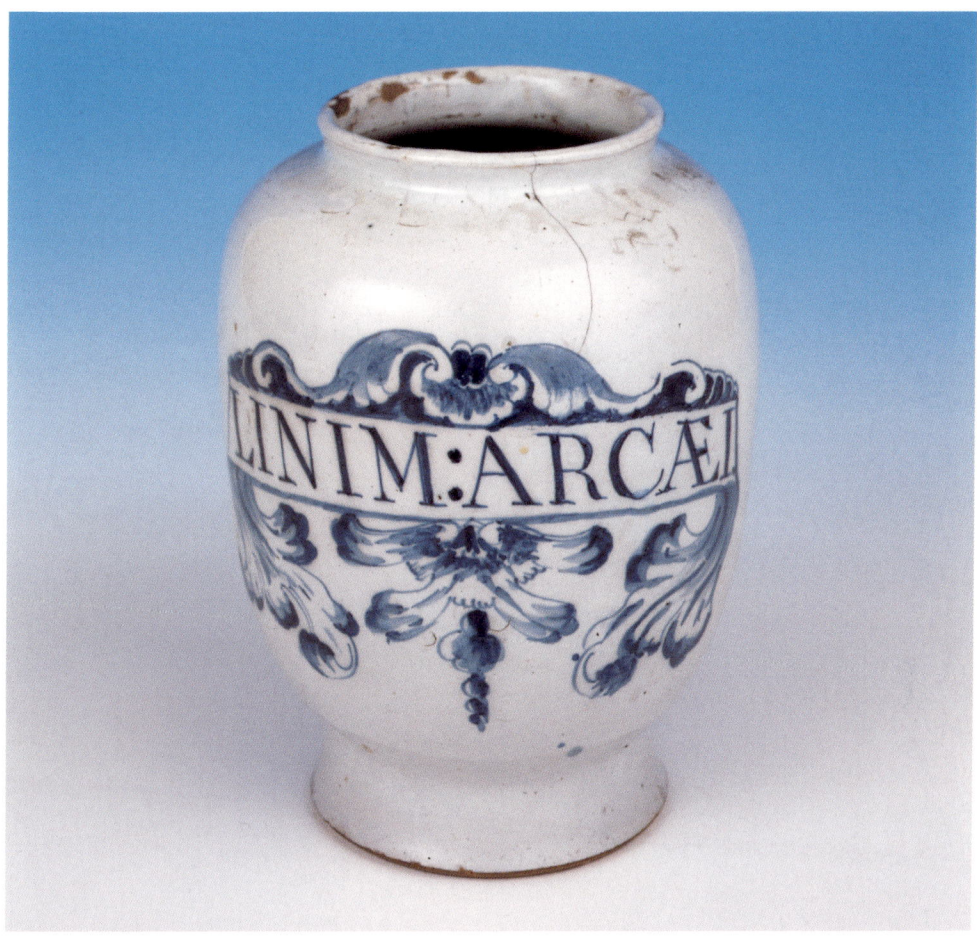

Wet drug jar (Cat.216)

ACCESSION NUMBER: KCE1

DESCRIPTION: Ovoid jar, tapering slightly towards base. White glaze with bluish tinge and design in blue. Label panel curved slightly upwards, outlined with leaf design. Neck everted with glazed rim, concave and glazed base, with unglazed rim.

DESIGN: Stylised acanthus leaf scrolls

INSCRIPTION: LINIM:ARCAEI

MEANING OF INSCRIPTION: *Linimentum arcei,* astringent, liniment for cleaning and 'digesting' wounds

CONTEMPORARY ACCOUNT: "'Take Gum Elemi and Turpentine, ana ʒ iss, old Sheep's Suet ʒ ii. Lard ʒ i. Mix and make them into an Ointment S.A.

"This is troublesome to make, because there can be procured none of the *Gum Elemi*, but with so much Dross as to make it necessary to strain it. This is reckon'd a better Dressing in fresh Wounds than *Basilicon*; because it does not incarn too fast, and is so warm and detersive, as to make it useful even in Ulcers of some standing. This is now much us'd in Surgery; but it generally goes under the Appellation of *Linimentum Arcei*." (J. Quincy, *A*

Compleat English Dispensatory, 1718, p. 455)

DATE OF MANUFACTURE: c. 1750–1770

PLACE OF MANUFACTURE: Probably Liverpool

DIMENSIONS: Height 180 mm, maximum width 143 mm

PROVENANCE: Bought in 1959.

CONDITION: Good; crack descending from neck, glaze crazed and flaked on rim of neck.

Miscellaneous and transitional designs

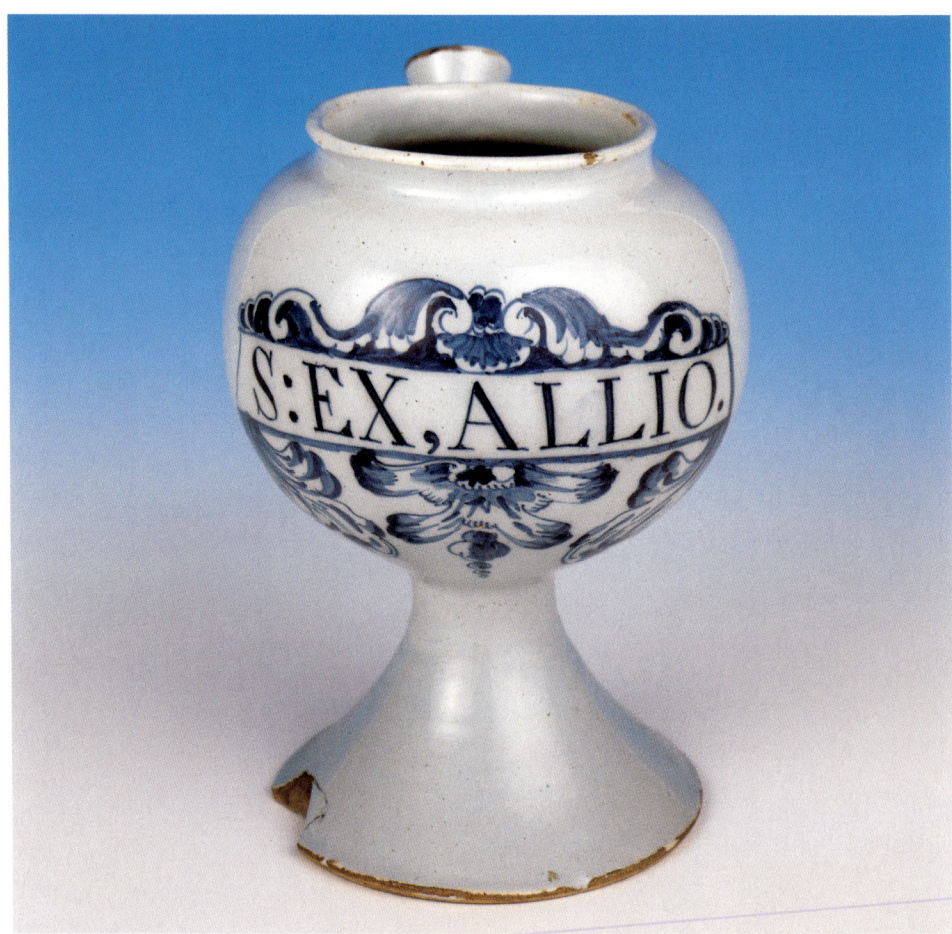

Wet drug jar (Cat.217)

ACCESSION NUMBER: KDY4

DESCRIPTION: Bulbous jar on spreading foot, with spout only (on opposite side to label). White glaze with bluish tinge and design in blue. Label panel straight with even outline. Neck ridged with glazed rim, flared spout, hollowed and glazed base, with unglazed edge.

DESIGN: Stylised acanthus leaf scrolls

INSCRIPTION: S:EX,ALLIO.

MEANING OF INSCRIPTION: *Syrupus ex allio*, syrup of garlic (*Allium sativum*). Used in the treatment of bronchitis, pneumonia and nervous afflictions.

CONTEMPORARY ACCOUNT: "Take of the root of garlick sliced one pound, of boiling water a quart. Steep the garlick in the water twelve hours in a close vessel, and in the liquor strained dissolve a sufficient quantity of sugar, so as to make the syrup." (H. Pemberton, *The Dispensatory*, 1746, p. 291)

DATE OF MANUFACTURE: 1750–1770

PLACE OF MANUFACTURE: London or possibly Liverpool

DIMENSIONS: Height 185 mm, maximum width 145 mm

PROVENANCE: Bought in 1962.

CONDITION: Good; 3 cm chip from base, glaze crazed and flaked from rim of neck and spout.

COMMENT: There are 18 known jars with this design, 9 dry and 9 wet. One of the dry jars is inscribed C. PRUNR. SYL with W+M 1764 on the reverse.

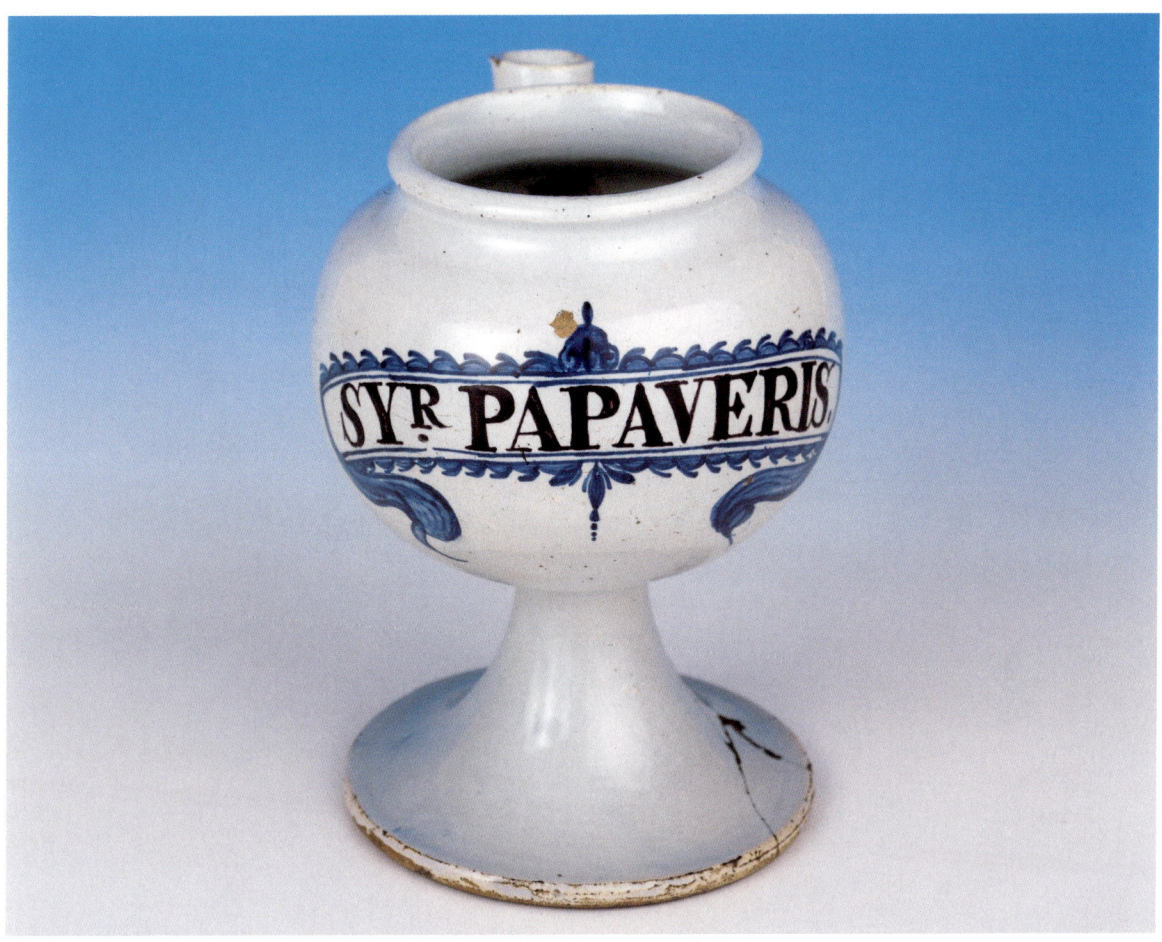

Wet drug jar (Cat.218)

ACCESSION NUMBER: KDY5

DESCRIPTION: Bulbous jar on spreading foot, with spout only (on opposite side to label). White glaze with bluish tinge and design in blue. Inscription in black. Label panel curved slightly upwards, framed in thin even line. Neck ridged with glazed rim, straight spout, hollowed and glazed base with unglazed edge.

DESIGN: Decorative variation on a ribbon cartouche with scalloped edge

INSCRIPTION: SYR PAPAVERIS

MEANING OF INSCRIPTION: *Syrupus papaveris*, syrup of poppy

CONTEMPORARY ACCOUNT: "Take of the fresh flowers of wild poppy four pounds, of boiling water four pints and a half. Set the water poured on the flowers over the fire, and stir the flowers in, till they are all throughly wet; and, as soon as ever the flowers are sunk, let them steep for a night; next day pour off, and press out the liquor, setting it by for another night, that its faeces may subside; then with a proper addition of double refined sugar make the syrup. Remark. The intent in setting the flowers over the fire is, that they may be a little scalded to cause them to shrink enough to be all immerged in the water; and without this artifice they can scarce all be got in: but they are no longer to be continued on the fire, than till this effect is produced, lest the liquor become too thick, and the syrup rendered roapy." (H. Pemberton, *The Dispensatory*, 1746, p. 298)

DATE OF MANUFACTURE: c. 1760–1780

PLACE OF MANUFACTURE: London

DIMENSIONS: Height 175 mm, maximum width 143 mm

PROVENANCE: Bequest, Saville Peck, 1955.

CONDITION: Poor; base damaged and repaired, glaze crazed and flaked on body and spout and base rims.

COMMENT: There are four delftware jars with this design: this jar, two at Colonial Williamsburg, and a cylindrical jar at the Wilkinson Collection at the Thackray Museum, Leeds. There is also a set of 13 goblet-shaped pale stoneware jars with this design in brown on a yellow background, also in the Thackray Museum, c. 1800.

PILL tiles

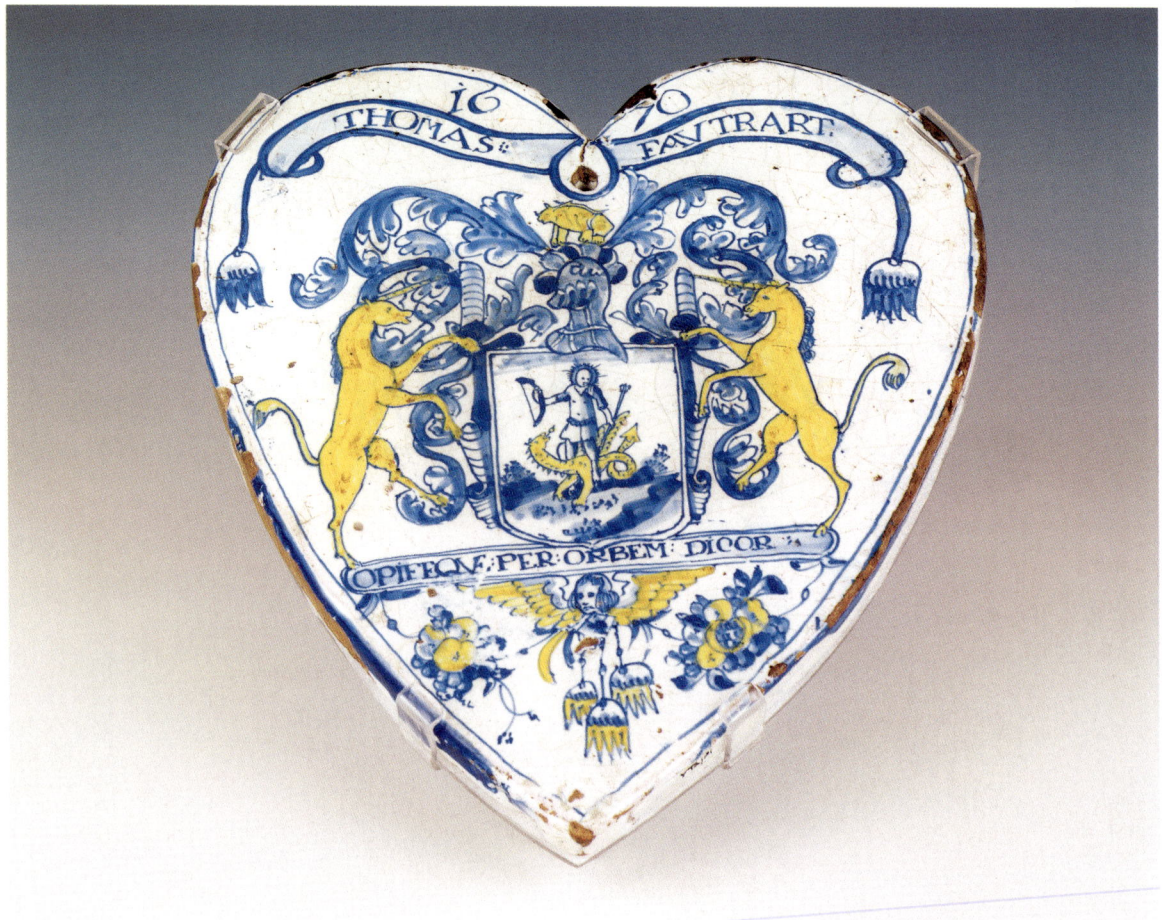

Pill tile (Cat.219)

ACCESSION NUMBER: YTA/P1

DESCRIPTION: Heart-shaped pill tile. White glaze and design in blue and yellow. One hole at top, for hanging.

INSCRIPTION: 1670 OPIFEQUE:PER:ORBEM:DICOR
THOMAS FAVTRART

MEANING OF INSCRIPTION AND DESIGN: The Worshipful Society of Apothecaries is a livery company formed in 1617. The arms feature Apollo (the god of healing) killing the dragon of disease, supported by two unicorns (from King James's royal arms), and a rhinoceros as the crest (the powdered horn was believed to be medicinal). The motto, from the first book of Ovid's 'Metamorphoses', translates: "I am spoken of all over the world as one who brings help."

DATE OF MANUFACTURE: 1670

PLACE OF MANUFACTURE: Southwark, London

DIMENSIONS: Height 280 mm, maximum width 248 mm

PROVENANCE: Bought in 1953.

CONDITION: Good; glaze flaked from edge.

COMMENT: Thomas Fautrart, presumed to be the original owner of this tile, has proved difficult to track down. He is likely to have been of Huguenot descent, and there was certainly a Fautrart family in Jersey in the 17th century. There appears to be no evidence that a Thomas Fautrart was a member of the Society of Apothecaries, or even apprenticed in the City of London. However, a Thomas Fautrart, born in St Helier in 1633 seems to be the most likely candidate for ownership of this tile.

REFERENCES: Britton, English Delftware in the Bristol Collection. p. 76.

Burnby, J. The Thomas Fautrart Pill Tile, Pharmaceutical Historian, 1977: 7(3), pp. 4–5.

Crellin, Medical Ceramics, p. 144.

Grigsby, The Longridge Collection of English Slipware and Delftware. catalogue number D410.

Lothian, Cherub Designs p. 609.

Lothian, English Delftware in the Pharmaceutical Society's Collection. p. 2 and Plate 2a.

Matthews, Antiques of the Pharmacy, p. 13.

Matthews, Apothecary Pill Slabs, p. 190.

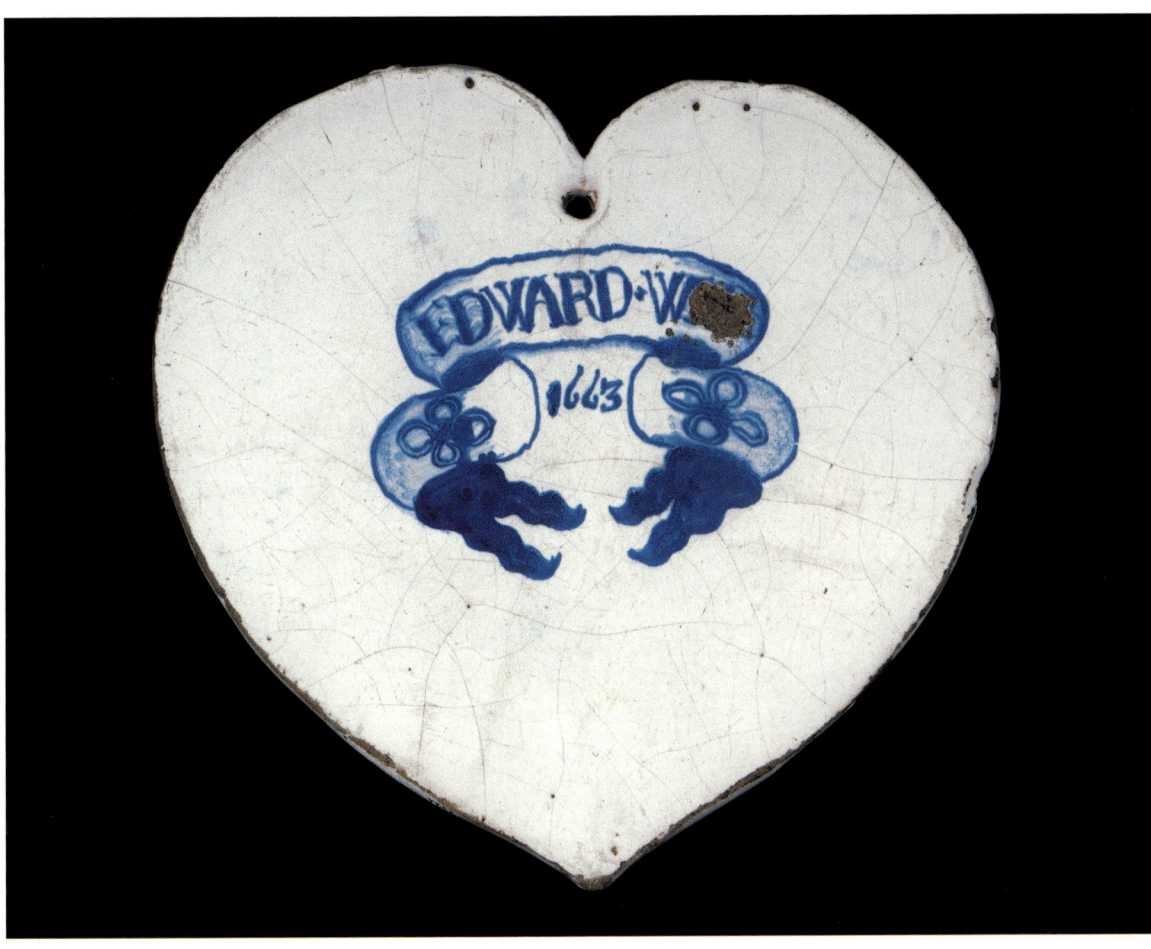

Pill tile (Cat.220)

ACCESSION NUMBER: YTA2

DESCRIPTION: Heart-shaped pill tile. White glaze with pinkish tinge and ribbon cartouche design in blue. One hole at top for hanging.

INSCRIPTION: EDWARD. W...1663

MEANING OF INSCRIPTION: Thought to be Edward Webb, assumed the original owner of the tile, although no further information is known.

DIMENSIONS: Height 260 mm, maximum width 270 mm

DATE OF MANUFACTURE: 1663

PLACE OF MANUFACTURE: Southwark, London.

PROVENANCE: Bought in 1965. From the collection of Mrs Freda Hicks, sold by Sotheby's, 9/2/1965 (lot 8). Previously Hemming Collection.

CONDITION: Good; glaze crazed and flaked on inscription and edge, glaze missing over inscription.

COMMENT: This is the earliest known dated heart-shaped pill tile (Grigsby D410).

REFERENCES: Britton, English Delftware in the Bristol Collection, p. 76.

Drey, Apothecary Jars. Plate 70A and p. 136.

Grigsby, The Longridge Collection of English Slipware and Delftware. catalogue number D410.

Hemming, Lambeth Delft. p. 195, Pl.I No.1.

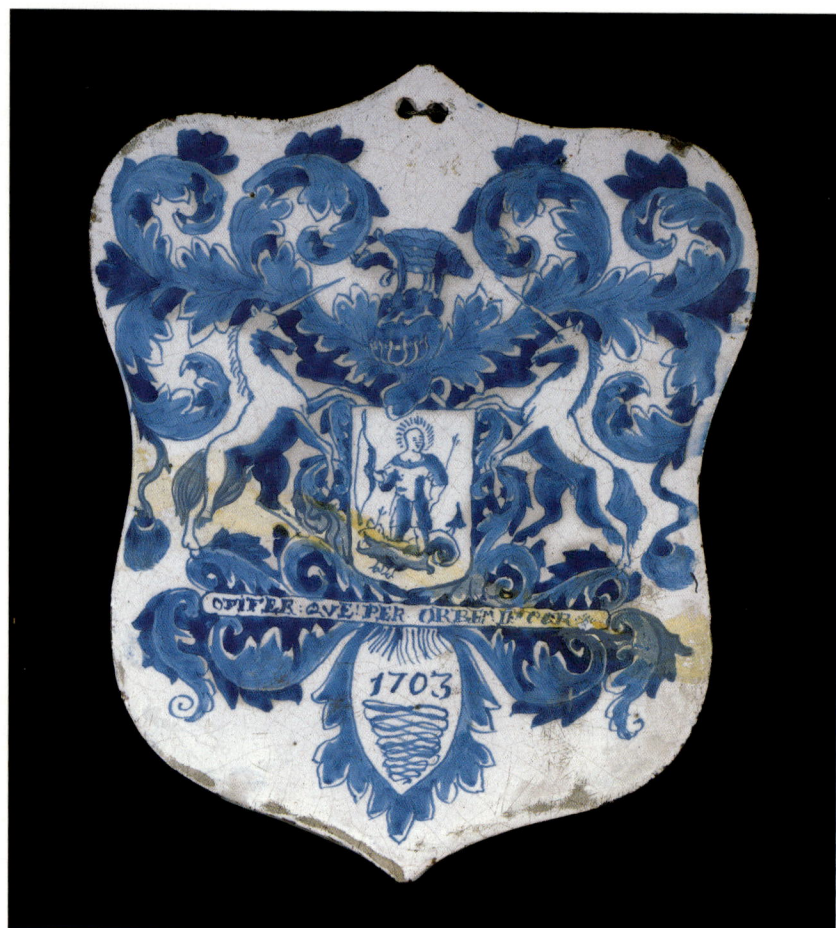

Pill tile (Cat.221)

ACCESSION NUMBER: YTA3

DESCRIPTION: Shield-shaped pill tile. White glaze and design in blue. Two holes at top for hanging.

DESIGN: Coat of arms of the Worshipful Society of Apothecaries, surrounded by foliage

INSCRIPTION: OPIFER: QVE: PER. ORBEM. DICOR 1703

MEANING OF INSCRIPTION AND DESIGN: The Worshipful Society of Apothecaries is a livery company formed in 1617. The arms feature Apollo (the god of healing) killing the dragon of disease, supported by two unicorns (from King James's royal arms), and a rhinoceros as the crest (the powdered horn was believed to be medicinal). The motto, from the first book of Ovid's 'Metamorphoses', translates: "I am spoken of all over the world as one who brings help."

DIMENSIONS: Height 300 mm, maximum width 255 mm

DATE OF MANUFACTURE: 1703

PLACE OF MANUFACTURE: London

PROVENANCE: Bought in 1957, Howard Collection. Formerly Lomax Collection.

CONDITION: Fair; has been repaired, glaze crazed and flaked from edges.

COMMENT: This is the only known dated shield-shaped tile, of a total of eight known dated tiles.

REFERENCES: Britton, English Delftware in the Bristol Collection, p. 76.

Crellin, Medical Ceramics, p. 144.

Howard, English Delftware Drug Jars, p. 40 and No. 62A.

Lothian, English Delftware in the Pharmaceutical Society's Collection. p. 2 and Plate 2b.

Lothian, The Armorial Delft of the Worshipful Society of Apothecaries, pp. 23 and 25.

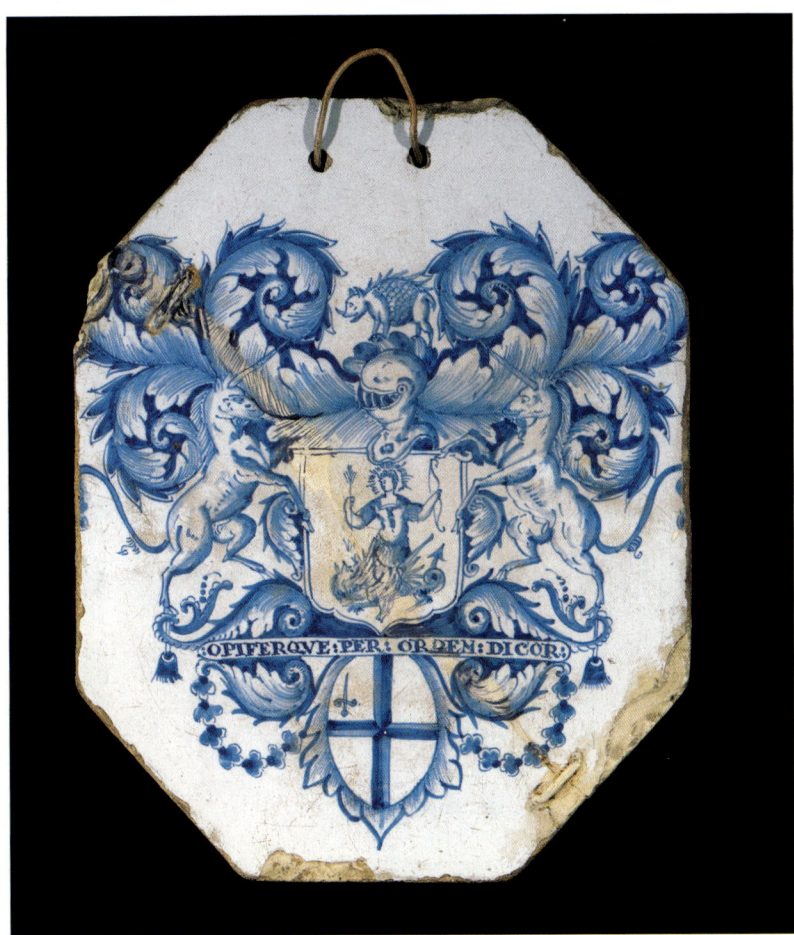

Pill tile (Cat. 222)

ACCESSION NUMBER: YTA6
DESCRIPTION: Octagonal pill tile. White glaze with bluish tinge and design in blue. Two holes at top for hanging.
DESIGN: Coat of arms of the Worshipful Society of Apothecaries, and City of London arms, surrounded by foliage
INSCRIPTION: OPIFEREQUE: PER: ORBEM: DICOR:
MEANING OF INSCRIPTION AND DESIGN: The Worshipful Society of Apothecaries is a livery company formed in 1617. The arms feature Apollo (the god of healing) killing the dragon of disease, supported by two unicorns (from King James's royal arms), and a rhinoceros as the crest (the powdered horn was believed to be medicinal). The motto, from the first book of Ovid's 'Metamorphoses', translates: "I am spoken of all over the world as one who brings help."

The arms of the City of London are said to have been adopted in the 14th century. They depict the cross of St George with the red Sword of St Paul. Another interpretation is that the sword is representative of that which killed Wat Tyler and ended the Peasants' Revolt of 1381.

DIMENSIONS: Height 300 mm, maximum width 245 mm
DATE OF MANUFACTURE: 1680–1750
PLACE OF MANUFACTURE: London
PROVENANCE: Bought from Mrs Ernest Saville Peck in 1956. Peck had stated that it was "Given to me by Mr Holder, Fitzwilliam Museum."
CONDITION: Very poor; has been repaired with rivets, all edges chipped.
REFERENCE: Archer, Delftware. p. 397 and catalogue K.12.

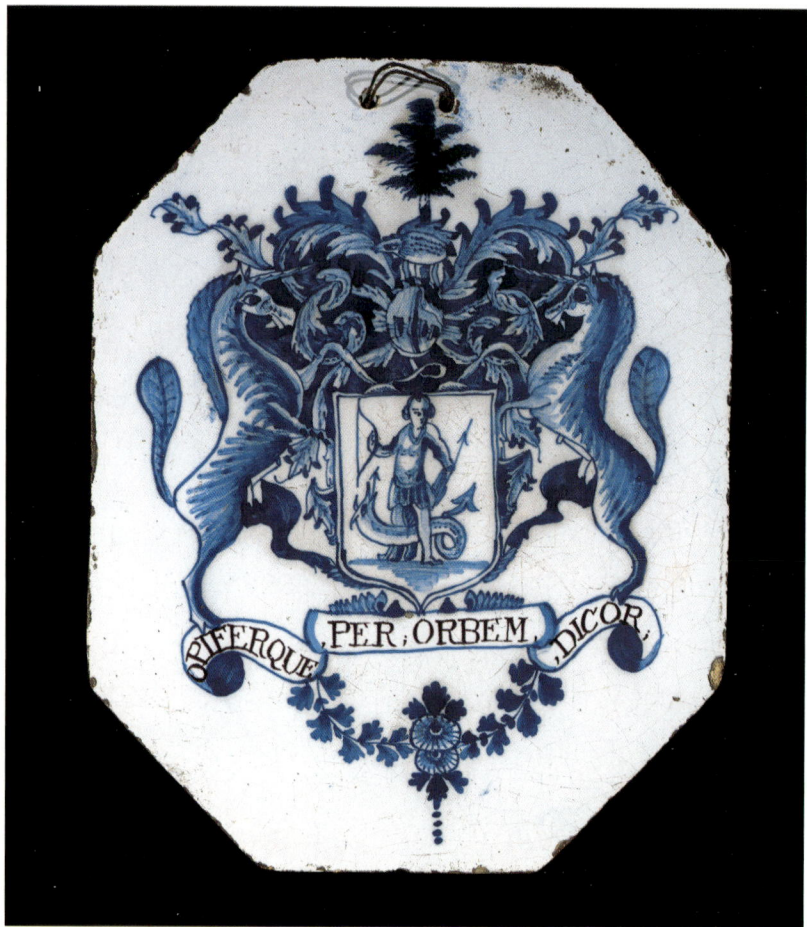

Pill tile (Cat. 223)

ACCESSION NUMBER: YTA4
DESCRIPTION: Octagonal-shaped pill tile. White glaze and design in blue. Inscription in black. Two holes at top for hanging.
DESIGN: Arms of the Apothecaries Company, with tree
INSCRIPTION: OPIFERQUE, PER; ORBEM, DICOR;
MEANING OF INSCRIPTION AND DESIGN: The Worshipful Society of Apothecaries is a livery company formed in 1617. The arms feature Apollo (the god of healing) killing the dragon of disease, supported by two unicorns (from King James's royal arms), and a rhinoceros as the crest (the powdered horn was believed to be medicinal). The motto, from the first book of Ovid's 'Metamorphoses', translates: "I am spoken of all over the world as one who brings help."
DIMENSIONS: Height 300 mm, maximum width 242 mm
DATE OF MANUFACTURE: 1690–1740
PLACE OF MANUFACTURE: Probably Mortlake, London.
PROVENANCE: Donation, Mr Hampton, date unknown.
CONDITION: Good; edge chipped, glaze crazed and flaked from edge.

COMMENT: It has been suggested that the tree in this design represents one of the first four cedar trees to be planted in Britain at the Society of Apothecary's Physic Garden in Chelsea. The trees were planted in 1683, and appear to have become a feature of tiles made in London.
REFERENCES: Drey, Apothecary Jars, Plate 70C and pp.136 and 139.

Matthews, Antiques of the Pharmacy. p. 14.
Sloane, *Early Modern Industry and Settlement.* p.71.

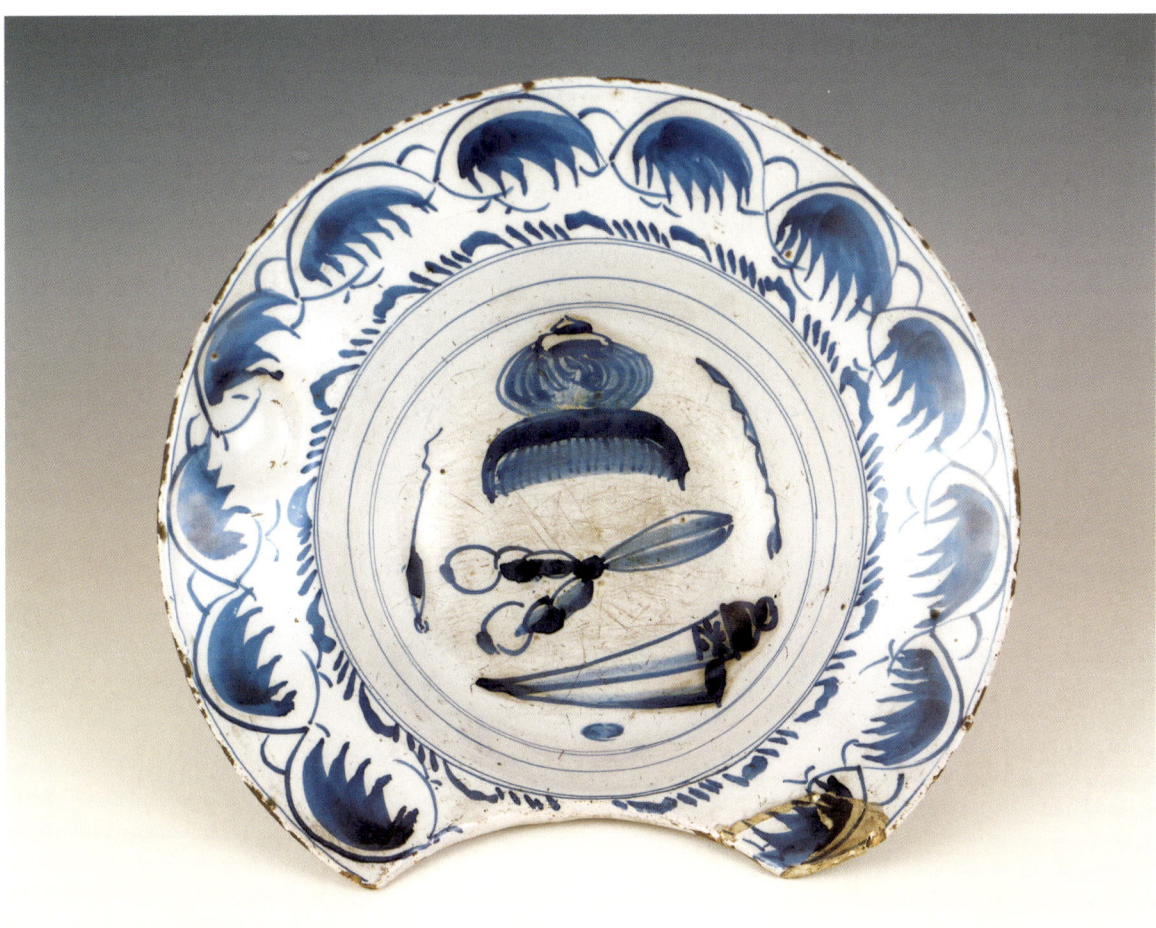

Barber's bowl (Cat.224)

ACCESSION NUMBER: YBB1
DESCRIPTION: Circular barber's bowl with space for neck and
circular depression on rim. White glaze with pinkish tinge and
design in blue. Recessed base.
DESIGN: Scallop design on rim, comb, scissors, razor and two
lancets on bowl
DIMENSIONS: Height 87 mm, maximum width 260 mm
DATE OF MANUFACTURE: 1680–1760
PLACE OF MANUFACTURE: Probably London
PROVENANCE: Bought in 1957, Howard Collection.
CONDITION: Good; rim repaired, glaze flaked on edge of rim.
COMMENT: Barbers' bowls are all of a typical shape, circular
with a semicircular section removed from the wide rim in order to
accommodate the neck of the person being shaved. They may also
have been used for bleeding, as the lancets decorating this bowl
would suggest. Some bowls have a circular depression in the rim
which may have held a ball of soap, or perhaps was a thumb hold.
REFERENCE: Howard, English Delftware Drug Jars, p. 41 and
No. 63A.

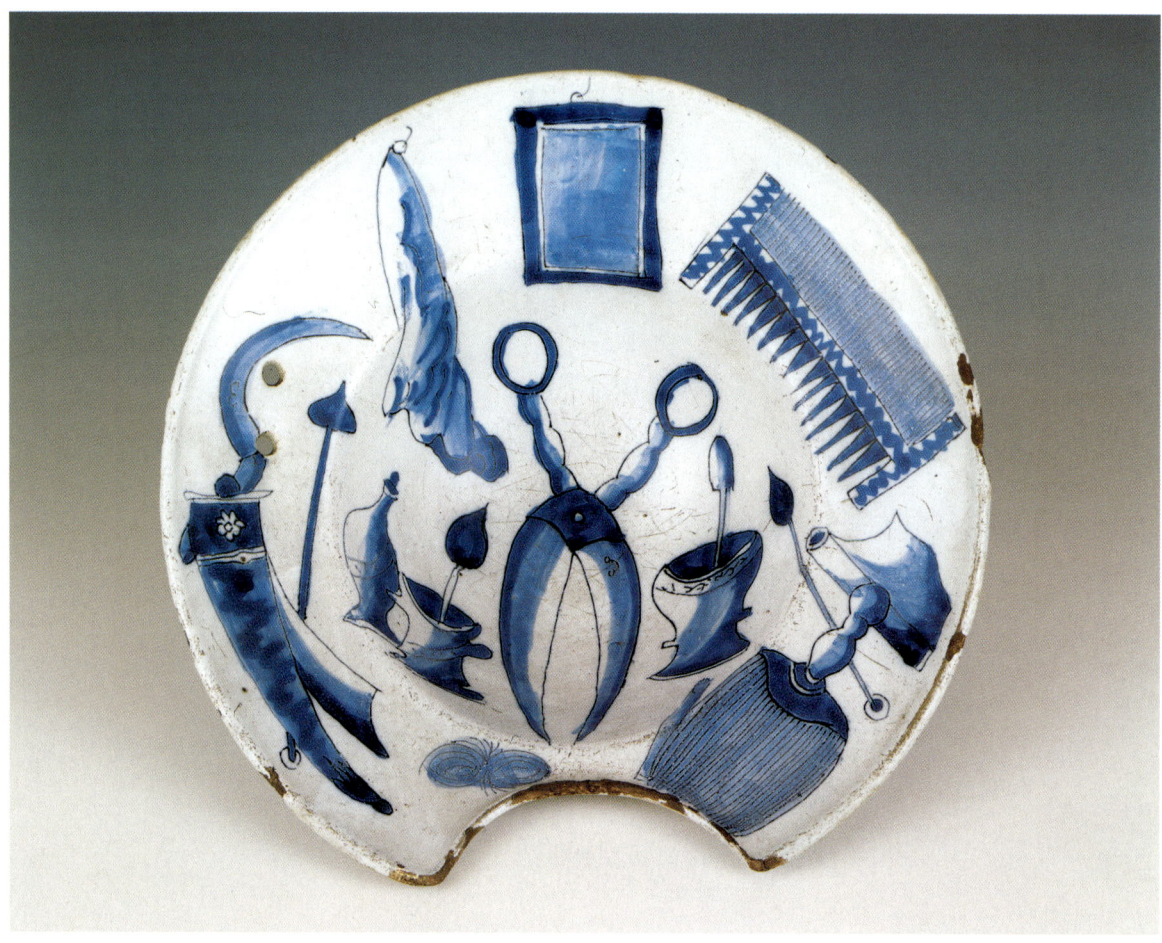

Barber's bowl (Cat.225)

Collection. p. 4 and Plate 7b.

ACCESSION NUMBER: YBB2

DESCRIPTION: Circular barber's bowl with space for neck on rim. White glaze with pinkish tinge and design in blue. Two holes on rim for hanging. Recessed base.

DESIGN: Combs, scissors, razor, storage pot, mirror and two mortars on bowl and rim

DIMENSIONS: Height 90 mm, maximum width 300 mm

DATE OF MANUFACTURE: 1690–1730

PLACE OF MANUFACTURE: Probably London. Possibly Bristol

PROVENANCE: Bought in 1957, Howard Collection.

CONDITION: Good; foot rim pierced with hole, glaze flaked on rim.

COMMENT: Barbers' bowls are all of a typical shape, circular with a semicircular section removed from the wide rim in order to accommodate the neck of the person being shaved. They may also have been used for bleeding.

REFERENCES: Grigsby, The Longridge Collection of English Slipware and Delftware. catalogue number D412.

Lothian, English Delftware in the Pharmaceutical Society's

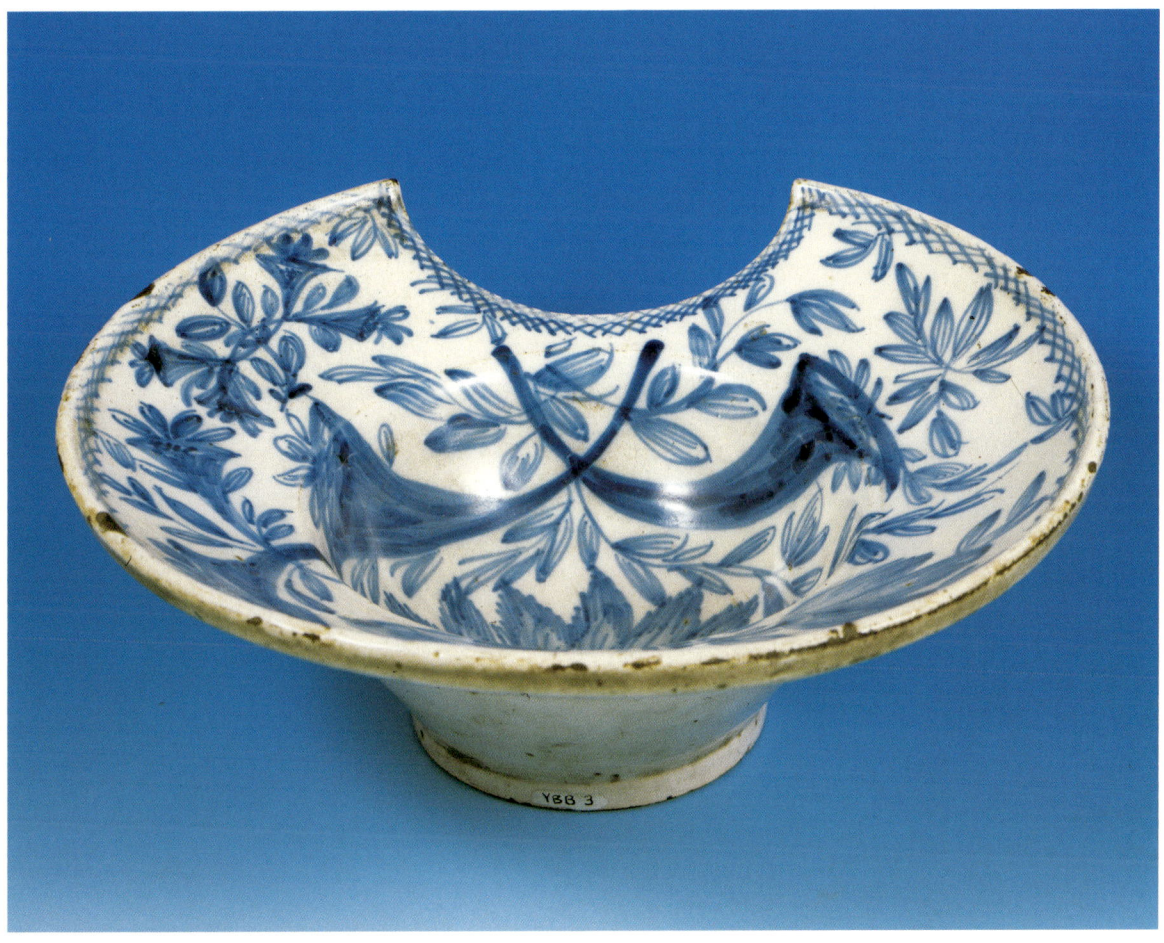

Barber's bowl (Cat.226)

ACCESSION NUMBER: YBB3

DESCRIPTION: Circular barbers' bowl with space for neck. White glaze with yellowish tinge and design in blue. Two holes in rim for hanging. Recessed base.

DESIGN: All-over design of flowers and leaves on bowl and rim

DIMENSIONS: Height 95 mm, maximum width 275 mm

DATE OF MANUFACTURE: 1700–1800

PLACE OF MANUFACTURE: London

PROVENANCE: Unknown

CONDITION: Good; glaze flaked on rim.

COMMENT: Barbers' bowls are all of a typical shape, circular with a semicircular section removed from the wide rim in order to accommodate the neck of the person being shaved. They may also have been used for bleeding.

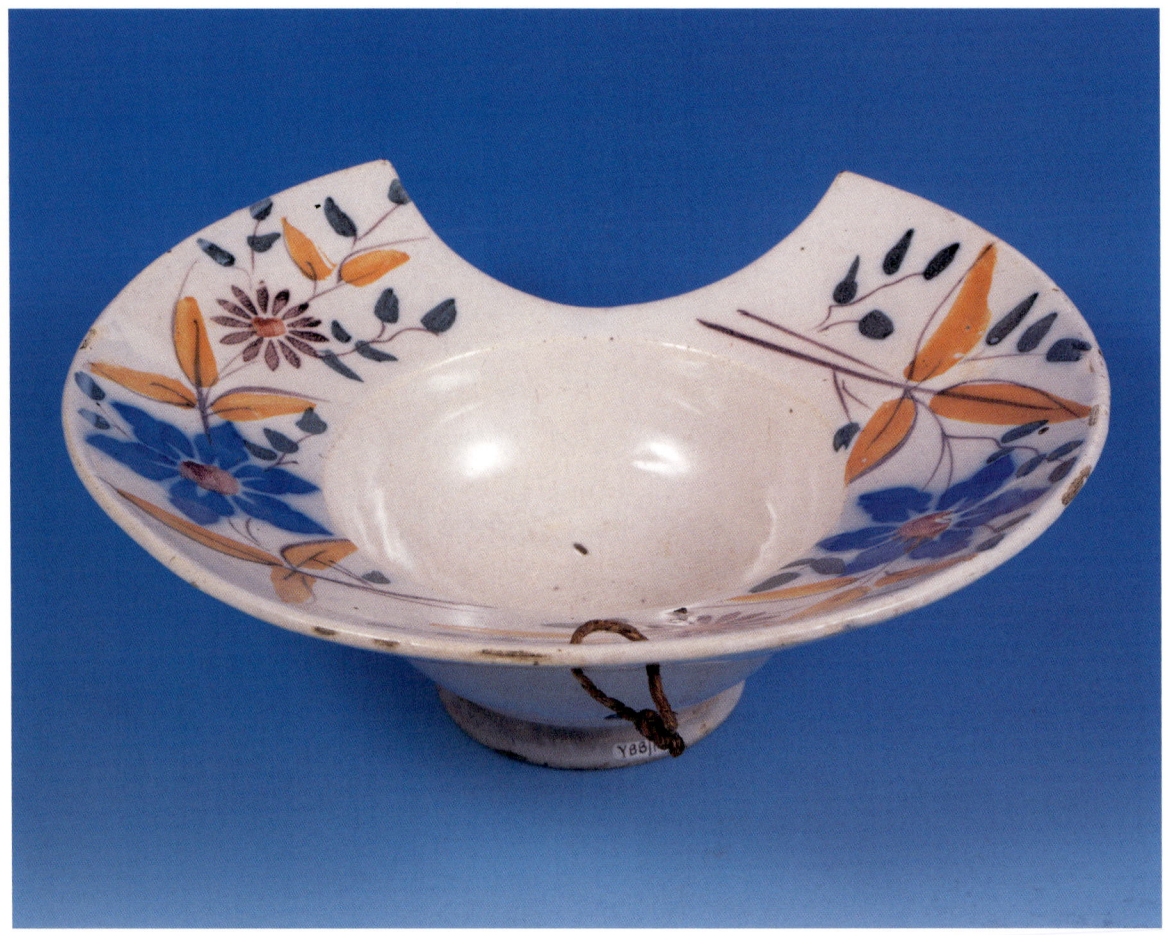

Barber's bowl (Cat.227)

ACCESSION NUMBER: YBB/P4
DESCRIPTION: Circular barber's bowl with space for neck.
White glaze with yellowish tinge and design in green, blue, yellow
and mauve. Two holes in rim for hanging. Recessed base.
DESIGN: Flowers and leaves on rim only
DIMENSIONS: Height 85 mm, maximum width 260 mm
DATE OF MANUFACTURE: 1700–1800
PLACE OF MANUFACTURE: London
PROVENANCE: Unknown
CONDITION: Good.
COMMENT: Barbers' bowls are all of a typical shape, circular
with a semicircular section removed from the wide rim in order
to accommodate the neck of the person being shaved. They may
also have been used for bleeding.

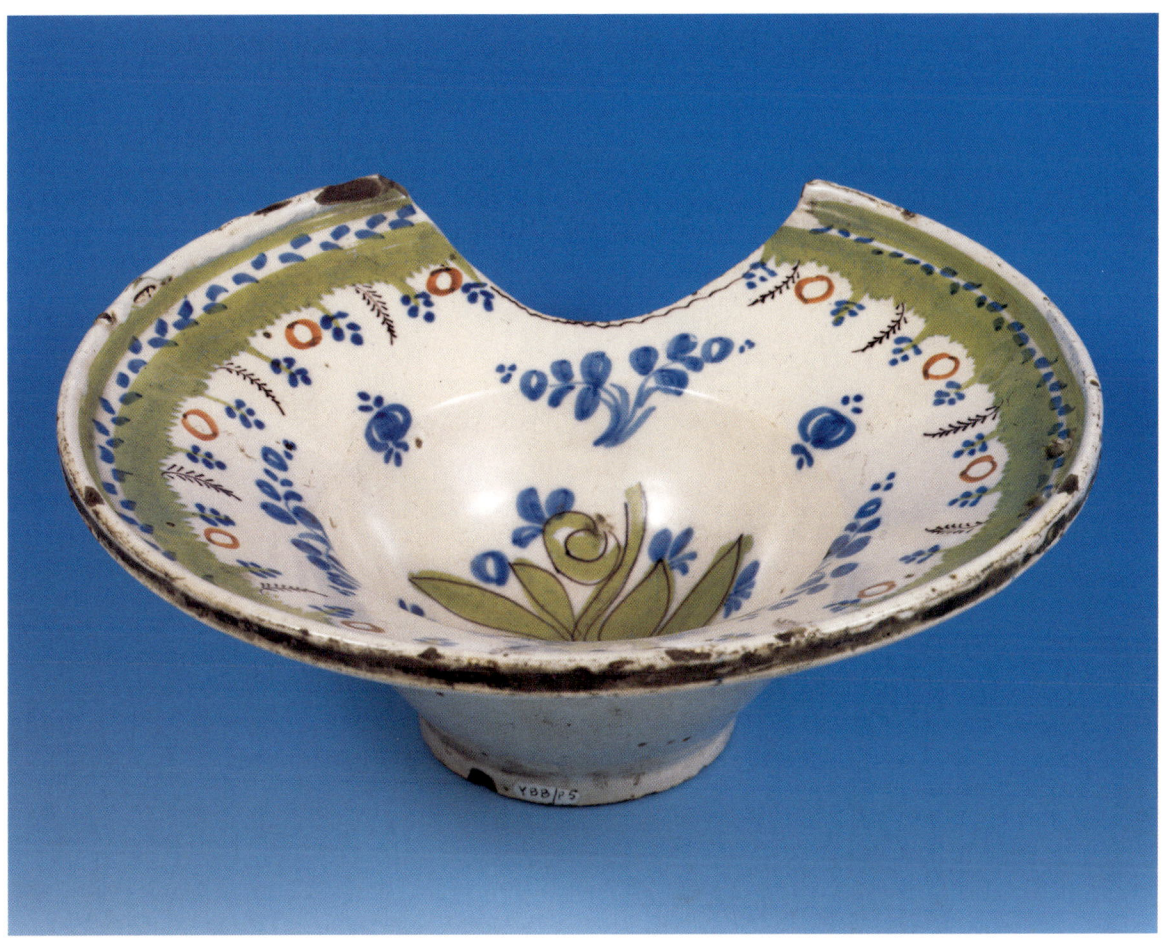

Barber's bowl (Cat.228)

ACCESSION NUMBER: YBB/P5

DESCRIPTION: Circular barber's bowl with space for neck. White glaze with yellowish tinge and design in green, blue, brown and black. Two holes in rim for hanging. Recessed base.

DESIGN: Flowers, leaves and grass on rim and bowl

DIMENSIONS: Height 100 mm, maximum width 270 mm

DATE OF MANUFACTURE: 1700–1800

PLACE OF MANUFACTURE: London

PROVENANCE: Unknown

CONDITION: Good; rim chipped, glaze flaked from edge of rim.

COMMENT: Barbers' bowls are all of a typical shape, circular with a semicircular section removed from the wide rim in order to accommodate the neck of the person being shaved. They may also have been used for bleeding.

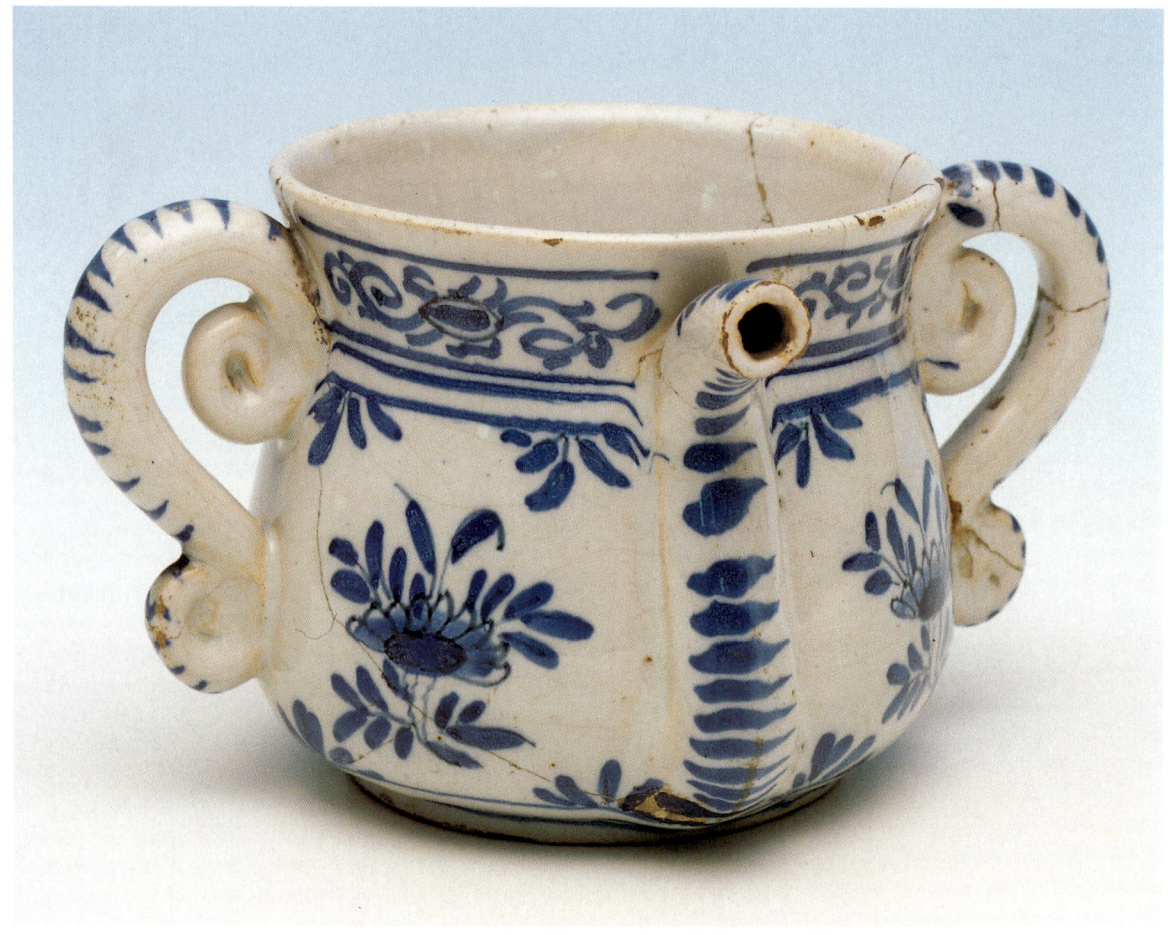

Posset pot (Cat.229)

ACCESSION NUMBER: GPA1

DESCRIPTION: Bulbous posset pot with two curled strap handles and spout. White glaze with pinkish tinge and design in blue.

DESIGN: Flowers and leaves, with blue stripes on handle and spout

DIMENSIONS: Height 78 mm, maximum width 138 mm

DATE OF MANUFACTURE: 1690–1720

PLACE OF MANUFACTURE: Probably Bristol

PROVENANCE: Bought in 1949.

CONDITION: Poor; major cracks and poor previous repairs.

COMMENT: Posset is a spiced, hot drink made from milk mixed with ale or wine. Posset pots generally take this two-handled, spouted form, and usually have a lid.

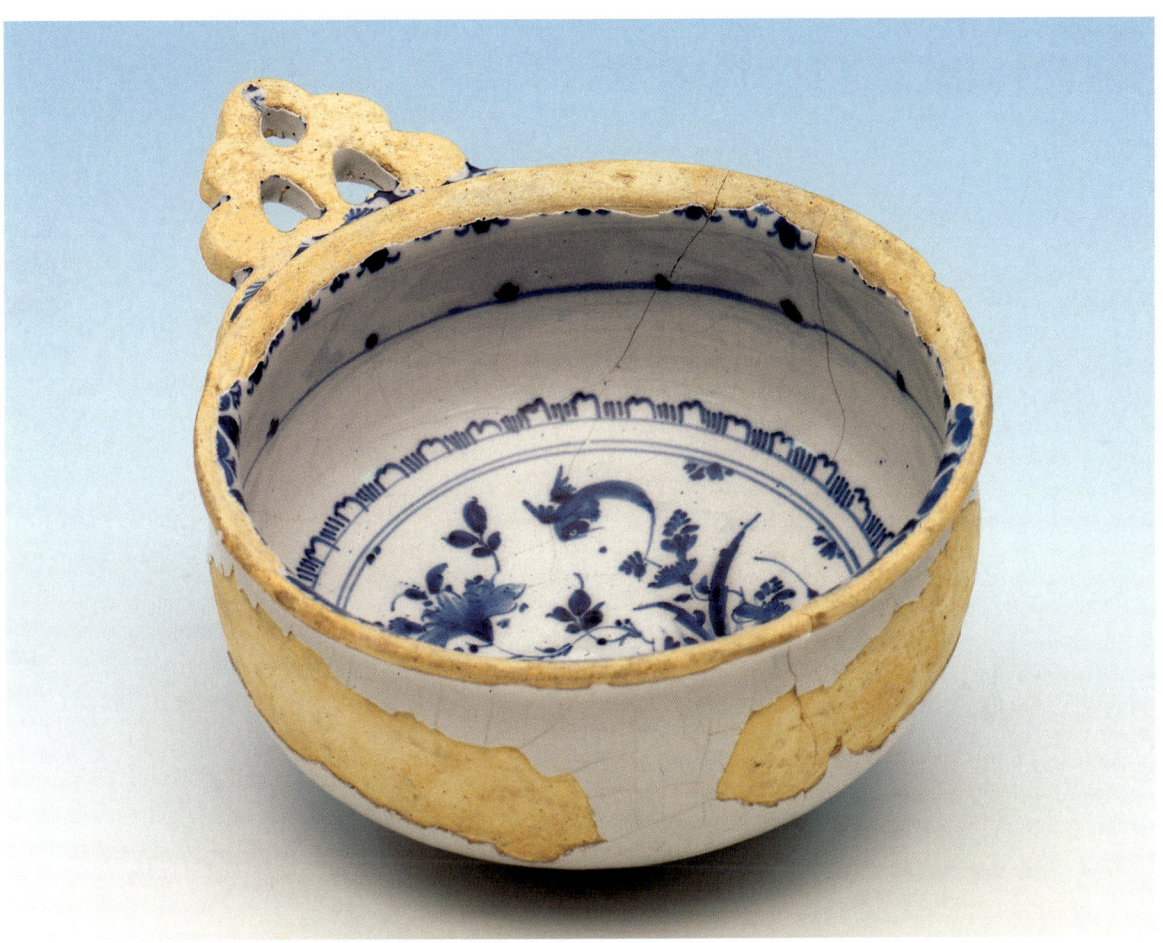

Porringer (Cat.230)

ACCESSION NUMBER: TR.1988.32
DESCRIPTION: Bowl with one flat 5-lobed handle. White glaze with design in blue.
DESIGN: Flowers and bird. B.S.1730
DIMENSIONS: Height 83 mm, maximum width 192 mm
DATE OF MANUFACTURE: 1730
PLACE OF MANUFACTURE: Probably London, but possibly Bristol
PROVENANCE: Bought in 1988.
CONDITION: Poor; significant loss of glaze, and cracked glaze.
COMMENT: It has been suggested that this is a bleeding bowl. There seems to be no evidence to confirm either use for any known bowls of this type, although some think that bowls with one handle, like this one, were bleeding bowls, while those with two handles were porringers. Porringers were used to serve broth and other liquid foods, or semi-liquid foods, such as porridge or pottage.

Bibliography

English and related delftware: General sources

Archer, Michael. *Delftware: The Tin Glazed Earthenware of the British Isles: A Catalogue of the Collection of the Victoria and Albert Museum*. London: The Stationery Office, 1997.

Archer, M. *Irish Pottery and Porcelain*. Dublin: Eason & Son Ltd, 1979.

Austin, John C. *British Delft at Williamsburg*. Williamsburg, VA: The Colonial Williamsburg Foundation, 1994.

Bedford, J. *Delftware*. London: Cassell & Co Ltd, 1966.

Black, J. *British Tin-Glazed Earthenware*. Princes Risborough: Shire Publications Ltd, 2001.

Britton, Frank. *English Delftware in the Bristol Collection*. London and New Jersey: Philip Wilson Publishers Ltd and Sotheby Publications, 1982.

Britton, Frank. *London Delftware*. London: Jonathon Horne, 1987.

Garner, F. H. and Archer, Michael. *English Delftware*, 2nd edn. London: Faber & Faber, 1972.

Grigsby, Leslie B. *The Longridge Collection of English Slipware and Delftware. Volume 2: Delftware*. London: Jonathan Horne Publications, 2000.

Hodgkin, John Eliot. *Examples of Early English Pottery, Named, Dated and Inscribed*. London: Cassell and Co., 1891.

Lipski, L. L. and Archer, M. *Dated English Delftware Tin-Glazed Earthenware 1600–1800*, London and Scranton Pennsylvania, published for Sotheby Publications by Philip Wilson Publishers Ltd and Harpers & Row Publishers Inc, 1984.

Ray, Anthony. *English Delftware Pottery: in the Robert Hall Warren Collection Ashmolean Museum Oxford*. London: Faber & Faber, 1968.

Ray, A. *English Delftware in the Ashmolean Museum*, Oxford and London: Ashmolean Museum in association with Jonathon Horne Publications, 2000.

Sloane, B., Hoad, S., with Cloake, J., Pearce, J. and Stephenson, R. *Early Modern Industry and Settlement. Excavations at George Street, Richmond, and High Street, Mortlake, in the London Borough of Richmond upon Thames*. London: Museum of London Archaeology Service, 2003.

Drug jars: Books

Crellin, J. K. *Medical Ceramics A Catalogue of the English and Dutch Collections in the Museum of the Wellcome Institute of the*

History Medicine, Volume 1 (no further volumes published), London: Wellcome Institute of the History of Medicine, 1969.

Drey, R. E. A. *Apothecary Jars: Pharmaceutical Pottery and Porcelain in Europe and the East 1150–1850*. London & Boston: Faber & Faber, 1978.

Howard, Geoffrey Eliot. *Early English Drug Jars*. London: The Medici Society, 1931. Includes a description of the author's personal collection, of which a substantial part is now held by the Museum of the Royal Pharmaceutical Society.

Matthews, Leslie G. *Antiques of the Pharmacy*. London: G. Bell and Sons, 1971.

Negus, V. *Artistic Possessions at the Royal College of Surgeons of England*. Edinburgh and London: E & S Livingstone Ltd, 1967.

Rackham, B. *Catalogue of the Glaisher Collection of Pottery and Porcelain in the Fitzwilliam Museum Cambridge*, 2 volumes, Woodbridge, Suffolk: Antique Collectors' Club Ltd, with the consent of Cambridge University Press, 1987. First published by Cambridge University Press, 1935.

Delftware and drug jars: Journal articles

Anon. An English Delft Mithridatium Jar. *The Pharmaceutical Journal*. February 1955; 94.

Anon. Drug Jar, All Our Yesterdays No 20. *Hobbypharm*. 1983; 4(3): 5. This illustrates a 'clobbered' drug jar – one to which polychrome decoration had been added, probably more than 100 years after its manufacture.

Archer, Michael. Irish Delftware: an exhibition at Castletown House. *The Connoisseur*. October 1971;178 (716): 99–107.

Burnby, J. The Thomas Fautrart Pill Tile. *Pharmaceutical Historian*. 1977; 7(3):4–5.

Chamberlain, L. J. A group of English drug jars: typical designs of 1650-1750. *Pharmacy Digest: incorporating The Alchemist*. January 1960.

Chamberlain, L. J. Drug Jars as a Pharmacist's Hobby. *The Chemist and Druggist*. August 1953:170-172

Hampson, M. Apothecaries' Jars. *World Medicine*. December 1974: 27–31.

Hemming, C. Lambeth Delft. *The Connoisseur*. December 1918: 193–203.

Hoffbrand, A. Victor and Cook, Dee. The Victor Hoffbrand Collection of 17th and 18th Century English Apothecary Drug Jars and Some of Their Original Owners, *Apothecary*, 2004: 30–35.

Jackson, W. A. Is The Man Depicted on Early English Drug Jars Really Smoking a Pipe? *The Pharmaceutical Journal*. December 2001: 918–919.

Lothian, Agnes. Drug jars and their inscriptions. *The Chemist and Druggist*. June 1950; 153: 805–807.

Lothian, Agnes. 'Observables' at the Royal College of Surgeons: English Delft drug jars bequeathed to the College by Sir St Claire Thomson in 1943. *Annals of the Royal College of Surgeons of England*. December 1950; 7: 497–502.

Lothian, Agnes. The Armorial London Delft of the Worshipful Society of Apothecaries, *The Connoisseur*, with which is incorporated International Studio, Vol. 127, March 1951: 21–26.

Lothian, Agnes. Vessels for Apothecaries. English Delft Drug Jars. Reprinted from *The Connoisseur Year Book*, 1953: 1–9.

Lothian, Agnes. Bird designs on English drug jars. *The Chemist and Druggist*. June 1954; 161: 672–677.

Lothian, Agnes.The pipe smoking man on seventeenth century English Delft drug jars. *The Chemist and Druggist*. May 1955; 163: 566–568.

Lothian, Agnes. Angels in the design of seventeenth century English Delft drug jars. *The*

Chemist and Druggist. June 1955; 163: 732–736.

Lothian, Agnes. Cherub designs on English Delft apothecary ware. *The Chemist and Druggist.* June 1956;165: 608–613.

Lothian, Agnes. English Delftware in the Pharmaceutical Society's collection: a paper read by Agnes Lothian at 17 Bloomsbury Square, London on November 12th 1958. *Transactions of the English Ceramic Circle.* 1960; 5(1).

Lothian, Agnes. 'The John Austen Collection' in Austen, John. *Historical Notes on Old Sheffield Druggists.* J. W. Northend Ltd: Sheffield, 1961: 95–100.

Lothian, Agnes. Two centuries of dated drug jars. *The Chemist and Druggist.* June 1962; 177: 722–725.

Lothian, Agnes. English drug jars in Sir Harry Jephcott's collection: part 1: the seventeenth century. *Bulletin International: the Glaxo Group quarterly.* Christmas 1968; 8: 24-25.

Lothian, Agnes, English drug jars in Sir Harry Jephcott's collection: part 2: the eighteenth century. *Bulletin International: the Glaxo Group quarterly.* Spring 1969; 9: 15-17.

Lothian Short, Agnes. Apothecary Jar Inscriptions – Their Interpretation. *Proceedings of the Royal Society of Medicine,* Vol. 63, February 1970: 145–147.

Lothian, Agnes. Seventeenth century English history reflected in pharmaceutical antiques. Publisher unknown, printed text held in RPSGB Library collection, n.d: 7–8.

Lothian, A. and Short, G. R. A. Angel Design Drug Jars. *Pharmaceutical Historian.* March 1977; 7(1): 1.

Matthews, L. G. Green-Glazed English Albarellos. *Post Medieval Archaeology.* 1972;6: 202–206.

Matthews, Leslie G. Apothecary Pill Slabs. *Antique Collector.* December 1989:190.

Tait, H. Southwark (alias Lambeth) Delftware and the potter, Christian Wilhelm. *The Connoisseur.* August 1960; 146, 587: 36-42.

Walker, Henry, Ancient pharmacy jars: with illustrations from examples in the possession of Mr James Prior, Chemist, Stamford, *The Connoisseur,* April 1908, pp. 251–254.

Wilkinson, John F. Apothecaries jars. *The Antique Collector.* March 1974; 45(1): 51-55.

Wilkinson, John F. Old English apothecaries' drug jars. *Proceedings of the Royal Society of Medicine.* February 1970; 63:137–144.

Wilkinson, John F. Early English apothecaries' drug jars: part 1 sixteenth and seventeenth centuries. *Art and Antiques.* March 1981; 44(6):26-29.

Wilkinson, John F. Early English apothecaries' drug jars: part 2 eighteenth century. *Art and Antiques.* March 1981; 44(7):27-29.

Wilkinson, John F. Early English apothecaries' drug jars: part 3 Bristol and Liverpool Delftware. *Art and Antiques.* March 1981; 44(8): 16-18.

Wilkinson, John F. English apothecaries' drug jars of the 16th to 18th centuries. *Journal of the Antique Collectors' Club.* July 1978;13(3): 24-29.

Reports of sales

The Pharmaceutical Journal contained numerous illustrated reports on the sales of pharmaceutical antiques, including many drug jars from 1970 to 2000.

Exhibitions

Anon. Exhibition of Ointment Jars. *The Pharmaceutical Journal.* September 1952: 188.

Anon. Jars and Mortars in a Pharmacy. *The Chemist and Druggist.* October 1953: 399.

Anon. 30 Years of Drug Jars. *Hobbypharm.* February 1983;4(1):4.

Legge, Margaret. The apothecary's shelf: drug jars

and mortars 15th-18th century. Melbourne, Victoria, Australia: National Gallery of Victoria, 1986.

17th and 18th century medicinal preparations

Primary sources (the editions stated are those used for research for this publication)

Culpeper, N. *Pharmacopoeia Londinensis or a physical directory or a translation of the London Dispensatory made by the College of Physicians in London*, London, 1649 and 1653.

Culpeper, N. *The Complete Herbal and English Physician Enlarged*, London, 1653.

Healde, T. *The Pharmacopoeia of the Royal College of Physicians of London*, 7th edition, London. G. Woodfall for T. Longman, 1796.

Lewis, W. *The New Dispensatory 1770*, 3rd edition, London, J. Nourse, 1770.

Pemberton, H. *The Dispensatory of the Royal College of Physicians, London.* Translated into English with Remarks, &c. London. Printed for T. Longman and T. Shewell, and J. Nourse, 1746.

Quincy, J. *Pharmacopoeia Officinalis & Extemporanea or A Complete English Dispensatory in Four Parts.* London. Printed for A. Bell, T. Varnam, J. Osborn, and W. Taylor, 1718 and 1728.

Salmon, *Pharmacopoeia Londinensis or The New London Dispensatory.* London. Printed by J. Dawks for M. Wotton, J. Walthoe, G. Conyers, J. Nicholson, J. Sprint, D. Midwinter, and T. Ballard, 1716

Secondary sources

Drey, R. E. A. *Apothecary Jars: Pharmaceutical Pottery and Porcelain in Europe and the East 1150-1850*. London & Boston:Faber & Faber, 1978. Includes a glossary of terms used in apothecary jar inscriptions.

Estes, J. W. *Dictionary of protopharmacology: therapeutic practices, 1700-1850.* Canton: Science History Publications, 1990.

Harrod, D. Appendix. Inscriptions and Recipes in Lipski, L. L. & Archer, M. *Dated English Delftware Tin-Glazed Earthenware 1600-1800*, London and Scranton Pennsylvania, published for Sotheby Publications by Philip Wilson Publishers Ltd and Harpers & Row Publishers Inc, 1984: 393-402.

Appendix

Museums and other organisations with pharmaceutical delft collections in Great Britain

Ashmolean Museum
Beaumont St, Oxford OX1 2PH
Warren Collection

Birmingham Museum and Art Gallery
Chamberlain Square, Birmingham B3 3DH

Bridewell Museum
Bridewell Alley, Norwich NR2 1AQ

Bristol City Museum and Art Gallery
Queen's Road, Bristol BS8 1RL

British Museum
Great Russell Street, London WC1B 3DG

Canterbury City Museums
Royal Museum and Art Gallery, 18 High Street, Canterbury, Kent CT1 2RA

Cheltenham Art Gallery and Museum
Clarence Street, Cheltenham, Gloucestershire GL50 3JT

Cuming Museum
155/157 Walworth Road, London SE17 1RS

Curtis Museum and Allen Gallery
High Street, Church Street, Alton, Hants GU34 1BA

Fitzwilliam Museum
Trumpington Street, Cambridge CB2 1RB
Glaisher Collection

Grosvenor Museum
27 Grosvenor Street, Chester, Cheshire CH1 2DD

Guildhall Museum
High Street, Rochester, Kent ME1 1PY

Harris Museum and Art Gallery
Market Square, Preston, Lancashire PR1 2PP

Ipswich Museum
High Street, Ipswich, Suffolk IP1 3QH

Liverpool Museum
William Brown Street, Liverpool L3 8EN

Manchester Art Gallery
Mosley Street, Manchester M2 3JL
Greg Collection

Museum of the History of Science
Broad Street, Oxford OX1 3AZ

Museum of London
London Wall, London EC2Y 5HN

National Museums of Scotland
Edinburgh EH1 1JF

National Museums and Galleries of Wales
Cathays Park, Cardiff CF1 3NP

New Walk Museum and Art Gallery
53 New Walk, Leicester LE1 7EA

Northampton Museum and Art Gallery
Guildhall Road, Northampton, Northamptonshire
NN1 1DP
Manfield Collection

Plymouth City Museum and Art Gallery
Drake Circus, Plymouth PL4 8AJ

The Royal College of Surgeons of England
35–43 Lincoln's Inn Fields, London WC2A 3PE
Sir St Claire Thomson Collection

Royal Cornwall Museum
River Street, Truro, Cornwall TR1 2SJ

Saffron Walden Museum
Museum Street, Saffron Walden, Essex CB10 1JL

Salford Museum and Art Gallery
Peel Park Crescent, Salford M5 4WU

Salisbury and South Wiltshire Museum
The King's House, 65 The Close, Salisbury SP1 2EN

Shakespeare Birthplace Trust
The Shakespeare Centre, Henley Street, Stratford
upon Avon, Warwickshire CV37 6QW

Sheffield Museums and Galleries Trust
Leader House, Surrey Street, Sheffield, South
Yorkshire S1 2LH

Spalding Gentlemen's Society Museum
Broad Street, Spalding, Lincolnshire PE11 1TB

Swansea Museum
Victoria Road, Swansea SA1 1SN

Thackray Museum
Beckett Street, Leeds, West Yorkshire LS9 7LN
Wilkinson Collection

University of Manchester Medical School Museum
Stopford Building, Oxford Road, Manchester
M13 9PT

Victoria and Albert Museum
Cromwell Road, South Kensington, London
SW7 2RL

Wellcome Museum of the History of Medicine at the Science Museum
Exhibition Road, London SW7 2DD

Winchester City Museum
The Square, Winchester, Hampshire SO23 9EX

The Worshipful Society of Apothecaries of London
Apothecaries' Hall, Blackfriars Lane, London
EC4V 6EJ

York Castle Museum
Castle Area, Eye of York, York YO1 9RY

York Medical Society
23 Stonegate, York YO1 2AW

Yorkshire Museum
Museum Gardens, York YO1 7FR

Index